WJ 141 mum

Management of Urological Emergencies

Edited by

Faiz Mumtaz MBBS FRCS(Eng) MD FRCS(Urol)
Consultant Urological Surgeon & Honorary Senior Lecturer
Barnet and Chase Farm Hospital NHS Trust
Hertfordshire, UK

Christopher R J Woodhouse MB FRCS FEBU
Reader in Adolescent Urology and Honorary Consultant Urologist
Institute of Urology
Middlesex Hospital
London, UK

Jack W McAninch MD
Professor of Urology
Urology Service
San Francisco General Hospital
San Francisco CA, USA

Dennis L Cochlin MB BCh FRCR
Consultant Radiologist
Department of Radiology
Cardiff Royal Infirmary
Cardiff, UK

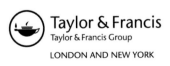

Taylor & Francis
Taylor & Francis Group
LONDON AND NEW YORK

A MARTIN DUNITZ BOOK

© 2004 Taylor & Francis, an imprint of the Taylor & Francis Group
First published in the United Kingdom in 2004
by Taylor & Francis, an imprint of the Taylor & Francis Group, 11 New Fetter
Lane, London EC4P 4EE

Tel.:   +44 (0) 20 7583 9855
Fax.:   +44 (0) 20 7842 2298
E-mail: info@dunitz.co.uk
Website: http://www.dunitz.co.uk

Although every effort has been made to ensure that drug doses and other
information are presented accurately in this publication, the ultimate responsi-
bility rests with the prescribing physician. Neither the publishers nor the
authors can be held responsible for errors or for any consequences arising
from the use of information contained herein. For detailed prescribing information or instructions on the use of any product or procedure discussed
herein, please consult the prescribing information or instructional material
issued by the manufacturer.

A CIP record for this book is available from the British Library.

Library of Congress Cataloging-in-Publication Data

Data available on application

ISBN 1 84184 177 3

Distributed in North and South America by
Taylor & Francis
2000 NW Corporate Blvd
Boca Raton, FL 33431, USA

Within Continental USA
Tel.: 800 272 7737; Fax.: 800 374 3401

Outside Continental USA
Tel.: 561 994 0555; Fax.: 561 361 6018
E-mail: orders@crcpress.com

Distributed in the rest of the world by
Thomson Publishing Services
Cheriton House
North Way
Andover, Hampshire SP10 5BE, UK
Tel.: +44(0)1264 332424
E-mail: salesorder.tandf@thomsonpublishingservices.co.uk

Composition by Wearset Ltd, Boldon, Tyne and Wear
Printed and bound in Spain by Grafos SA

Contents

List of contributors

Mark Emberton MD, FRCS (Urol)
Senior Lecturer & Consultant Urologist
Institute of Urology
Middlesex Hospital
London, UK

Giles O Hellawell DM, FRCS
Specialist Registrar in Urology
The Royal Hospital NHS Trust
London

Masood Khan MD, FRCSI
Urology Resident
James Buchanan Brady Urological Institute
Johns Hopkins Hospital
Baltimore, MD, USA

Chris Laing MBChB, MRCP
Specialist Registrar in Nephrology
Institute of Urology and Nephrology
Middlesex Hospital
London, UK

Marc Laniado MD, FRCS(Urol), FEBU
Consultant Urological Surgeon
Heatherwood and Wrexham Park Hospitals
Berkshire, UK

Leon Lilas FRCS(Urol)
Specialist Registrar in Urology
Department of Urology
Guys & St Thomas Hospital NHS Trust
London, UK

Gregory J Malone MBBS, FRACS(Urol)
Visiting Urologist
Princess Alexandra Hospital
Woolloongabba, Brisbane
Queensland
Australia

Jack W McAninch MD, FACS
Professor of Urology
Chief of Urology
San Francisco General Hospital
San Francisco, CA, USA

Michael J Metro MD
Associate Professor
Clinical Assistant Professor of Surgery, Urology
Albert Einstein Medical Center, Philadelphia and
Temple University Medical Center
Philadelphia, PA, USA

Gerald Mingin MD
Assistant Professor of Surgery/Urology
Department of Urology
University of California
San Francisco, CA, USA

Finn Morgan FRCS
Specialist Registrar in Urology
Department of Urology
Barnet and Chase Farm Hospital NHS Trust
Barnet, Hertfordshire, UK

Robert J Morgan MA, FRCS
Consultant Urologist
Department of Urology
Royal Free Hampstead NHS Trust
London, UK

Larry Mulleague MB, BCh, FRCA
Consultant in Anesthetics & Intensive Care Hospitals
Epsom & St Helier's NHS Hospitals
London, UK

Faiz Mumtaz MBBS, FRCS(Eng), MD, FRCS(Urol)
Consultant Urological Surgeon & Honorary Senior
Lecturer
Department of Urology
Barnet and Chase Farm Hospital NHS Trust
The Ridgeway, Middlesex, UK

Anthony R Mundy MS, FRCP, FRCS
Professor of Urology
Director, The Institute of Urology and Nephrology
Medical Director, UCL Hospitals NHS Trust
Institute of Urology
London, UK

Tim Nathan FRCS(Urol)
Specialist Registrar
Institute of Urology and Nephrology
Middlesex Hospital
London, UK

Guy Neild MD, FRCP
Professor of Nephrology,
Head of Clinical Nephrology & Transplantation
Institute of Urology and Nephrology
Middlesex Hospital
London, UK

David L Nicol MBBS, FRACS(Urol)
Director of Urology and Renal Transplantation
Princess Alexandra Hospital
Woolloongabba, Brisbane
Queensland
Australia

Hiep T Nguyen MD
Department of Urology
University of California
San Francisco, CA, USA

Kiaran J O'Malley MCh, FRCS(Urol)
Fellow in Reconstructive Urology
The Institute of Urology and Nephrology
Middlesex Hospital
London, UK

Alan W Partin MD, PhD
Bernard L Schwartz Distinguished Professor of
Urology Oncology
James Buchanan Brady Urological Institute
The Johns Hopkins Hospital
Baltimore, MD, USA

David Ralph BSc, MS, FRCS(Urol)
Consultant Uro-Andrologist and Honorary Senior
Lecturer
Institute of Urology
Middlesex Hospital
London, UK

Steve Shaw MB, BS, FRCA
Consultant Intensivist
Intensive Care Unit
Royal Free Hospital
London, UK

Mark E Sullivan BSc, MD, FRCS(Urol)
Consultant Urologist
Department of Urology
Churchill Hospital
Oxford, UK

Christopher RJ Woodhouse MB, FRCS, FEBU
Reader in Adolescent Urology and Honorary
Consultant Urologist
The Institute of Urology and Nephrology
Middlesex Hospital
London, UK

Foreword

It is timely that a textbook of urological emergencies should be published. This book is of particular value because it covers all types of emergencies, from acute renal failure to trauma and much else besides. It is unusual to see a textbook which takes all of these emergency situations together and, because of this, the reader can use this as a very valuable reference textbook. The editor in his preface state that this book will be essential reading for urological trainees preparing for exit examinations; this is definitely correct but it will also be valuable reading for the practicing urologist.

The authors have international reputations in the investigation and management of genito-urinary trauma and reconstruction and because of this they have been able to get together an excellent list of contributors. Because of the wide scope of the book the authors, who are all well known contributors to the literature, come from a wide range of urological subspecialties. The majority come from the United Kingdom but there is representation from the United States of America as well. I would like to congratulate them all on a clearly presented and practical textbook which will, I feel, become the leading reference textbook in urological emergencies.

John M Fitzpatrick MCh, FRCSI, FC, Urol (SA), FRCSGlas, FRCS
Consultant Urologist and Professor of Surgery
Department of Surgery, Mater Misericordiae Hospital
and University College Dublin

Preface

Currently, the literature on the management of urological emergencies is predominantly available in general urological textbooks. This book presents in a single volume a clear, practical account of all urological emergencies for the benefit of trainees/residents and practising urological surgeons. The principles relevant to decision-making and clinical management of all types of urological emergencies are discussed in detail. Management of Urological Emergencies is expected to be used as a quick reference guide on the wards and emergency rooms to provide effective and safe treatment of patients.

The chapters include the detailed management of all aspects of upper and lower urinary tract trauma, obstruction and infections. The book also includes separate chapters on scrotal, penile and oncological emergencies. In addition, the management of septic shock, renal failure and medical co-morbidities associated with urological emergencies are discussed. Chapters are supported by algorithm charts that will allow rapid instigation of the relevant investigations and treatment. Each chapter contains a list of key references for further reading. This book will form an essential read in the preparation for the FRCS (Urol) and other equivalent end-of-training exit examinations.

I would like to express my thanks to Dennis Cochlin for providing excellent radiological images. I also thank all the contributors for trying to inform rather than persuade, and to the editors for their support and encouragement.

Faiz Mumtaz MBBS, FRCS (Eng), MD, FRCS (Urol)
Consultant Urological Surgeon & Honorary Senior Lecturer

1. Co-morbidity in urological emergencies

Finn Morgan and Faiz Mumtaz

'How is that renal colic that came in last night?'

Any junior who has worked on a busy urology unit will have heard questions like that on the morning ward round. And yet, written down, it is easy to see the absurdity – renal colics don't come into hospital, people do. And people often have other 'annoying' illnesses that complicate their urological management. This can make life difficult for the junior doctor who is expected to manage not only the urological condition at hand but also the patient's comorbidities at the same time. Of course help is available from other inpatient specialist teams but this may not be available immediately. Besides, the medical management of some conditions may need to be altered in the surgical context.

The purpose of this chapter is to outline a few of the fundamentals of management of some comorbidities that may be present in emergency patients. Conditions have been chosen for discussion either because they are commonly encountered or because they present a particular challenge. It is not possible to include every medical condition. Those excluded are conditions in which there is little that the urology junior can do to optimize the situation. It is also not our purpose to provide comprehensive information on management of non-urological conditions; it is a doctor's duty to seek specialist help when it is needed.

RENAL FAILURE

Patients with chronic renal failure (CRF) are particularly vulnerable to further renal injury. This is important because the quality of life of a patient with renal impairment who is just about getting along with a serum creatinine of 350 µmol/l can be ruined by having to go on dialysis. Avoid further renal injury by:

- **Paying close attention to fluid balance to avoid dehydration**. Find out how much urine the patient normally passes. Most CRF patients lack concentrating ability and may continue to pass this amount of urine even when dehydrated. Keep a low threshold for central venous monitoring.
- **Avoiding nephrotoxic drugs**. Everyone remembers aminoglycosides; many forget that intravenous contrast is highly nephrotoxic. Take care and always refer to Appendix 3 of the *British National Formulary* (*BNF*).

CRF patients are usually on a multitude of drugs and have serious comorbidities, especially hypertension and diabetes, which are often the cause of the renal failure in the first place. Early liaison with the renal team is highly advisable and is **absolutely essential** if the patient is on any form of dialysis so that they can arrange appropriate time on a dialysis machine.

Acute renal failure (ARF) is sometimes a presenting feature in urological emergencies. If the cause is obstructive, the best treatment is relief of the obstruction. Provided the patient has good premorbid renal function, the serum creatinine should fall swiftly; in these circumstances you should watch for postobstructive diuresis which may require vigorous salt and water replacement in the first 24 hours.

Some patients with ARF may require emergency hemofiltration. The three **primary indications** for emergency hemofiltration are easy to remember:

- too much potassium (hyperkalemia)

- too much intravascular volume (pulmonary edema).
- too much acid (acidosis).

A high serum creatinine on its own is not an indication for emergency hemofiltration.

EMERGENCY TREATMENT OF RAISED SERUM POTASSIUM

This is important as hyperkalemia can have serious cardiac consequences and treatment should be initiated if serum $K^+ > 6.5$ mmol/l or if electrocardiographic (ECG) changes are present (peaked T-waves or widened QRS complexes). Treatment consist of:

- Insulin 15 U in 100 ml 20% dextrose intravenous (IV) over 30 min
- 20 ml 10% calcium gluconate IV slowly
- 100 ml 4.2% bicarbonate IV to correct acidosis
- Polystyrene sulfonate resin 15 g qds orally or one 30 g enema
- 5 mg salbutamol nebulizer
- Emergency hemofiltration

CARDIOVASCULAR DISEASE

HYPERTENSION

Emergency patients are often hypertensive when they first present to hospital; they are anxious. If possible base your management of their hypertension on repeated measurements following admission and especially after pain relief.

Hypertensive patients can be divided into three groups:

- Well-controlled hypertensive patients are patients already on antihypertensives and their diastolic blood pressure is less than 100 mmHg. These patients are not high-risk.
- Moderately controlled hypertensive patients have a diastolic blood pressure of 100–115 mmHg. These patients should be considered high risk if they have evidence of hypertensive nephropathy or retinopathy or if there is coronary artery disease.
- All patients with a diastolic blood pressure greater than 115 mmHg should be considered high risk.

Avoid listing high-risk patients for surgery if possible. They have a significantly increased risk of perioperative stroke, myocardial infarction (MI) and renal failure. Ideally they should be referred for medical investigation and treatment of their hypertension.

ISCHEMIC HEART DISEASE

Patients with ischemic heart disease present very different risks depending on the severity of their disease. Therefore it is vital to take **a good history**.

Your primary objective in managing surgical patients with ischemic heart disease is to avoid a perioperative myocardial infarct – a highly dangerous condition. Of these, 60% are 'silent', presenting only as a circulatory disturbance or dysrhythmia without chest pain. This results in late diagnosis and contributes to the poor survival figures; only 40–60% of patients survive.

In angina, determine if the patient has stable or unstable angina. In stable angina, perioperative risk correlates closely with the patient's exercise tolerance. If your patient has difficulty climbing stairs then consider all but the most minor of procedures to be high-risk surgery and think of getting a cardiology opinion before operating (or not operating at all). Patients who have had their angina treated successfully with a coronary artery bypass graft are at no more risk than a patient without ischemic heart disease. Patients with unstable angina are extremely risky candidates for surgery: there is an 80% risk of perioperative completed myocardial infarct. The benefit of surgery must be compelling to justify taking such a risk.

Patients with a history of previous MI have a

greater risk of having another one at the time of surgery, but this risk decreases over time. The risk is 80% if the surgery is carried out within 3 weeks of the MI but this reduces to 40% at 3 months, 15% at 6 months and 5% after 6 months. So, if you can temporize the situation with a stent or a catheter, do so and bring the patient back another day.

Outcome in ischemic heart disease can be improved by avoiding swings in blood pressure, heart rate and oxygen saturation that may lead to myocardial ischemia. Therefore consider a period in a high-dependency unit (HDU) postoperatively and certainly give supplemental oxygen for 24–72 hours after surgery.

HEMATOLOGICAL DISORDERS

ANEMIA

Causes of anemia:

- blood loss
- bone marrow infiltration or suppression
- hemolysis
- anemia of chronic disease
- B_{12} or folate deficiency.

If your patient is anemic on admission, it will at some stage be necessary to determine the cause. Ask for serum iron, total iron binding capacity, ferritin, B_{12} and folate. Do this before the patient receives any transfusion or the results will be altered.

There is no hard evidence to support a particular hemoglobin concentration below which a patient should be transfused. Clinical judgment must weigh strongly in your decision and should take into account the following:

- Is the patient manifesting symptoms of anemia such as shortness of breath or chest pain?
- Does the patient have a condition (such as ischemic heart disease) that will be worsened by anemia?

- Can the cause of the anemia be readily treated?
- Is the patient well enough to restore their hemoglobin level to normal?
- Is the patient heading for surgery in which there may be significant blood loss?

In an **emergency**, crossmatched blood will take 30 min to prepare if the lab does not already have a 'group and save'. Most hospitals keep a supply of O negative blood for emergencies, although a slightly safer option is to ask for group-specific blood which can be available in 10 min. Do not use these emergency blood transfusions unless it is absolutely necessary; you are risking a life-threatening transfusion reaction.

ANTICOAGULATION

The number of patients on long-term anticoagulation continues to grow and these patients can present a dilemma for surgeons who must balance the risks of stopping anticoagulation with the risks of surgical bleeding. The indications for warfarin can be divided into two groups:

- venous thromboembolism (deep vein thrombosis (DVT) and pulmonary embolism (PE))
- Arterial thromboembolism (atrial fibrillation and mechanical heart valves).

These two groups should be treated differently because arterial thromboembolism is much more likely to result in death or serious disability than venous thromboembolism. For most operations, warfarin should be stopped 4 days before surgery and restarted immediately afterwards. In the run-up to surgery, patients who are within 1 month of a thromboembolic event should be given supplementary intravenous heparin while their international normalized ratio (INR) is less than 2. This can be stopped 3 hours prior to surgery. Twelve hours postoperatively all anti-coagulated patients should be considered for subcutaneous low molecular weight heparin at the DVT treatment dose. This should be continued until the INR is greater than 2. Patients who have recently had a thromboembolic event should be on intravenous heparin at this time. However, all postoperative anticoagulation must be balanced against the risk of bleeding and this risk may make anticoagulation impossible in individual cases.

If a **warfarinized patient needs emergency surgery** consult the hematology department immediately for advice. The warfarin can be reversed with fresh frozen plasma and intravenous vitamin K, but expect the patient to be difficult to re-anticoagulate later.

JEHOVAH'S WITNESSES

Jehovah's Witnesses are a Christian movement with about six million members worldwide. Their teachings and beliefs are based upon a very literal interpretation of the Bible and it is from this interpretation that they draw their firm belief that blood transfusions are against God's law. Usually Jehovah's Witnesses will refuse blood transfusions in all circumstances. This refusal extends to most (but not all) blood products and may also include cell salvage procedures and autotransfusions. Individual patients vary in how radically they interpret the ban. Fortunately most will make your life easier by presenting you with a document that clearly states which treatments are acceptable to them and which are not.

Respect the wishes of Jehovah's Witnesses even if you do not agree with their views. Failure to do this may result in criminal charges being brought against you for assault. All patients have the right to refuse treatment that they object to, even if it endangers their life. In an emergency situation where the patient is unable to indicate their consent you must act in the best interests of the patient, transfusing blood if necessary. Only compelling evidence of the patient's desire to avoid transfusion should be accepted (such as a formal written advance directive).

Jehovah's Witnesses do not have an absolute right to prevent their children (under the age of 16 years) from receiving blood transfusions where such transfusions are necessary to prevent death or serious injury. It is possible for the hospital to apply for a court order to allow transfusion against the wishes of the parents. In a dire emergency it is your duty to proceed even without a court order and transfuse to save life if necessary; this action is defensible in court later.

Jehovah's Witnesses have a hospital liaison committee whose members can provide advice and help in mutual understanding between Jehovah's Witness patients and doctors. In any situation of real conflict it is imperative that the hospital management is involved. Keep meticulous records!

METABOLIC DISORDERS

DIABETES MELLITUS

Be cautious when treating patients with diabetes mellitus; as well as requiring specific diabetic management they are prone to other serious illnesses as a consequence of their diabetes. These include the following:

- infections
- renal impairment
- hypertension
- ischemic heart disease
- cerebrovascular disease.

Insulin requirements are not the same in health and disease. The stress of acute illness or surgery will increase a patient's basal metabolic rate, increasing insulin requirements. Thus even the most well-controlled diabetic patients can have very unstable blood sugar levels when admitted to hospital as an emergency. The safest course of action in such patients is to take them off their usual diabetic regimen and prescribe an intravenous glucose/potassium/insulin sliding scale. Hospitals will usually have a local policy describing how the sliding scale should be prescribed. Sliding scales are safe because they are easy to use and achieve the primary aims of diabetic management during illness and surgery, which are:

- avoiding wide swings in blood glucose
- providing insulin to avoid ketoacidosis
- maintaining blood glucose in the range 6–10 mmol/l
- avoiding hypokalemia.

The time to reinstate the patient back on their normal diabetic regimen is when they are recovering – in the light of day and when the diabetic support team are around.

GLUCOCORTICOIDS

When a patient is exposed to the stresses of surgery or illness, serum cortisol levels are known to rise. Some patients who are on steroid therapy will be unable to mount this physiological cortisol response because of suppression of the hypothalamic–pituitary–adrenal axis. Cases have been described of addisonian crisis occurring in such patients leading to death. For this reason some patients need to be given extra steroids at times of surgical stress.

Take a full drug history from the patient, going back 3 months as their drug treatment may have changed in the recent past. Steroid potencies can be compared easily with the following drugs taken to be equivalent to prednisolone 5 mg:

- hydrocortisone 20 mg
- triamcinolone 4 mg
- cortisone acetate 25 mg
- methylprednisolone 4 mg
- deflazacort 6 mg
- betamethasone 750 µg
- dexamethasone 750 µg

Patients who are taking less than 10 mg prednisolone a day require no special management. Patients who are taking more than this (or who have been during the preceding 3 months) should be managed as follows:

- The normal dose of steroid is given in the preoperative period.
- At induction 25 mg hydrocortisone IV is given.
- After minor surgery the patient can go back to the normal dose of steroid postoperatively.
- After intermediate or major surgery 25 mg hydrocortisone IV should be given every 6 h for 24–72 hours depending on the magnitude of the surgery.
- Patients on high-dose immunosuppression must be given their usual dose of steroid by the intravenous route until they are well enough to go back on oral therapy.

PULMONARY DISEASE

The two most frequently encountered pulmonary diseases are asthma and chronic obstructive airways disease (COAD). These conditions share some features and many aspects of the management are common to both. In addition, many patients who have COAD will state that they are suffering from asthma.

ASTHMA

Asthma has a wide range of severity. Some patients may only wheeze after heavy exercise and are otherwise well – they may own an inhaler but almost never use it. In contrast, some patients have severe life-threatening disease.

Remember that asthma strikes as **acute asthma attacks** and that a patient who appears completely well may still have severe disease. It is essential to determine the severity of the asthma by taking **an adequate history**. Patients who have life-threatening disease are likely to have the following features in their history:

- multiple courses of oral steroids
- repeated hospital admissions
- admission to intensive care unit (ITU).

Further assessment can be made by doing peak expiratory flow rates (looking for diurnal variability, response to bronchodilator therapy and compare with predicted values) and spirometry.

Patients with severe asthma should be considered for additional steroid therapy prior to surgery and should be reviewed by the respiratory physicians as early as possible. All patients should have their inhaled bronchodilators switched to nebulizers prior to surgery and should have nebulized salbutamol with their premedication.

Postoperatively:

- continue regular nebulized salbutamol
- give supplemental oxygen (humidified if possible) for 72 h
- nurse the patient sitting up
- arrange early chest physiotherapy
- mobilize as soon as possible.

CHRONIC OBSTRUCTIVE AIRWAYS DISEASE

Assess the severity of disease by taking a history. Particular markers of severity include:

- poor exercise tolerance
- multiple hospital admissions
- home oxygen therapy.

Further assessment of the patient can be made by formal spirometry (which will also yield information on reversibility of airways obstruction) and by doing arterial blood gases (provides a useful baseline as well as identifying CO_2-retaining patients).

Ask for a preoperative review by the respiratory team. This should focus on maximizing treatment of any reversible disease and also optimizing treatment of any cardiac failure

which may be accompanying the COAD. Patients with severe COAD may need to go to ITU postoperatively; liaise with the anesthetists early. Switch inhaled bronchodilators to nebulizers preoperatively.

Postoperatively:

- continue regular nebulized salbutamol and ipratropium
- give supplemental oxygen*
- nurse the patient sitting up
- arrange early chest physiotherapy
- mobilize as soon as possible
- ensure adequate pain relief – ask acute pain team to review daily.

*As every medical student knows, some patients with COAD have a high arterial P_{CO_2}. These patients' respiratory drive depends on their arterial P_{O_2} and therefore giving these patients high-flow oxygen may worsen their respiratory failure. **Only a very small proportion of COAD patients fall into this category**; they are usually very sick and have severe right-sided heart failure. Oxygen therapy in these patients needs to be managed in the light of serial arterial blood gas measurements. Don't allow this rare condition to frighten you out of giving necessary oxygen to other patients with pulmonary disease.

NEUROLOGICAL CONDITIONS

EPILEPSY

Your primary aim in epilepsy is to **maintain epileptic control**. This means that you have to interfere as little as possible with the therapeutic regimen that has been keeping the patient (hopefully) fit-free at home. Do this as follows:

- Assess the patient. Patients who have been seizure free for a year are probably low risk and are likely to tolerate a bit of interference with their drug regimen. Other patients are much more brittle. Take a proper history and put in an urgent request for the old notes.

- Keep antiepileptic drugs going right up until surgery. Even patients who are nil by mouth can take their pills with a sip of water.
- Anticonvulsant drugs need a gastrointestinal tract to absorb them so aim to disturb the gut as little as possible (e.g. spinal anesthesia is preferable to general anesthesia).
- If you expect a significant period of gastrointestinal disturbance then you must plan ahead for a nasogastric or parenteral anticonvulsant regimen. Take specialist advice on this.
- Liaise with the neurologists, preferably those who already know the patient.

If your patient has a fit:

- don't panic
- position the patient on their side and in such a way as to avoid injury
- give high-flow oxygen
- do a finger-prick test to rule out hypoglycemia.

Most fits do not last long. If the fit is not stopping after ten minutes, try to place a Guedel or a nasopharyngeal airway. Try to stop the fit with a dose of intravenous lorazepam or diazepam. Call for specialist help.

CEREBROVASCULAR DISEASE

Patients with cerebrovascular disease present with three different clinical syndromes:

- multi-infarct dementia
- transient ischemic attack
- major stroke.

Patients in the third category are easy to recognize as high risk for surgery but patients in the first two can appear surprisingly well! Be aware of this because **all patients with cerebrovascular disease are high risk**. This is important – any patient in the first two categories can end up in the third postoperatively. This risk needs to be considered when consenting patients for surgery.

- Try to avoid surgery on patients suffering from transient ischemic attacks until they have been assessed by a vascular surgery team with carotid Doppler. It may be that the patient would benefit from a carotid endarterectomy.
- Surgery within 6 weeks of a stroke is associated with a 20-fold increase in risk of a postoperative stroke so avoid surgery in these patients if possible.
- Patients with cerebrovascular disease should remain on aspirin if at all possible and should be kept normotensive at all times.

FURTHER READING

Association of Anaesthetists of Great Britain and Ireland. *Management of Anaesthesia for Jehovah's Witnesses.* London: Association of Anaesthetists of Great Britain and Ireland, 1999.

Burke JF, Francos GC. Surgery in the patient with acute or chronic renal failure. [Review] *Med Clin North Am* 1987; **71:** 489–97.

Smith MS, Muir H, Hall R. Perioperative management of drug therapy. *Drugs* 1996; **51:** 238–59.

Spandorfer J. The management of anticoagulation before and after procedures. [Review] *Med Clin North Am* 2001; **85:** 1109–16.

Turner M, Haywood G. Preoperative assessment of cardiac risk for non-cardiac surgery. *J R Coll Phys Lond* 1998; **32:** 545–7.

2. Sepsis: recognition and management

Larry Mulleague and Steve Shaw

Sepsis occurs in approximately one in five of all hospital admissions and is the leading cause of death in intensive care. There are an estimated 700 000 cases of severe sepsis in the USA every year resulting in the death of 200 000 patients. Its incidence is increasing reflecting an increasingly aging population, changes in antibiotic use, cancer and immunosuppression treatments and the increased use of indwelling devices. Once organ failure is established, mortality ranges from 20 to 80% and upwards. Early recognition and aggressive therapy can improve survival, and greater understanding of the complex pathophysiology of sepsis has led to new treatment options.

DEFINITIONS

To aid its early recognition it is important to define the problem. The terms sepsis, septic shock, septicemia and bacteremia are often used interchangeably and this can be confusing. In 1991, at the American College of Chest Physicians and Society of Critical Care Medicine Consensus Conference physicians sought agreement on a set of definitions that could be applied to patients with sepsis and its sequelae (Table 2.1).[1] It was also an attempt to improve homogeneity between putative treatment trials. The conference proposed a new term – systemic inflammatory response syndrome (SIRS) to describe the widespread inflammation that occurs following a wide variety of insults that may be independent of infections.

Table 2.1 Definitions of sepsis and associated terms

Infection
> Invasion of microorganisms into a normally sterile site, often associated with an inflammatory host response

Systemic inflammatory response syndrome (SIRS)
> A systemic inflammatory response to a variety of clinical insults, consisting of two or more of the following:
> - temperature >38 °C or <36 °C;
> - heart rate >90 beats/min;
> - respiratory rate >20 breaths/min or $Paco_2$ <4.3 kPa
> - white blood cell count > 12 000/mm³, <4000 cells/mm³, or >10% immature cells

Sepsis
> The systemic inflammatory response to infection. SIRS caused by infection.

Severe sepsis
> Sepsis associated with organ dysfunction:
> - hypotension/hypoperfusion
> - oliguria
> - alteration in mental status
> - lactic acidosis
> - coagulopathy

Septic shock
> Sepsis with hypotension despite adequate fluid resuscitation
> Hypotension defined as systolic blood pressure <90 mmHg or a reduction of >40 mmHg from baseline

(Reproduced with permission from Bone et al. *Chest* 1992; 101: 1644–55.[1])

RISK FACTORS

A variety of host factors, both exogenous and endogenous, predispose to the development of sepsis. They include extremes of age, immunosuppression, malignancy, multiple trauma, diabetes mellitus, malnutrition, alcoholism, prolonged hospitalization, renal and/or hepatic failure, indwelling catheters/devices and prolonged antibiotic use.

PATHOPHYSIOLOGY OF SEPSIS

Although incompletely understood, sepsis can be seen as a cascade of events or network that is initiated by a focus of infection or injury and ends with severe endothelial damage, profound hemodynamic derangement and often death. Sepsis results from a generalized inflammatory and procoagulant host response to infection.

Septic shock has traditionally been recognized as a consequence of Gram-negative bacteremia, but it is also caused by Gram-positive organisms, toxins, fungi, viruses and parasites. Endotoxin, also known as lipopolysaccharide (LPS), is exclusive to and an integral component of the cell wall of Gram-negative bacteria and has a protective role against host defense factors. It is the LPS that is the primary initiator of Gram-negative septic shock. Gram-positive bacteria produce an exotoxin or cause an inflammatory reaction via a component of the cell wall.

Infection activates plasmatic (complement, coagulation and kallikrein-kinin systems) and cellular (neutrophils, monocytes/macrophages and endothelial cells) elements in the host, which lead to the release of a number of mediators and molecules (cytokines, chemokines and acute phase proteins) that orchestrate the host inflammatory response to infection.

The production of proinflammatory cytokines, vasoactive mediators and reactive oxygen species in the immuno-inflammatory process is common to both SIRS and sepsis. Proinflammatory cytokines are soluble immunoregulatory peptides, the most important of which are interleukin (IL)-1, tumor necrosis factor (TNF), IL-6, IL-8 and IL-10. Released by the host in response to bacteria or bacterial products they can stimulate the release of other proinflammatory cytokines promoting endothelial cell leukocyte adhesion, activation of clotting factors, release of proteases and induction of cyclooxygenase. Host response to infection also involves the anti-inflammatory cytokines, which antagonize or modulate the proinflammatory response. Cytokine production in the blood results in widespread endothelial cell activation with expression of adhesion molecules, activation of the coagulation cascade and further production of chemokines and cytokines.

The activation and adhesion of circulating neutrophils to the endothelium result in loss of vascular integrity and consequent failure to maintain blood pressure. IL-1 and TNF act synergistically causing the induction of cyclooxygenase, platelet activation factor and NO synthase to induce hypotension, increased vascular permeability and platelet aggregation. TNF and IL1 also depress myocardial function directly. Refractory shock with leakage of fluid (edema) and the failure of organs with large capillary beds (lungs and kidneys) leads to death.

Recent advances indicate that inflammation and coagulation are intimately linked and that the hemostatic system participates in the pathophysiology of severe sepsis and associated acute organ dysfunction. Abnormal activation of coagulation is due in part to expression of tissue factor (TF) on intravascular cells in response to cytokines including IL-1β and TNF leading to thrombosis and disseminated intravascular coagulopathy (DIC). Other factors include deficiency of protein C (which is associated with increased mortality in sepsis) and an impaired fibrinolytic response. New treatment strategies are seeking to address the imbalance in all three of the major processes that drive sepsis – coagulation, inflammation and suppressed fibrinolysis.

PATHOPHYSIOLOGY OF MULTIORGAN DYSFUNCTION SYNDROME

It is believed that multiorgan dysfunction syndrome (MODS) develops as a result of tissue hypoxia, hypoperfusion, abnormal tissue blood flow and abnormal cellular metabolism.

CARDIOVASCULAR DYSFUNCTION

Sepsis has a profound effect on the cardiovascular system, the dominant hemodynamic feature being peripheral vascular failure. Expression of nitric oxide and cyclooxygenase products result in quite profound microcirculatory changes:

- vasodilatation
- arteriovenous shunting
- decreased oxygen extraction
- increased capillary permeability with interstitial edema.

The initial response is characterized by vasodilation, increased cardiac output, and provided hypovolemia is corrected, initially, a maintained blood pressure. As vasodilation continues blood pressure decreases.

Myocardial depression is a common feature of sepsis. It may result from a combination of direct myocardial depressant effect of TNF or other factors that include acidosis, hypoxemia and myocardial edema. There may be reduction in ejection fraction and reversible left and right ventricular segmental wall abnormalities.

The principal function of the circulation is to deliver oxygen to respiring tissue.

Oxygen delivery (DO_2)	= cardiac output $\times$ arterial oxygen content = 500–700 ml/min/m^2 (600 ml/min)
Oxygen consumption (VO_2)	= cardiac output $\times$ arterial-venous oxygen content = 120–160 ml/min/m^2 (250 ml/min)

As oxygen delivery falls a critical point is reached after which oxygen consumption also falls representing anaerobic tissue respiration leading to lactic acidosis and tissue damage. Increasing oxygen delivery may help improve survival but this is the subject of some debate.

RESPIRATORY DYSFUNCTION

Respiratory failure is a common manifestation of sepsis and 25% of patients present with or develop acute respiratory distress syndrome (ARDS) or acute lung injury (ALI) (Figure 2.1). The primary cause is pulmonary capillary endothelial dysfunction resulting in interstitial and alveolar edema of protein-rich exudative fluid leading to hypoxemia – 'leaky lungs'.

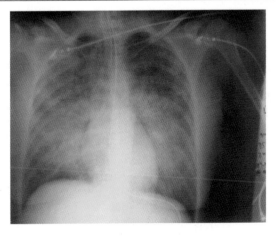

Figure 2.1
A chest radiograph of a patient with acute respiratory distress syndrome (ARDS).

Reduction in pulmonary blood flow and perfusion pressure leads to ventilation–perfusion inequalities (V/Q mismatch) producing hypoxemia. An important pathogenic mechanism of lung destruction is the recruitment and degranulation of neutrophils. Therapeutic agents that may prevent this primary pathophysiological process, e.g. neutrophil elastase inhibitors, are currently being investigated.

RENAL DYSFUNCTION

Acute renal failure is a common complication (approximately 50%) of sepsis and is thought to be secondary to a combination of factors – changes in distribution of renal blood flow, hypoperfusion, hypovolemia and loss of autoregulation.

GASTROINTESTINAL DYSFUNCTION

Hypoperfusion of the gut predisposes to ischemic injury of gut mucosa, which once described as the 'motor' of sepsis now probably serves more as the fuel. The resulting translocation of bacteria or bacterial products such as endotoxins helps to amplify the inflammatory process.

HEMATOLOGICAL DYSFUNCTION

Cytokine-mediated activation of the clotting system can result in DIC which predisposes to both bleeding and microvascular thrombi and worsening of MODS. Circulating levels of protein C and antithrombin III are reduced in severe sepsis and may prognosticate survival. Neutrophils and platelet counts are frequently depressed as a result of marrow suppression and endothelial adherance. The prothrombin time is prolonged and fibrin/fibrinogen degradation products (FDPs) are elevated.

CENTRAL NERVOUS SYSTEM DYSFUNCTION

Cerebral dysfunction is a common feature of sepsis. Septic encephalopathy results in agitation, confusion and a decrease in Glasgow Coma Scale (GCS) score. It can progress to coma. The etiology is multifactorial – toxins, metabolic and electrolyte disturbances and reduced cerebral perfusion.

CLINICAL FEATURES OF SEPSIS

Septic shock is an emergency. The diagnosis is often difficult and a high index of suspicion is required. The manifestation of sepsis may be slow and insidious or rapid and immediately life-threatening. Timely intervention is the key to positive patient outcome. Resuscitation should not be delayed whilst trying to establish an accurate diagnosis. A detailed history may help to identify factors that predispose to development of sepsis as outlined in Table 2.2.

INVESTIGATIONS

Commence with a detailed examination and history. Bacterial cultures of blood and urine should be done for all septic patients. A low white blood cell (WBC) count with left shift suggests severe sepsis. At least two sets of blood cultures should be taken from a fresh venepuncture site soon after the onset of rigor or fever. Positive blood cultures are the accepted proof of serious infection, but blood cultures are positive in approximately 30% of patients only. A chest radiograph is part of the basic routine investigations in these patients. Where there is cough with productive sputum culture of secretions should be done. Where intra-abdominal sepsis is suspected an upright abdominal radiograph should be obtained in the first instance. Elevated bilirubin and alkaline phosphatase suggests biliary obstruction. Ultrasound is the modality of choice for investigating suspected pathologies of the gallbladder, kidneys and pelvis (Figures 2.2 and 2.3). It is non-invasive and feasible to perform at the bedside. When ultrasound is difficult or not diagnostic or if the collection is

Table 2.2 Key systemic features predisposing to the development of sepsis

Temperature: pyrexia >38 °C but also hypothermia <36 °C
rigors/sweating

Hemodynamic: sinus tachycardia
hypotension
warm extremities/rapid capillary
refill/bounding pulse

Respiratory: tachypnea
respiratory alkalosis
hypoxemia

Metabolic: metabolic acidosis
increased lactate
hyperglycemia/or in severe cases
hypoglycemia

Hematological: leukocytosis/leukopenia/
leukemoid reaction
thrombocytopenia
prolonged prothrombin time
increased fibrin degradation
products (FDPs)

Hepatic: abnormal liver function tests
jaundice

Renal: oliguria

Neurological: confusion
restlessness
stupor/coma

Gastrointestinal: nausea/vomiting
hypoalbuminemia

retroperitoneal more sophisticated imaging technologies such as helical computed tomography (CT), magnetic resonance and scintographic methods should be considered. Pyuria and WBC casts suggest renal origin. Helical CT is the main initial study in acute renal infection (Figure 2.4) and useful for identifying small stones and perinephric fluid collections.

Collections identified by radiology should, where technically possible, be aspirated and drained and samples sent for microbiological analysis and Gram staining.

When a central venous catheter (CVC) or other indwelling device is suspected to be the source of infection, the diagnosis may be made by blood cultures or evidence of infection of the skin site. When the potential risk outweighs the benefit of leaving the catheter in place the catheter should be removed.

When definitive identification of the source of infection is difficult, lumbar puncture for cerebrospinal fluid (CSF) analysis, transthoracic or transeosphageal echocardiogram for suspected bacterial endocarditis and facial sinus radiograph for occult sinusitis should be considered.

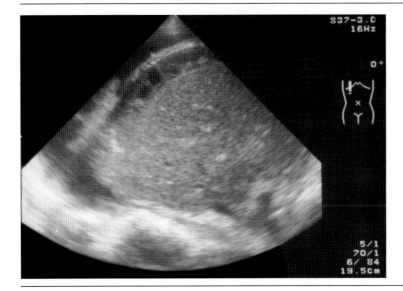

Figure 2.2

Ultrasound scan showing a thick-walled chronic perinephric collection as the source of acute sepsis.

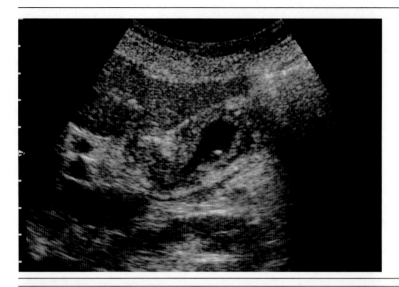

Figure 2.3

Ultrasound scan showing a thick walled and swollen gallbladder with calculus as the source of acute sepsis.

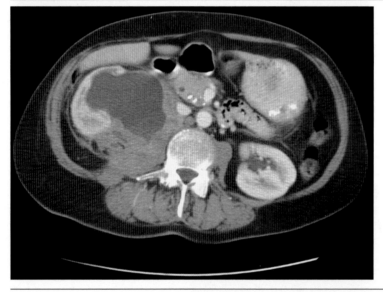

Figure 2.4

A computed tomography (CT) scan identifying a large intra-renal abscess as the source of acute sepsis.

TREATMENT

Therapy of sepsis, despite years of clinical trials, is primarily supportive. Multimodal therapies aimed at the several immunological and physiological disturbances occurring simultaneously have met with limited success. Simple but critical measures remain the best. The first impor-

tant step is recognition and assessment of severity. An astute assessment including checking for vital signs, level of consciousness, laboratory tests and hemodynamic status is critical to planning interventions for optimum outcome. Treatment is based on the following principles:

- Identification of source and control of infection.

- Early and appropriate antibiotics to eliminate the pathogens.
- Support of failing organs.

CONTROL OF INFECTION

Half of all cases of septic shock in most ICUs are caused by infections requiring urgent surgical management. Pus filled cavities (abscess, empyema), necrotic tissue and infected tissue or gross tissue contamination (open wounds, peritonitis) will need surgical treatment at the earliest opportunity. The initial management of well-defined and accessible abscesses should be percutaneous drainage. Laparotomy should be reserved for those circumstances in which there is a suspicion of necrotic tissue, or collections are not well defined or amenable to percutaneous drainage or there is a significant risk of ongoing peritoneal contamination or bowel ischemia. There is a limited role for empirical laparotomy. Suspected infected catheters should be removed and tips sent for culture.

CHOICE OF ANTIBIOTICS

Presumed infection that threatens life or major organ dysfunction warrants empirical antibiotic therapy. If a patient is hospitalized the potential is greater. The suspected site of infection and probable microbe, host factors, immuno-suppression and hospitalization, and local antibiotic resistance patterns dictate the antibiotic choice.

Retrospective studies have shown that early administration of appropriate antibiotics reduces mortality in patients with bloodstream infections caused by Gram-negative organisms. This is also likely for patients with Gram-positive-induced sepsis. Table 2.3 outlines some recommendations for choice of agent in certain infections. Where doubt exists expert microbiological advice should be sought.

Table 2.3 Some recommendations for empirical antibiotic therapy in sepsis

Disease/common pathogens	Empirical therapy
Pneumonia Commmunity acquired, e.g. *Streptococcus pneumoniae, Haemophilus influenzae, Staphylococcus aureus*	Co-amoxiclav or cefotaxime + erythromycin
Hospital acquired, e.g. *S. aureus, Klebsiella* and *Pseudomonas* spp.	Ceftazidime alone or piperacillin + gentamicin
Intra-abdominal sepsis/ biliary tree sepsis *Enterobacter* spp., *S. aureus*, anaerobes	Cefuroxime + metronidazole or piperacillin + gentamicin
Urinary tract Commuinity acquired, e.g. *Escherichia coli* and *Klebsiella*	Co-amoxiclav or cefotaxime
Hospital acquired *Enterobacter, Serratia* and *Pseudomonas*	Ceftazidime or piperacillin + gentamicin
Skin and soft tissues *S. aureus*, group A streptococci	Co-amoxiclav or amoxycillin + flucloxacillin
Febrile neutropenic patient *P. aeruginosa, K. pneumoniae, E. coli, S. aureus*	Cephalosporin, aminoglycoside + anti-fungal/antiviral

---

Third and fourth generation cephalosporins and carbapenem antibiotics are equally effective as empirical therapy in patients with severe sepsis. Indiscriminate use of glycopeptide antibiotics (e.g. vancomycin and teicoplanin) for presumed Gram-positive infections in patients with severe sepsis should be avoided. However, they are appropriate in severely ill patients with catheter-related infections or in certain circumstances where MRSA (methicillin-resistant *Staphylococcus aureus*) predominates.

The immunocompromised patient and the intensive-care patient with significant underlying disease or organ failure are at risk of fungal infections, most often with *Candida* spp., but also increasingly *Aspergillus* spp. Antifungals are recommended for patients with proved candidemia. Intravenous administration is generally preferred and results in rapid therapeutic concentrations at the site of the infection.

Emergence of resistant strains and cross-infections are common in the ITU; these may be prevented by appropriate infection control measures and a strict antibiotic policy.

SUPPORT OF FAILING ORGANS

Management of septic shock is similar for all patients in shock. Assessment and resuscitation should proceed simultaneously beginning with Airway, Breathing and Circulation (ABC). The goals of management are to restore tissue perfusion and oxygen delivery as well as metabolic support and treatment of the source of sepsis.

MONITORING

The need for close monitoring of the hemodynamic, respiratory, renal, neurological and metabolic endpoints of resuscitation warrants early referral to critical care staff. Early referral improves chances of recovery.

Invasive monitoring is especially important in patients with serious myocardial, pulmonary or renal dysfunction, or in those unresponsive to low-dose vasopressor/inotropic agents. Arterial catheters allow beat to beat assessment of blood pressure and frequent arterial blood gas analysis. Central venous pressure (CVP) readings are useful to assess volemic status but be aware that ventricular compliance and peripheral vascular tone can be significantly altered by changes in temperature, vasopressor drugs, sedatives and mechanical ventilation. Pulmonary artery catheters which provide measurements of right and left-sided heart function may be indicated to assist in the diagnosis and management of severe sepsis, helping to differentiate cardiogenic from septic shock. Furthermore, they may help guide the use of inotropic agents, intravenous fluids and vasoconstrictor therapy. The routine use of these devices has recently been questioned.[2]

Non-invasive techniques for assessing cardiac function include aortic Doppler ultrasound and echocardiography. Stroke volume as measured by esophageal Doppler has been demonstrated to be a very useful guide to endpoint resuscitation.

The importance of adopting a quick and aggressive approach to resuscitation cannot be overemphasized. The response to resuscitation should be monitored closely by frequent reassessment of tissue perfusion.

GENERAL SUPPORTIVE MEASURES
- Establish large bore intravenous (IV) access (minimum 2 × 16 G cannula)
- Administer oxygen
- Insert urinary catheter
- Measure pulse oximetry
- Send blood for investigations/cultures/arterial blood gas
- Chest radiograph

CARDIOVASCULAR SUPPORT
The primary goal of cardiovascular support is to rapidly normalize tissue perfusion and optimize oxygen delivery. Efforts to drive oxygen delivery to supranormal values – goal-directed therapy – has been the subject of longstanding controversy. However, recent literature suggests there may be some benefit of early goal-directed therapy.

A number of studies have shown that aggressive volume resuscitation is one of the mainstays of treatment of septic shock. Adequate volume resuscitation is not easily determined and should be titrated to multiple clinical endpoints, which include blood pressure, heart rate, urine output, mentation, skin perfusion and lactic acidosis. Fluids should be administered until an optimal cardiac output is achieved. Because of vasodilatation and capillary leakage in septic shock most patients require a minimum of 1–2 l of colloid or 4–8 l of crystalloid to restore circulating volume in the early period of resuscitation. A fluid challenge – by definition in adults – involves the administration of 250 ml of fluid over 10 minutes thus allowing assessment of the hemodynamic response. The aim is to restore the mean arterial blood pressure (MAP) to sustain adequate end-organ perfusion indicated by improved mentation, urine output and reduced acidosis. The goal of MAP 70 mmHg is often quoted but this may not be appropriate in certain situations such as a premorbid history of hypertension or a rapidly changing clinical condition. The type of fluid used probably has no significant clinical impact on outcome as long as appropriate clinical endpoints are used. Crystalloids and colloids have been found to be equally effective when titrated to the same hemodynamic endpoint.

In patients who remain hypotensive despite adequate fluid resuscitation an inotrope and/or vasopressor is required. Due to the presence of inflammatory mediators a raised cardiac output often accompanies a low systemic vascular resistance (SVR) in fluid-resuscitated septic patients. Inotrope selection will depend to some extent on the etiology of the septic shock. The high cardiac output, peripherally vasodilated patient who is often typical of septic shock will benefit from a vasopressor agent such as norepinephrine. Dopamine has also traditionally been used but is a relatively weak vasoconstrictor in septic shock and has a dose-dependent range of actions.

The effects of some commonly used agents on blood pressure, vascular resistance and cardiac output are summarized in Table 2.4.

RESPIRATORY SUPPORT

Respiratory failure in sepsis is common. ARDS is the pulmonary manifestation of multiple organ failure (see Figure 2.1). Respiratory support begins in the conscious patient with high-flow oxygen therapy followed by continuous positive airways pressure (CPAP). This is a mechanical means whereby a high-flow air–oxygen mixture is delivered to the patient who exhales against a valve. In this way a positive pressure is continually produced keeping the alveoli open during expiration and preventing atelectasis. This improves oxygenation, reduces the work of breathing and lowers right ventricular preload. When CPAP fails or if the level of consciousness falls, or exhaustion threatens the airway the patient must be intubated

---

Table 2.4 Effects of some therapeutic agents used for cardiovascular support in septic shock

	Blood pressure	Cardiac output	SVR
Epinephrine (0.01–0.2 µg/kg/min)	+	++	+
Norepinephrine (0.03–0.8 µg/kg/min)	++	+/−	++
Dopamine			
low dose (0.5–2.5 µg/kg/min)	+/−	+	−
high dose (2–10.0 µg/kg/min)	++	++	++
Dobutamine (2.5–10 µg/kg/min)	−/+	++	−
Vasopressin (0.02–0.1 U/min)	++	+/−	++

+, increase; −, decrease; +/−, no significant change.

and mechanical ventilation commenced. Respiratory failure may manifest itself as either a low Pao_2 and/or high $Paco_2$. A respiratory rate >30 breaths/min, hypoxemia requiring an inspired oxygen concentration (FiO_2) of 50% or above and a pH <7.2 are all indications of impending respiratory failure requiring mechanical ventilation. Controversy surrounds almost all aspects of mechanical ventilation of patients with ARDS and is beyond the scope of this discussion. However, a recent multicenter study using lower tidal volumes demonstrated a clear outcome benefit.[3]

RENAL SUPPORT

No single therapy has been shown to prevent or reverse renal failure but optimal volume resuscitation and maintenance of adequate blood pressure are universally accepted goals. The use of 'low-dose' dopamine to preserve renal function is not supported by current evidence. Potentially nephrotoxic agents should be avoided where possible. Renal replacement is now provided by continuous hemofiltration.

GASTROINTESTINAL SUPPORT

Again, fluid resuscitation and adequate blood pressure serve to prevent mesenteric hypoperfusion. The optimal timing, mode of replacement, composition and level of nutritional replacement is subject to debate. Timely provision of enteral replacement is generally preferred to intravenous replacement. Stress ulcer prophylaxis includes the above plus the use of either an H_2-blocker or sucralfate.

COAGULATION

DIC may require correction with fresh frozen plasma, activated clotting factors and cryoprecipitate. Thrombocytopenia is not routinely corrected unless there is a risk of hemorrhage or the platelet count is less than 20 000/mm³.

OTHER SUPPORTIVE MEASURES

All patients should receive prophylaxis against the development of DVT. Unless contraindicated fixed dose unfractionated heparin, low-molecular weight heparins or venous-compression devices should be used.

Unless contraindicated, a hemoglobin level between 7 g/dl and 9 g/dl is associated with better ITU survival.

CONTROVERSIAL MEASURES

Recent therapies that have yet to receive widespread approval in the treatment of sepsis include recombinant activated protein C (rAPC), anticytokine therapy, low dose steroids, early goal-directed treatment and tight glycemic control.

SUMMARY

Severe sepsis occurs when the physiological response to infection leads to impaired function of vital organs. Sepsis is a major cause of morbidity and mortality in hospitals and its incidence is increasing. The development of specific therapies continues, but for now, early recognition and prompt treatment is essential to prevent disease progression.

REFERENCE

1. Bone RC, Balk RA, Cerra FB et al. Definitions for sepsis and organ failure and guidelines for the use of innovative therapies in sepsis. The ACCP/SCCM Consensus Conference Committee. American College of Chest Physicians/Society of Critical Care Medicine. *Chest* 1992; **101**: 1644–55.
2. Connors A, Speroff T, Dawson N, et al. The effectiveness of right heart catheterization in the initial care of critically ill patients. *JAMA* 1996; **276**: 889–97.
3. The ARDS network. Ventilation with lower tidal volumes as compared with traditional volumes for acute lung injury and the acute respiratory distress syndrome. *N Engl J Med* 2000; **342**: 1301–8.

FURTHER READING

Bersten AD, Soni N. Oh's Intensive Care Manual, 5th edn. Oh TE (ed). Oxford: Butterworth Heinemann, 2003.

Corke CF. *Practical Intensive Care Medicine – Problem Solving in the ICU*. Oxford: Butterworth-Heinemann Ltd, 2000.

Hinds CJ, Watson D (eds). *Intensive Care – A Concise Textbook*, 2nd edn. London: WB Saunders Co. Ltd, 1996.

Llewelyn M, Cohen J et al. Diagnosis of infection in sepsis. *Intensive Care Med* 2001; 27 (Suppl 1): S10–32.

Webb AR, Shapiro MJ, Singer M, Suter PM (eds) *Oxford Textbook of Critical Care*, 1st edn. Oxford, Oxford Medical Publications, 1999.

3. Acute renal failure

Chris Laing and Guy Neild

Acute renal failure (ARF) is a common medical emergency occurring, in some estimates, in up to 10% of hospital admissions. It may cause death if untreated but even with optimal management results in significant morbidity and mortality. Established ARF necessitates renal replacement therapy, which is a scant resource in many healthcare settings, presents logistical problems, is expensive and may be hazardous. Management of ARF is therefore an important subject for clinicians in the secondary care setting but is of particular interest to the urologist. Urological disease may present with obstructive nephropathy resulting in ARF while many urological interventions may compromise renal function. There is a relatively high incidence of background renal insufficiency in urology patients, particularly the elderly, and such cases may be rendered clinically anephric by relatively minor renal insults. We advocate early involvement of the renal physician in the management of ARF, however specialist nephrology input is not always immediately available. We therefore hope this chapter will serve as a primer in ARF for the non-nephrologist.

PATHOPHYSIOLOGY OF ACUTE RENAL FAILURE

Kidney function is essential for normal homeostasis and maintenance of the *internal milieu*. Each human kidney contains around one million nephrons, each of which comprises a glomerulus and renal tubule. The glomeruli filter the renal blood and this filtrate is then modified by the renal tubule, where reabsorption and excretion of solutes and water take place under hormonal influence. Filtered bicarbonate is reabsorbed in the proximal tubule while net acid is excreted in by the distal tubule. As a conse-

quence, the kidney is able to maintain electrolyte, osmolar, circulating volume and acid–base homeostasis. The kidney also secretes erythropoietin (which is required for erythropoiesis), renin (which stimulates the renin–angiotensin cascade to preserve circulating volume and blood pressure) and hydroxylates vitamin D, thereby facilitating calcium homeostasis.

The glomerular filtration rate (GFR) is a measurement of the volume of blood which can be filtered in a given time (ml/min) and provides an overall measure of renal excretory capacity. To maintain the GFR the kidney must have adequate renal blood flow, intraglomerular pressure and the structural integrity of the glomerulus must be maintained, and the filtrate must pass through the tubule without intrarenal or more distal obstruction. When the aforementioned conditions are adversely affected, e.g. in a number of disease processes, renal failure occurs.

ETIOLOGY OF ACUTE RENAL FAILURE

Causes of ARF are traditionally divided into prerenal, renal and postrenal. In prerenal causes of ARF renal blood flow is compromised because of reduced total or effective circulating volume or by renal arterial disease. Renal causes of ARF include a number of specific disease processes that result in glomerular or tubular damage or intrarenal obstruction. The most common is acute tubular necrosis (ATN) – ischemic injury of the renal tubular epithelium caused by a number of insults which result in intrarenal tubular obstruction. In postrenal ARF urine outflow is compromised resulting in tubular back-pressure and reduced filtration. One recent study reported on etiology of ARF in a secondary care setting; 45% were due to ATN, 21% prerenal, 13% acute on chronic, 10% due to obstruction, 4% due to glomerulonephritis or vasculitis, 2% due to interstitial nephritis and 1% due to atheroemboli. The causes of ARF are summarized in Tables 3.1–3.3. Specific disease processes are described in more detail later in the chapter.

COMPLICATIONS OF ACUTE RENAL FAILURE

As GFR falls clearance of uremic toxins (the breakdown products of catabolism) accumulate in the circulation. This leads to the 'uremic' syndrome – a condition of non-specific ill health – with malaise, lethargy, anorexia and vomiting. Uremic encephalopathy may ensue. In its early stages this encephalopathy may be manifest by subtle personality change, disturbance of

Table 3.1 Prerenal causes of acute renal failure

Cause	Examples
Hemorrhage	Trauma
	Surgery
	Gastrointestinal hemorrhage
	Ruptured abdominal aortic aneurysm
	Hematuria
Dehydration	Gastrointestinal losses (vomiting, diarrhoea)
	Gastrointestinal obstruction
	Excessive diuresis
	Glycosuria
	Pyrexia and hyperpyrexia
	Third space fluid losses (e.g. acute pancreatitis)
	Excessive exertion
	Confusion and immobility
Decreased effective blood volume	Sepsis
	Anaphylaxis
	Hepatic failure
	Nephrotic syndrome and other hypoalbuminemic states
Cardiogenic shock	Cardiac arrhythmia
	Myocardial infarction
	Cardiomyopathy
	Myocarditis
	Valvular heart disease
	Cardiac tamponade
	Pulmonary embolism
Renovascular disease	Complete renal artery occlusion in atherosclerotic renal artery stenosis
	Dissecting abdominal aortic aneurysm
	Renal artery thrombosis
	Renal thromboembolism
Hepatorenal syndrome	Acute hepatitis with fulminant hepatic failure
	Decompensated chronic liver disease

Table 3.2 Renal causes of acute renal failure

Cause	Examples
Acute tubular necrosis	Shock
	Systemic sepsis
	Drug toxicity
	Iodine contrast
Acute interstitial nephritis	Drugs
	Pyelonephritis
	Idiopathic
	Sarcoidosis
	Autoimmune (Sjögren's syndrome)
	Systemic bacterial infection (leptospirosis, streptococcosis)
	HIV infection
	Hypercalcemia
Rapidly progressive glomulonephritis/renal vasculitis	Anti-GBM disease
	Post-infectious
	Wegener's granulomatosis
	Churg–Strauss syndrome
	Microscopic polyangiitis
	Systemic lupus erythematosus
Thrombotic microangiopathy	Idiopathic
	Escherichia coli O157:H7 associated
	Malignant hypertension
	Pregnancy
	Drugs
	Antiphospholipid antibodies
Intrarenal obstruction	Cast nephropathy
	Myoglobinuria (rhabdomyolysis)
	Crytalluria (tumor lysis syndrome)

Table 3.3 Postrenal causes of acute renal failure

Cause	Examples
Pelviureteric and ureteric obstruction	Stone
	Blood clot
	Neoplasm
	External compression from neoplasm or lymph nodes
	Retroperitoneal fibrosis
Bladder obstruction	Prostatomegaly
	Bladder neoplasm
	External compression from neoplasm

sleep–wake cycle and proprioceptive deficits (demonstrable by a uremic 'flap' of the out-stretched hands). In advanced uremic encephalopathy there is confusion, drowsiness, coma and death. Uremia can also lead to acute gastritis resulting in gastrointestinal hemor-rhage and uremic pericarditis, which rarely causes cardiac tamponade, and hemodynamic compromise. It also causes disordered platelet function and therefore increases risk of bleed-ing.

In renal failure there is reduced proximal tubular bicarbonate reabsorption and distal tubular proton secretion. This results in meta-bolic acidosis with reduced serum bicarbonate and a compensatory reduction of P_{CO_2} through hyperventilation. This compensatory mecha-nism may be inadequate to maintain pH within normal limits and genuine acidemia may ensue. This is deleterious to cellular function and, per-haps most significantly, can lead to decreased myocardial contractility. In ARF, due to severe illness (such as sepsis or cardiogenic shock) the acidosis may be exacerbated by a superimposed lactic acidosis from reduced tissue perfusion.

Failure to excrete potassium in ARF may result in hyperkalemia. The excretory deficit in ARF is often compounded by metabolic acido-sis, which increases extracellular potassium as well as catabolism and tissue breakdown, which increase the potassium load. The increase in extracellular potassium results in reduced intra-cellular to extracellular potassium concentration gradient, reduced cell membrane excitability and hence neuromuscular and cardiac conduc-tion problems. Severe hyperkalemia will lead to T-wave peaking on the electrocardiogram (ECG), broadening of the QRS complexes, bradycardia and cardiac asystole.

Hyperphosphatemia is common and may result in a profound itch. Phosphate binds cal-cium leading to hypocalcemia which is further exacerbated by reduced renal 1-hydroxylation of vitamin D. In the longer term renal hypocal-cemia will be countered by secondary hyper-parathyroidism. The coexistent acidosis in ARF usually maintains ionized calcium within near normal limits and symptomatic hypocalcemia (with tetany) is unusual.

Reduced natriuresis in the face of a main-tained fluid intake will result in hypervolemia and increased pulmonary capillary hydrostatic pressure. This causes a movement of fluid from the intravascular compartment to the interstitial space and finally into the alveoli. As this fluid retention progresses left ventricular dilatation and failure may occur, particularly in those with underlying cardiac disease, and this further exacerbates pulmonary venous hypertension. As pulmonary edema develops, lung compli-ance reduces and alveolar diffusion capacity is reduced resulting in hypoxia (type I respiratory failure). In severe pulmonary edema and exhaustion the P_{CO_2} may start to rise resulting in type II respiratory failure.

CLINICAL ASSESSMENT OF THE PATIENT WITH ACUTE RENAL FAILURE

As outlined above, ARF is a medical emergency leading to serious neurological, cardiovascular and respiratory complications. The initial assessment should therefore be as for all criti-cally ill patients. The patency of the airways should be ascertained followed by an assess-ment of respiration and circulatory status. A full set of observations including pulse, blood pres-sure, oxygen saturation and formal assessment of conscious level should then be taken and documented.

The more detailed clinical assessment of the ARF patient should then focus on assessment of fluid status, presence of complications and determination of the likely causes of the ARF. With this information an appropriate plan of investigation and management can be formu-lated. This assessment is reliant on thorough history taking, examination and rigorous review of the patient's medical notes and charts with particular emphasis on premorbid levels of renal function, rate of deterioration of function, drug administrations, vital signs, urinalysis, fluid balance and urine output.

ASSESSMENT OF VOLUME STATUS

Assessment of fluid status should determine whether the patient is euvolemic, hypovolemic or hypervolemic. In hypovolemia there may be malaise, lethargy and subjective sensation of thirst. On examination there will be cooling of the peripheries and reduced skin turgor. The jugular venous pressure will not be visible and there will be general emptying and collapse of the peripheral veins. Peripheral measurements of oxygen saturation may be reduced (due to decreased capillary perfusion rather than hypoxia). Tachycardia will normally be present, however, the pulse should be interpreted with caution in patients who are beta-blocked. Postural hypotension – determined by blood pressure measurement in the supine then upright or standing posture – is highly suggestive of hypovolemia, however, other causes of orthostatic hypotension such as vasodilator drug therapy or autonomic failure should be considered. Once the compensatory mechanisms of chronotropy and peripheral vasoconstriction have been overcome, hypotension will ensue and reduced organ perfusion may result in alteration of the conscious level, oliguria and cardiac complications such as chest pain or arrhythmias.

In hypervolemia patients will generally be hypertensive, however, in severe uremia (and hence acidosis) or in patients with cardiovascular comorbidity this may not be the case. The jugular venous pressure will generally be elevated. Pulmonary edema will present with dyspnea, orthopnea, wheeze and pink sputum and clinical examination will reveal expiratory ronchi, bibasal effusions, bibasal crepitations and a third heart sound on auscultation of the precordium. Raised venous hydrostatic pressure may result in peripheral edema, however, in bed-bound patients this may accumulate around the waist and sacrum rather than the ankles or feet. The presence of edema secondary to hypoalbuminemia can be misinterpreted as evidence of fluid overload when, in fact, such patients may be intravascularly depleted. In critically ill patients, or in patients where determination of volume status is difficult, ultrasonographic or invasive arterial and venous monitoring may be undertaken. This will be discussed later.

ASSESSMENT OF URINE OUTPUT

Oliguria is a good early marker of impaired renal function and should be regarded as significant when the urine output is persistently less than 30 ml/h. Complete anuria is uncommon but may be seen in obstructive ARF, vascular occlusion or very aggressive forms of glomerulonephritis such as Goodpasture's syndrome.

Severe renal impairment may occur in the presence of normal or even increased urine volumes. This is chiefly dependent on relative glomerular and tubular dysfunction. Around 90% of the water filtered in the glomerulus is reabsorbed in the renal tubule. If the tubule's water reabsorption capacity is significantly reduced, urine volume may be normal or even increased in the face of drastic reductions in GFR.

Polyuric ARF can occur in acute tubular disease such as acute interstitial nephritis and is often seen in the recovery phase of ATN. Urinary obstruction leads to increased intrarenal tubular pressures, reduced glomerular filtration, tubular dysfunction and downregulation of distal tubular aquaporins. The latter facilitate tubular water reabsorption and the reduced tubular reabsorptive capacity may result in polyuric ARF secondary to partial obstruction.

CLINICAL MANIFESTATIONS AND COMPLICATIONS OF UREMIA

The clinical manifestations of uremia are variable but include anorexia, nausea, vomiting, malaise and lethargy. The conscious level and lucidity of the patient should be noted, as should the presence or absence of a uremic flap (see above). Metabolic acidosis may be evident as breathlessness. A deep, sighing respiratory pattern described as 'Kussmaul's respiration' is characteristic of the compensatory hyperventilation of a profound metabolic acidosis. There may be an itch (related primarily to hyperphosphatemia) and hiccups. Uremic pericarditis is a rare complication of uremia resulting in chest pain (often pleuritic), fever, a pericardial rub on auscultation of the precordium and occasionally cardiac tamponade with hypotension, pulsus paradoxus and jugular venous distension increased on inspiration. Hyperkalemia may present clinically with muscle weakness and bradycardia.

CLINICAL ASSESSMENT OF THE CAUSE OF ARF

In prerenal ARF there may be a clear clinical history of hypovolemic insult such as vomiting, diarrhoea or recent administration of diuretics. Perioperative surgical patients are particularly vulnerable and fluid losses may be underestimated in conditions such as bowel obstruction, pancreatitis, high outputs from stomas or other diversions or in any presentation of sepsis. The elderly, due to problems with mobility, may be unable to replenish their fluid losses in dehydration while the very incapacitated may be unable to perceive or complain of symptoms of dehydration. Hemorrhage sufficient to cause ARF will usually be apparent, however, in covert intra-abdominal blood loss (from, for example, ruptured aortic aneurysm or spleen) and long bone fractures such losses may be underestimated.

Renal arterial disease is a significant risk factor for ARF regardless of the cause. Acute renal artery occlusion from thrombosis, dissection or complete stenosis may cause ARF when bilateral. Pointers to the presence of renal artery disease are a history of small or large vessel disease

or cardiovascular risk factors. Acute thrombosis, or occlusion resulting in infarction, will normally present with loin pain and hematuria.

ATN usually presents in the context of severe systemic illness, sepsis or drug administration. Direct drug toxicity may be determined from a thorough assessment of the relevant timing of drug administration and the onset of ARF as well as drug levels. Drug-induced interstitial nephritis is more idiosyncratic and may present in association with a drug-associated rash or other symptoms of drug allergy such as wheeze or angioneurotic edema. In rhabdomyolysis there may be an obvious history of hypothermic insult, burns, seizures, direct trauma or immobilization.

Features suggesting glomerular disease in the history are edema, macroscopic hematuria, frothy urine (suggesting proteinuria) or hypertensive symptoms such as headache. Acute or rapidly progressive glomerular nephritis resulting in ARF may be associated with systemic autoimmune or vasculitic disease and, thus, particular attention must be paid to symptoms such as arthralgia, joint swelling, rashes, headaches, pleuritic or pericarditic pains and respiratory symptoms. The crescentic rapidly progressive glomerular nephritis (RPGN) of Goodpasture's disease may be preceded by dyspnea and hemoptysis from pulmonary hemorrhage, particularly in smokers. Pulmonary hemorrhage may also be seen in severe systemic lupus erythematosus, Churg–Strauss syndrome or Wegener's granulomatosis. Hemolytic–uremic syndrome may be preceded by acute gastrointestinal upset while thrombotic, thrombocytopenic purpura may present with purpura, hemorrhage, thrombosis or neurological symptoms.

Many patients with postrenal ARF may be entirely asymptomatic; however, a previous history of obstruction or urological history such as stone disease is particularly relevant. Loin pain may suggest upper urinary tract obstruction while bladder outflow obstruction may present with frequency, urgency, nocturia or dysuria.

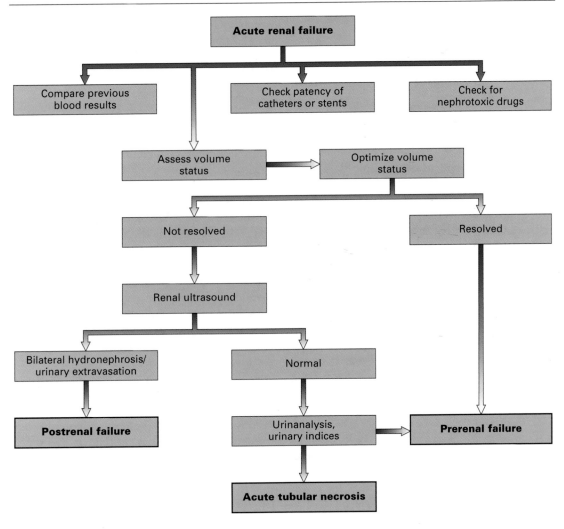

Figure 3.1

Algorithm for clinical assessment of acute renal failure.

Frank hematuria, though present in some glomerulonephritides, should alert the clinician to the possibility of urological disease. Oliguria or anuria, though more common, is by no means a universal feature of acute obstructive nephropathy as shall be discussed later. Renal, bladder, pelvic or gynecological masses raise suspicion of obstruction. A rectal examination is advised as is a gynaecological examination in females with suspected obstruction.

An algorithm for clinical assessment of acute renal failure is shown in Figure 3.1.

INVESTIGATION OF THE PATIENT WITH ACUTE RENAL FAILURE

BLOOD TESTS

Routine biochemical tests should include measurements of urea, creatinine, electrolytes, liver function tests, calcium, phosphate, glucose, plasma bicarbonate and, if bicarbonate is reduced or the patient is breathless, arterial blood gases. Other blood tests are aimed at establishing the cause. Where the cause of ARF is unknown we recommend measurement of creatine kinase, immunoglobulins, immunoglobulin electrophoresis, antinuclear antibody, antiglomerular basement membrane antibody, antineutrophil cytoplasmic antibody, serum complement, blood film and hemolysis screen (lactate dehydrogenase, reticulocyte count and haptoglobins). Parathyroid hormone (PTH) assay levels may be useful to assess onset of renal failure as very high levels suggest established secondary hyperparathyroidism and therefore chronicity.

ESTIMATION OF RENAL FUNCTION

Serum creatinine is dependent on the muscle mass from which it is produced and excretion by the kidney. It is useful for tracking renal function, however, creatinine levels may vary widely between patients with the same GFR depending on their size. A common pitfall is therefore to overestimate kidney function in patients with low muscle mass. The Cockcroft–Gault formula goes some way to correct this but is only accurate if function is static.

The creatinine:GFR relationship is exponential such that small early rises in creatinine represent large falls in GFR In general when the creatinine becomes abnormal most patients will have lost nearly half of their GFR. Serum creatinine levels in the 100–220 μmol/l range are therefore highly significant. Twenty four-hour creatinine clearance measurement gives a better overall picture

of function if urine is collected accurately. An isotopic GFR measurement remains the gold standard but is not readily available.

URINALYSIS

Urinalysis is an extremely useful, non-invasive investigation in ARF and should be considered mandatory. It may not only yield diagnostic information but, in glomerular disease, may also help determine disease activity. A mid-stream specimen should be obtained and inspected within 60 min of collection. It should then be dipstick tested using one of the many available reagent-impregnated dipsticks available. The sample should then be centrifuged at 300 rpm for 5 min. The relative coloration of supernatant and sediment should be noted, the supernatant discarded and the sediment examined under a glass slide with light microscopy.

Normal urine is clear and yellow, the depth of this color reflecting urinary concentration. Cloudy urine indicates pyuria, chyluria or crystalluria. Red urine usually represents hematuria, less commonly hemoglobinuria, myoglobinuria or rare conditions such as acute intermittent porphyria. These may be differentiated by centrifugation then dipstick testing of the supernatant. In genuine hematuria only the sediment will be red. In myoglobinuria and hemoglobinuria the supernatant will be red and test positive for heme. In severe myoglobinuria the urine may appear brown-black. Drugs may induce color changes such as the orange appearance seen with rifampicin.

Dipstick proteinuria suggests the presence of negatively charged proteins, particularly albumin and become positive when excretion exceeds 500 mg/24 h. Bence Jones proteins, tubular proteins and immunoglobulins will not be detected. Heavy albuminuria is the hallmark of glomerular disease but proteinuria may be seen in acute tubular injury and interstitial nephritis. Dipstick hematuria will be present when there is the equivalent of three red cells per high-power field on microscopy. This may represent glomerular blood loss secondary to inflammatory renal disease when it is usually present with significant proteinuria. Microscopic hematuria with negative microscopy suggests hemoglobinuria or myoglobinuria. Glycosuria suggests hyperglycemia or reduced proximal renal tubular glucose reabsorption (as seen in Fanconi syndrome). Reagent dipsticks also usually measure ketones, pH and specific gravity but these have limited value in the diagnosis of ARF.

Urine microscopy (Table 3.4) may reveal crystals, red cells, white cells, casts, bacteria and uroepithelial cells which may be normal or dysplastic. Casts form when cellular or other debris accumulated in tubules 'cast' themselves in the tubular shape and then are excreted. Red cell casts are most significant as these imply glomerular bleeding and therefore glomerulonephritis. Granular casts are usually degenerate tubular cells and may be seen in ATN. Epithelial casts are non-specific but large numbers suggest tubular disease. Hyaline casts are not pathological. White cell casts may represent active pyelonephritis as distinct from lower urinary tract sepsis. All forms of urinary tract infection may result in pyuria. Calcium oxalate crystals will form in ethylene glycol poisoning while uric acid crystals will be present in tumor lysis syndrome.

Table 3.4 The various urinary abnormalities associated with acute renal failure

Urine microscopy	
Normal	Pre-renal/obstruction
Red blood cell casts	Acute glomerulonephritis/vasculitis
Eosinophils	Acute interstitial nephritis
Granular casts	Acute tubular necrosis

URINE BIOCHEMISTRY

Measurement of urinary sodium and osmolality has traditionally had a role in ARF in distin-

guishing prerenal failure from ATN. In prerenal failure there will be real or perceived hypovolemia, activation of the renin–angiotensin system and offloading of baroreceptors resulting in reduced secretion of atrial natriuretic peptide and increased secretion of antidiuretic hormone. The net result is concentrated urine with a low sodium content (<40 mmol/l). In acute tubular necrosis tubular concentrating ability and salt reclamation is disordered resulting in dilute urine of relatively high (>40 mmol/l) concentration. In practice urinary electrolytes rarely influence management as fluid optimization will be underway regardless. Renal salt losses may be determined more accurately by calculating the fractional excretion of sodium.

RENAL ULTRASONOGRAPHY

Ultrasound imaging of the kidneys is mandatory in all ARF in which the cause is not immediately clear or rapidly reversed. The first priority is to exclude obstruction demonstrated by bladder, ureteric or pelvicalyceal (PC) dilatation (Figure 3.2). Ureteric or PC dilatation may not be seen in very acute ureteric obstruction or where there is external compression (as seen in malignant infiltration or retroperitoneal fibrosis) while in some cases there may be chronic dilatation of the collecting systems without functional obstruction due to congenital dilatation or previous obstruction which has been ameliorated.

The second priority is to determine renal size. Many cases of presumed ARF are late presentations of chronic renal failure (CRF) and the presence of small (<9 cm), scarred kidneys is highly suggestive of chronicity (Figure 3.3). Any anatomical or congenital anomalies – cystic change, horseshoe kidney, single kidney – should be evaluated. Parenchymal changes, such as reduced corticomedullary differentiation, may suggest intrinsic renal disease such as glomerulonephritis but we do not consider these as reliable findings (Figure 3.4). Underlying renal arterial disease is suggested by renal asymmetry but such asymmetry may

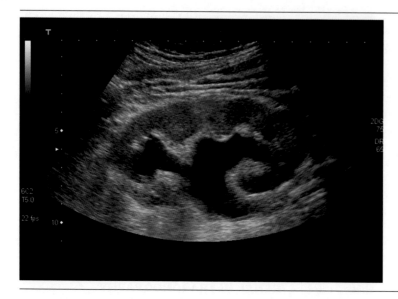

Figure 3.2

Ultrasound scan showing marked hydroureteronephrosis.

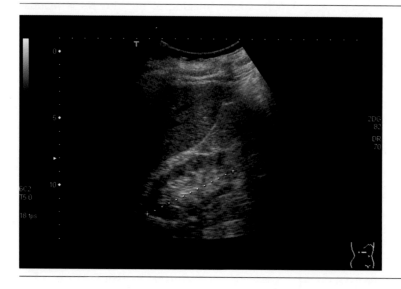

Figure 3.3

End stage shrunken right kidney.

be congenital or due to other unilateral disease such as chronic pyelonephritis or previous unilateral obstruction. Some information on renal blood flow may be obtained from the renal ultrasound but formal evaluation with duplex scanning is laborious, difficult and its sensitivity as an investigation is very user dependent (Figure 3.5).

ISOTOPE RENOGRAPHY

In a normal renogram the isotope is taken up rapidly and equally in both kidneys with uniform distribution and prompt excretion following diuretic administration. Isotope renography therefore gives useful information on renal

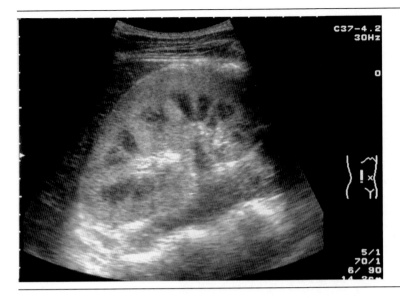

Figure 3.4

Ultrasound demonstrating reduced cortico-medullary differentiation indicative of intrinsic renal disease.

perfusion, divided function and drainage (Figure 3.6). It is particularly useful in screening for renal artery occlusion or stenosis (the sensitivity of the latter is enhanced by comparing perfusion traces before and after administration of captopril) (Figure 3.7). It is also particularly useful in determining whether obstruction is present in chronically dilated collecting systems or where there is a high index of suspicion of obstruction but no dilatation on the ultrasound scan (USS) (as in extrinsic ureteric compression) (Figure 3.8). ATN has a characteristic appearance and a renogram may be useful supportive evidence for this diagnosis when suspicion is high (Figure 3.9) but biopsy has not been done. Its use is limited in cases of severe renal failure regardless of cause as the uptake traces will be too weak to yield any useful information (Figure 3.10).

PLAIN ABDOMINAL RADIOGRAPH

The plain radiograph or KUB (views of kidneys, ureters and bladder) is not routinely done in ARF but when obstructive nephropathy secondary to nephrolithiasis is suspected it should be taken. The sensitivity is not as high as intravenous pyelography and radiolucent stones (e.g. urate stones) will not be detected.

INTRAVENOUS UROGRAPHY

The intravenous urogram was previously widely used to evaluate renal disease; this has led to an extensive vocabulary of pyelographic radiological signs. It still has a role in the diagnosis of specific chronic disorders such as medullary sponge kidney. Its usefulness in the investigation of ARF is, however, limited as it requires contrast administration and will add little that cannot be ascertained by ultrasonography or non-contrast computed tomography (CT).

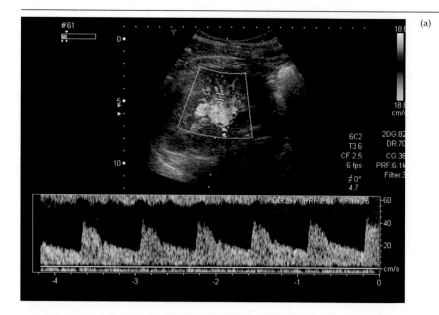

(a)

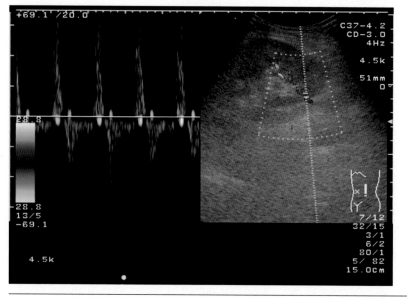

(b)

Figure 3.5

(a) A normal renal Doppler ultrasound scan.

(b) A renal Doppler ultrasound scan showing very little blood flow in the kidney in the diastolic phase suggesting renal vein thrombosis.

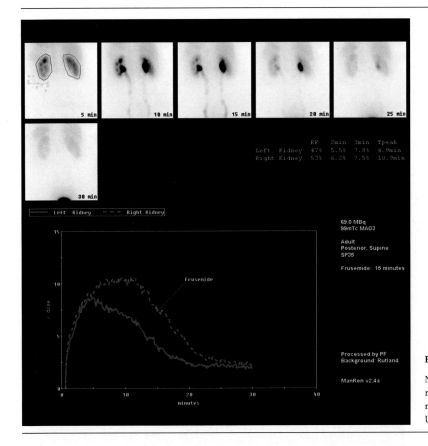

Figure 3.6

Normal MAG 3 scan with a normal response to furosemide (frusemide). (Courtesy of John Rees, University Hospital of Wales.)

COMPUTED TOMOGRAPHY

CT scanning is of particular value for more detailed evaluation of obstruction. A non-contrast study demonstrate renal anatomy, macroscopic irregularities and size (Figure 3.11). It will also detect the presence of stones, tumors in the renal tract or external compression as in widespread lymphadenopathy or retroperitoneal fibrosis. Renal perfusion may only be assessed with contrast administration and we prefer magnetic resonance (MR) scanning or MAG 3 renography for the formal assessment of renal blood flow. The disadvantages of a CT study are its relatively high cost and radiation exposure.

MAGNETIC RESONANCE IMAGING

MR imaging (MRI) gives valuable information on renal anatomy, size, perfusion, function and obstruction (Figures 3.12 and 3.13). Formal MR angiography requires no nephrotoxic contrast and is the principal non-invasive investigation used to assess renal blood flow and renal arterial anatomy. Though sensitivity is high, its specificity is lower and false positives may occur. For this reason it is often necessary to proceed to formal angiography if the MR angiogram is abnormal and intervention is considered.

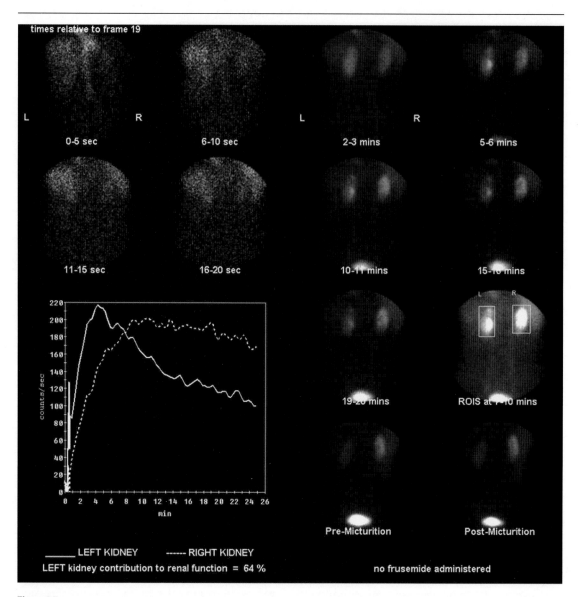

Figure 3.7

Post-captopril ^{99m}Tc MAG 3 study of right renal artery stenosis.

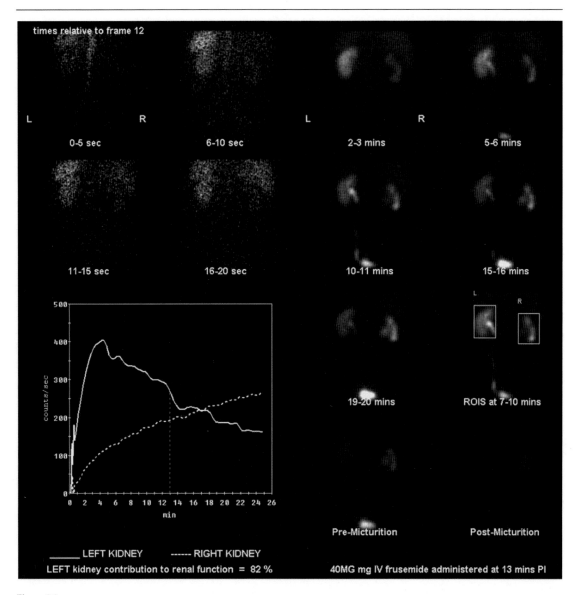

Figure 3.8

[99m]Tc MAG 3 study of right obstructive nephropathy. Upper left-hand panel: the dynamic phase shows slightly reduced perfusion of the right kidney compared with the left. Upper right-hand panel: the progress of activity from the renal parenchyma into the pelvicalyceal system from the right is slow and left is brisk. Lower right-hand panel: most of the activity from the left kidney has drained while the tracer is retained in the right kidney (kidney is more black). Lower left-hand panel: the time activity curve from the right kidney does not trend towards baseline as the left. (Courtesy of Dr J Bomanji, UCL, London.)

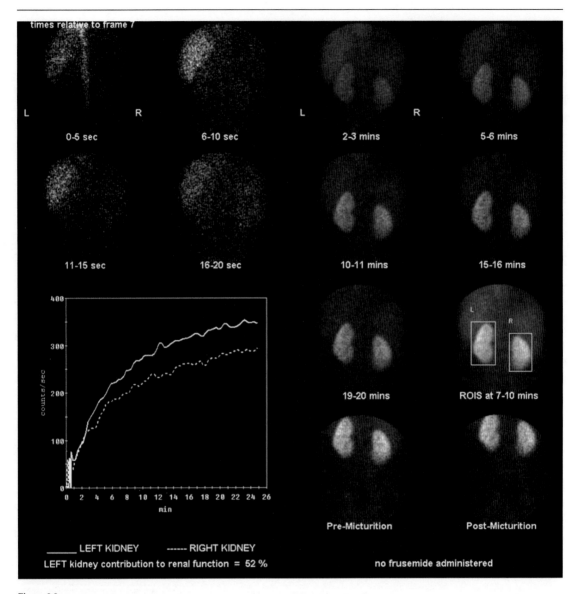

Figure 3.9

⁹⁹ᵐTc MAG 3 study in a patient with clinical suspicion of acute tubular necrosis. Upper left-hand panel: the dynamic phase shows perfusion of both kidneys. Upper right-hand panel: the activity accumulates in the renal parenchyma, but tracer is seen in the pelvicalyceal system. Lower right-hand panel: further accumulation in the renal parenchyma and no excretion of tracer. Lower left-hand panel: the time activity curve from the both kidneys which continues to rise and does not trend towards baseline. (Courtesy of Dr J Bomanji, UCL, London.)

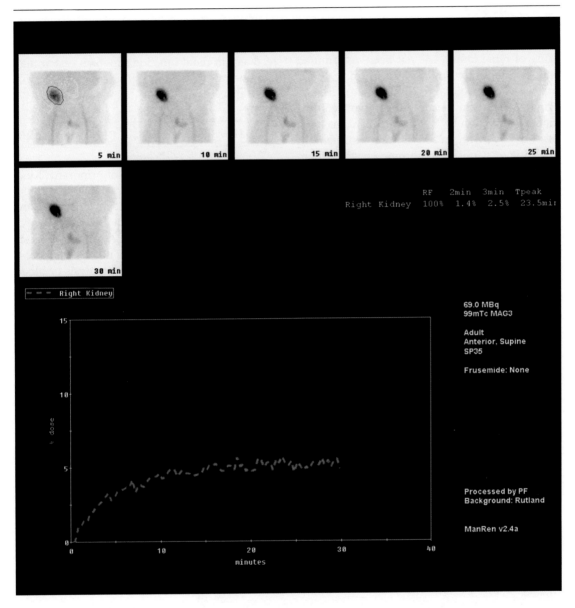

Figure 3.10

A MAG 3 renogram study indicative of acute tubular necrosis. (Courtesy of John Rees, University Hospital of Wales.)

RENAL BIOPSY

Renal biopsy is usually undertaken when the cause of renal failure has not been determined and is likely to be due to intrinsic renal parenchymal pathology (Figure 3.14). It may provide useful diagnostic and prognostic information and should be undertaken in most cases of ARF with an active urine sediment, in nephritic or nephritic syndrome or when there is clinical evidence of systemic autoimmune or vasculitic disease. In such instances there is is a strong possibility of a primary glomerulonephritis or renal vasculitis and renal biopsy will be essential to refine diagnosis, stage severity of disease and plan treatment. Renal biopsy is also required to firmly establish a diagnosis of thrombotic microangiopathy or acute interstitial nephritis. ATN is the most common intrinsic renal cause of ARF in the secondary care setting and if the clinical suspicion is high, e.g. in the intensive care patient with severe sepsis, multiorgan dysfunction and a bland urine sediment, a biopsy is often unnecessary. A biopsy may, however, be undertaken in ATN for prognostic reasons when there has been a slower than expected recovery in renal function in which case it may demonstrate irreversible ischemic damage or cortical necrosis.

ACUTE VERSUS CHRONIC RENAL FAILURE

When there is no knowledge of prior renal function it may be difficult to ascertain the chronicity of renal dysfunction. None of the biochemical parameters with the exception of PTH are discriminatory. Anemia suggests chronicity but only if there is no other apparent cause such as severe sepsis, hemolysis or blood loss. The most reliable indicator of chronic renal failure is significantly reduced renal size on ultrasonography.

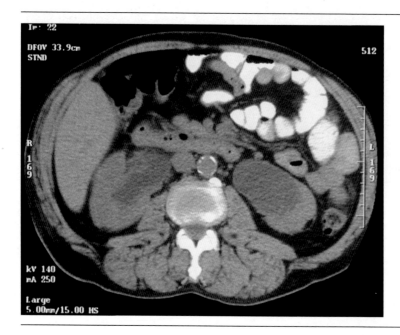

Figure 3.11

A non-contrast computed tomography (CT) scan demonstrating bilateral hydronephrosis.

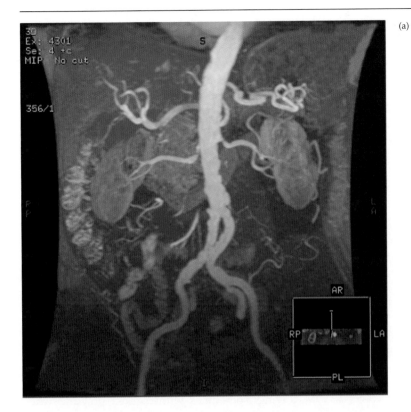

(a)

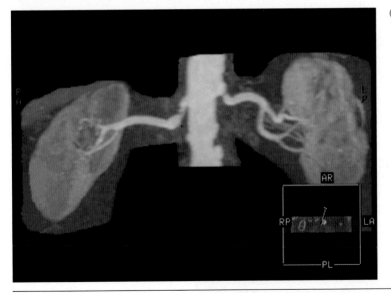

(b)

Figure 3.12

(a, b) MRI scan showing bilateral renal artery stenosis. (Courtesy of Andrew Wood, University Hospital of Wales.)

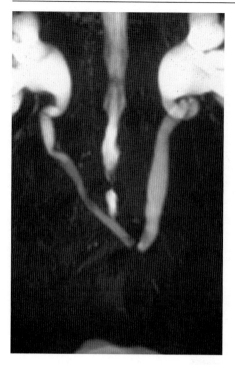

Figure 3.13

Magnetic resonance imaging (MRI) showing an obstruction at the ureteroileal junction on a T2 image.

MANAGEMENT OF ACUTE RENAL FAILURE

After the initial assessment there are four distinct phases in the management of ARF. In the first phase the clinician is presented with a patient who has evidence of incipient ARF with oliguria or a rising creatinine level. In this instance the aim of therapy is prompt diagnosis of the cause(s) of ARF and reversal with appropriate intervention. In the second phase the patient has clearly developed 'established' ARF and it is likely that there will be a period of severe renal dysfunction, often with profound oliguria, prior to renal recovery. Here the priority is to maintain health prior to recovery or transfer to an appropriate environment for renal replacement therapy. When it is clear that recovery will not occur in sufficient time to avoid serious complications of ARF, or when such complications are already present, the third or 'renal replacement' phase of management begins with dialytic or filtration techniques. The final 'recovery phase' is when function is recovering, sometimes with marked polyuria when specific physiological effects require considera-

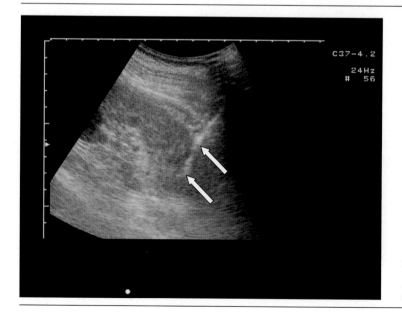

Figure 3.14

An ultrasound scan being used to localize a renal biopsy.

tion. Throughout the clinician must concentrate on treating the underlying causes and the complications of ARF.

GENERAL CONSIDERATIONS

When the clinician is presented with a patient with ARF a thorough clinical assessment should be followed by the essential basic investigations as outlined above. From this the following should be ascertained: The potential causes of ARF, the degree and duration of renal impairment, the volume status of the patient, whether or not there is any obstructive component and whether any complications of ARF are present. Pulse, blood pressure, oxygen saturation and respiratory rate should be recorded regularly and documented, and accurate fluid charts should be maintained. A daily estimation of weight is an effective way of assessing trends in hydration. In the acute phase of management urinary catheterization and measurement of urine volumes can be useful to assess response to therapy. In established ARF, with sustained oligoanuria, a urethral catheter adds little to management and is a conduit for sepsis and should be removed. Administration of oxygen to the hypoxic patient is a crucial part of general care, indeed, renal tubular ischemia is a common cause of ARF and many therefore advocate maximal oxygenation in all patients with incipient or established ARF.

Drug therapy must be completely reappraised. In some cases there will be a clear diagnosis of drug toxicity causing ARF and in such cases the offending agent should be withdrawn unless there are truly exceptional circumstances. Other commonly prescribed agents may be detrimental to renal function even if they have not been the source of the primary insult and such drugs should be withdrawn if possible. Angiotensin converting enzyme (ACE) inhibitors and angiotensin II antagonists limit the kidneys' ability to maintain GFR in the face of a renal insult due to reduction of efferent glomerular arteriolar tone. This effect is most marked in patients with underlying small or large vessel renovascular disease. We therefore recommend that patients are 'rested' from these agents if possible. They can be reinstituted on recovery of function. Non-steroidal anti-inflammatory drugs (NSAIDs) reduce renal blood flow and should similarly be withdrawn while diuretics should be withheld in hypovolemic patients. The hypoglycemic agent metformin can cause lactic acidosis in ARF and should be discontinued until kidney function has recovered. Potassium supplementation and potassium-sparing diuretics should also be withheld. Though drug therapy should be minimized, it may be necessary for the patient to continue with certain agents but dose adjustments may be required, particularly in antimicrobial or chemotherapeutic regimens. Here, accurate estimation of renal function is essential. Drug level monitoring is now available for many renally excreted antimicrobials such as gentamicin, vancomycin and teicoplanin and this should be done rigorously.

Maintaining adequate nutrition is crucial in ARF. Though ARF does not increase catabolism in itself, renal replacement therapy causes amino acid loss while the underlying cause of ARF (such as sepsis) may result in a highly catabolic state and therefore increase protein and calorie requirements. Vitamin and trace element requirements are also increased. Proper evaluation by a dietician is preferable but all clinicians should be able to make some assessment of nutritional adequacy and the need for supplementation. Self-administered oral supplements may be used but often enteral feeding via a nasogastric tube is required. In vomiting or gastrointestinal dysfunction parenteral nutrition may be necessary. Renally adjusted supplements and feeds should be prescribed by a dietician and, prior to the renal replacement phase, volume restriction may be necessary. Once replacement therapy is underway normal volume feeds may be given and ultrafiltration (fluid removal on dialysis) adjusted accordingly.

Sepsis is a common complication of ARF, particularly in patients undergoing invasive monitoring or other interventions. Scrupulous care must be taken in general nursing care to avoid hospital-acquired infection and intravenous lines, wounds drains and in-dwelling catheters should be regularly assessed for signs of infection. Uremic gastritis may result in upper gastrointestinal hemorrhage and routine prophylactic therapy with a proton-pump inhibitor or H_2-antagonist is recommended.

FLUID THERAPY

Hypovolemia should be managed by appropriate fluid resuscitation. In uncomplicated hypovolemia this may be at a rate of 50–100 ml/h in excess of ongoing losses; however, in ARF correction should be achieved as quickly as possible. In certain situations (such as hypovolemic shock) rapid transfusion of fluid via large bore peripheral venous cannulae will be required. Regular clinical reassessment with revision of fluid prescription is mandatory. Advance prescriptions of fluid may be practical in maintenance intravenous (IV) fluid management but they have little role in ARF when such prescriptions should be regularly adjusted. If there is doubt about the volume status small aliquots (e.g. 250 ml of colloid or normal saline) may be given and the response assessed.

Hemorrhage sufficient to cause ARF will normally require administration of packed red cells. Other blood products such as fresh frozen plasma, platelets and cryoprecipitate will also be required after rapid transfusion of large volumes of blood (usually in excess of 6 units) to maintain coagulation. This should be on the basis of laboratory coagulation measurements and according to specialist hematological advice. Delayed transfusion, prior to definitive surgical intervention, is an emergent theory in resuscitation which has some logic but is not yet widely used.

In non-hemorrhagic hypovolemia the choice remains between colloids and crystalloids. Colloids used are human albumin solution and the synthetic colloids of which several are available. Colloids are retained within the intravascular compartment prior to breakdown while crystalloids disperse throughout the extracellular fluid and interstitium. Roughly three times as much crystalloid as colloid will therefore have to be transfused to achieve a similar increase in circulating volume. Colloids therefore confer the theoretical advantage of improving circulating volume more rapidly for the same transfused volume. A further theoretical advantage is that they maintain plasma oncotic pressure and hence reduce the risk of peripheral and organ (particularly pulmonary) edema in hypoalbuminemic states such as severe sepsis. Recently, a large meta-analysis was unable to demonstrate any advantage of albumin over crystalloid while a further analysis suggested some harm from using synthetic colloid over crystalloid (a 4% increase in mortality). It would seem that colloids confer no real benefit over crystalloid unless transfusion rates are limited by venous access. They are also expensive, though the synthetic colloids are considerably cheaper than human albumin solution, the cost of which is prohibitive. In crystalloid therapy in ARF, normal saline is preferable to more complex solutions such as Hartmann's solution which often contains potassium. We recommend that if potassium is required it should be prescribed on a *per bag* basis as rebound hyperkalemia is an attendant risk in ARF. Half-strength saline (dextrose saline) may be used in severe hypernatremia while twice-strength saline has a role in some severe hyponatremic states. The use of alkaline fluids is discussed later.

In euvolemia only maintenance fluids are required. This amounts to insensible losses added to urine output and other losses (diarrhea, drains, etc.). Insensible losses (breathing, sweat, etc.) amount to around 500 ml of fluid loss per day though this will increase in tachypnea or pyrexia. An anuric patient with normal insensible losses will therefore only require 500 ml of fluid per day. This should be given orally if possible.

In hypervolemia fluid should be restricted until such time as euvolemia is achieved, however, this may require diuretic or renal replacement therapy as outlined below.

DIURETICS

Furosemide has been shown to be of no benefit in prophylaxis in ARF or for improving GFR in incipient or established ARF. It may promote a diuresis of salt and water. This will be of benefit if the patient is symptomatically hypervolemic but will not facilitate clearance of other solutes or uremic toxins. Some advocate its use to 'convert' oliguric to polyuric ARF which may ease the management but we believe this assertion only adds complexity to a therapeutic area which already causes considerable confusion among non-specialists. We therefore recommend furosemide only be given to hypervolemic patients with peripheral or pulmonary edema prior to initiation of dialysis. It may also be used in ARF secondary to cardiogenic shock where offloading may improve cardiac output. It should not, however, be used to 'rescue' renal function.

In hypervolemic ARF adequate doses must be administered. Reduction of GFR moves the furosemide dose–response curve to the right and hence higher doses are required to achieve diuresis. When estimated GFR <50% we would recommend a bolus dose of 80 mg followed by slow infusion of 250 mg, increasing to infusions of 500 mg and 1 g per 24 h if there is no response. If diuresis is not achieved with these doses loop diuretics are unlikely to be effective in reducing hypervolemia and renal replacement will be necessary.

The thiazide metolazone is a powerful diuretic, which, as it acts on the distal tubule as opposed to the loop of Henle, has complementary and synergistic actions when used in tandem with furosemide in hypervolemic, edematous states. It is only available as an oral preparation and should be given in daily or twice daily doses of 2.5, 5 and 10 mg according to response. Other diuretics such as the potassium-sparing diuretics spironolactone and amiloride are potentially hazardous in ARF and should be avoided.

RENAL DOSE DOPAMINE

Administration of 'renal' or 'low' dose dopamine (<5 µg/kg/min) has been used in prophylaxis and treatment of ARF. It activates DA_1 and DA_2 receptors and has renal diuretic and hemodynamic effects which have been the subject of considerable study in animals.

At doses of 0.5–5 µg/kg/min dopamine causes afferent and efferent glomerular arteriolar vasodilation. This reduces intrarenal vascular resistance and increases renal blood flow but does not increase intraglomerular pressure and therefore has no effect on GFR. Higher doses of dopamine induce renal arteriolar vasoconstriction. Dopamine also has non-hemodynamic diuretic effects. It inhibits the activity of both the Na-H and Na-K-ATPase proximal tubular transporters resulting in reduced sodium reabsorption and hence natriuresis.

Renal dose dopamine has not been shown to be of any benefit in prevention or treatment of ARF in clinical trials. It may have a role as a diuretic in hypervolemic ARF or refractory congestive cardiac failure but there is currently no evidence of benefit over and above conventional diuretics. It must be used through central venous access due to risks of extravasation, tissue necrosis and myocardial ischemia. On the basis of current evidence we do not recommend the use of dopamine in ARF in any circumstances.

INOTROPES

Inotropic support is indicated in persisting hypotension or reduced organ perfusion in spite of adequate fluid resuscitation. Dobutamine still has some use in cardiogenic shock due to its inotropic and chronotropic effects mediated via β-1 adrenoceptor agonism. It also causes some β-2 agonism resulting in peripheral vasodilation and reduced cardiac afterload. For this reason, however, it should not be used in septic shock. Low dose dopamine is discussed above. Intermediate doses of dopamine have similar effects to dobutamine, however, at high (>10 μg/kg/min) doses it is a vasoconstrictor via α adrenoceptor stimulation.

Norepinephrine is a more potent α receptor agonist and vasoconstrictor and, for many, the inotrope of choice in septic shock. Epinephrine induces inotropy, chronotropy (via β-1 agonism) and varying effects on systemic vascular resistance due to β-2 (vasodilator) and α-1 (vasonconstrictor) effects. Norepinephrine and epinephrine are now the most commonly used pressor agents in intensive therapy units but, due to the requirement for exacting titration and adjustment, should not be used on general wards.

MANAGEMENT OF HYPERKALEMIA

Hyperkalemia may be manifest by muscle weakness and ECG changes which include 'tall, tented' T-waves and broadened QRS complexes; if left untreated, bradycardia and asystolic cardiac arrest will ensue. Susceptibility to these varies between patients and hypocalcemia and acidosis increase the risk of cardiac complications.

Generally, potassium concentration above 6.5 mmol/l warrants urgent attention. This is obviously more serious if the patient's renal function is static or declining in which case the potassium is likely to continue to rise. Muscle weakness or ECG changes should be considered an emergency. In established ARF with rising creatinine and hyperkalemia emergency dialysis is indicated. Hyperkalemia should be managed medically while dialysis is being arranged and such conservative management may suffice if renal function is rapidly improving.

When ECG changes are present 10 ml of 10% calcium gluconate should be given by slow IV bolus injection. This antagonist improves membrane depolarization. An infusion of 15 IU Actrapid insulin in 50 ml% dextrose should then be administered as an infusion over 30 min with blood glucose monitoring. This drives potassium intracellularly, works after 30 min and lasts up to 4 h. This therapy does not increase potassium excretion so the same levels of total body potassium are maintained. Bicarbonate therapy is of benefit in hyperkalemia with acidosis as it also moves potassium into cells. In hyperkalemic acidosis a dose of 50 ml 8.4% sodium bicarbonate with repeat dosage after reassessment of acid–base status is recommended. Calcuim polystyrene sulfonate (Calcium Resonium) increases gut potassium excretion and may be given orally or rectally in a dose of 15 g three times daily. Salbutamol reduces extracellular potassium via β-agonism and should be given in a dose of 5 mg 4-hourly while life-threatening hyperkalemia is present. All these therapies should be discontinued when the patient is established on dialysis.

MANAGEMENT OF PULMONARY EDEMA

Pulmonary edema in ARF is generally an indication for renal replacement therapy. If, however, a good urine output is achieved and renal function is in recovery phase it may be possible to manage the patient without dialysis. There may be delays in arranging for dialysis and the patient should be optimally managed with pharmacological and other therapies. High-flow oxygen therapy with oxygen saturation and arterial blood gas monitoring is mandatory.

Diuretic therapy has been discussed above. Opiates are commonly used in cardiogenic pulmonary edema due to their anxiolytic and vasodilatory effects. They may have a role here; however, opiate metabolites tend to accumulate in ARF and their use should be restricted to very small doses (e.g. 2.5 mg diamorphine 4-hourly). Sublingual and intravenous nitrates reduce preload and are of benefit, particularly in hypertensive ARF. We would recommend a continuous intravenous infusion of glyceryl trinitrate at 1–10 mg/h in pulmonary edema associated with ARF while provisions for renal replacement are being made.

Continuous positive airways pressure (CPAP) via mask improves oxygenation in pulmonary edema and should be commenced in hypoxia resistant to oxygen therapy but should not delay efforts to reduce hypervolemia. In patients with severe respiratory failure or exhaustion intubation and invasive ventilation is required.

MANAGEMENT OF HYPOCALCEMIA AND HYPERPHOSPHATEMIA

Hyperphosphatemia may cause itching and discomfort in ARF. The phosphate also binds calcium and therefore induces hypocalcemia, which is compounded by failure of renal 1-hydroxylation of vitamin D. This is rarely a major clinical concern but calcium-based phosphate binders ('calcium-500', one tablet three times daily) and 1-hydroxylated vitamin D (alphacalcidol 0.25–1 µg once daily) may be given. In severe symptomatic hypocalcemia calcium chloride or calcium gluconate may be administered intravenously.

MANAGEMENT OF ACIDOSIS

Acidosis in ARF constitutes an indication for urgent renal replacement therapy. Infusion of bicarbonate may help temporarily stabilize the patient to commencement of dialysis. It may also be useful as a stop-gap if renal recovery is underway and dialysis is otherwise unnecessary. Although the use of bicarbonate in other forms of metabolic acidosis (such as ketotic and lactic acidosis) is controversial it should always be considered when the acidosis is primarily 'renal'. Dialysis itself results in movement of bicarbonate from the dialysate into the blood and is itself a *de facto* form of bicarbonate infusion. Withholding bicarbonate in severe, life-threatening acidosis with hyperkalemia is therefore illogical unless dialysis is immediately available.

Bicarbonate may be administered by small (50 ml) aliquots of 8.4% sodium bicarbonate via central venous access with the biochemical response assessed after each dose. In hypovolemia requiring transfusion of large amounts of crystalloid 1.26% sodium bicarbonate may be given as a substitute for normal saline provided the bicarbonate is measured after transfusion of each liter. Either strategy will be hazardous in profound hypervolemia or pulmonary edema when it will represent an intolerable volume challenge. In less severe renal failure with mild acidosis (serum bicarbonate >15 mmol/l) oral sodium bicarbonate may be given at a dose of 500 mg–1 g three times daily.

INVASIVE HEMODYNAMIC MONITORING

Insertion of a central venous catheter can be useful in ARF management. The right internal jugular vein is the most suitable vein for catheterization although the left internal jugular vein may also be used. Use of the subclavian veins has largely been phased out due to problems with subclavian vein stenosis. It is preferable for the catheter to be inserted under portable ultrasound guidance as there is considerable anatomical variation.

The cental venous pressure (CVP) reflects right ventricular filling and, in the absence of cardiac dysfunction, volume status providing measurements are taken in the context of pulse, blood pressure and peripheral vasoconstriction. It is of value particularly in ensuring adequate resuscitation in hypovolemia (when the response to boluses of fluid may be assessed) and in preventing overresuscitation in oliguric ARF. A CVP of 10–15 cmH$_2$O (7.4–11 mmHg) represents adequate fluid loading and if this is achieved there is unlikely to be any benefit from continued fluid resuscitation but a risk of fluid overload.

When the patient is clearly hypervolemic CVP monitoring will add little to patient management and should not be inserted. CVP lines generally have fine bore lumens of considerable length and will transfuse less rapidly than large bore peripheral venous cannulae. They are, however, useful when peripheral cannulation is difficult or when multiple intravenous infusions are required and for sampling of venous blood.

Pulmonary artery catheterization may be more informative as it provides measurements of pulmonary artery pressure (and hence left atrial pressure) as well as measurements of cardiac output, pulmonary and systemic vascular resistance (SVR). Insertion is difficult and hazardous and the impact of this procedure on survival is a matter of ongoing controversy. Transesophageal echocardiographic assessment of cardiac output and SVR is less invasive and, in combination with CVP monitoring, is now used instead of pulmonary artery catheterization in many intensive care units.

OTHER AGENTS

Therapy of ATN with insulin growth factor-1 (IGF-1), atrial natriuretic peptide and thyroid hormone have been the subject of clinical trials in ARF. There is currently no evidence of benefit with these agents and they cannot be recommended.

DISEASE-SPECIFIC THERAPY

The underlying causes of renal failure – prerenal, renal and postrenal – should be addressed at all times during management and specific treatment given depending on the aetiology. This will be discussed in the section on specific causes of ARF (see below).

RENAL REPLACEMENT THERAPY IN ACUTE RENAL FAILURE

Indications for renal replacement therapy include:

- symptomatic uremia
- uremic encephalopathy
- uremic pericarditis or gastritis

- persistent hyperkalemia >6.5 mmol/l
- acidosis (pH <7.2)
- fluid overload
- uncontrolled hypertension.

INTERMITTENT HEMODIALYSIS

Dialysis in its purest sense is the movement of solutes down a concentration gradient from one fluid compartment to another across a membrane. In hemodialysis this is provided by establishing an external circuit of blood and dialysate which are passed through an artificial kidney in opposing directions separated by semipermeable membranes. The dialysate is osmotically balanced and its composition modified according to the requirements and includes a buffer (usually bicarbonate). Solutes and bicarbonate will equilibrate due to diffusion during a dialysis session, purifying the blood and normalizing the pH. Removal of water, or ultrafiltration, is achieved through establishing a hydrostatic pressure gradient between the blood and dialysate. The diaylsate is then discarded. The external blood circuit requires rapid blood flows of 150–250 ml/min. To achieve this a large bore venous catheter is inserted into a great vein (usually the internal jugular or femoral vein) and left in situ. Longer courses of treatment may be served with tunneled 'Permacath' catheters to reduce risk of infection. Systemic anticoagulation (with intravenous heparin or prostacyclin) is administered during the dialysis session.

Intermittent hemodialysis is highly efficient and provides for the rapid clearance of solutes and, with ultrafiltration, water. It also provides rapid elimination of some drugs in self-poisoning. It is the principal modality of renal replacement therapy used in acute renal units. The main drawbacks are: it is technically difficult to administer; and due to the rapid circulation of venous blood, it may not be tolerated in patients with hemodynamic instability or severe cardiac disease. Its high efficiency can lead to over-rapid solute clearance, a positive osmotic gradient between systemic and cerebral blood across the blood–brain barrier and hence cerebral edema. The latter phenomenon is known as dialysis disequilibrium.

Intermittent hemodialysis in ARF will usually be initiated with daily, short (2 h) sessions for 3 days building up to 4–5-hourly sessions on alternate days according to catabolic requirements. Ultrafiltration requirements will vary but large volumes (2–3 l) may be removed at each session if necessary.

CONTINUOUS HEMOFILTRATION

In hemofiltration no dialysis occurs. Instead an external blood circuit is passed through a hemofilter which removes water and solutes. A replacement fluid is then simply added to the circuit prior to the return of the blood to the patient. The composition of this replacement fluid is modified according to requirements but includes bicarbonate. The most common form of this treatment is continuous venous–venous hemofiltration (CVVH) although continuous arterio–venous hemofiltration (CAVH), in which arterial pressure rather than an external pump drives the circuit, has also been used. In CVVH venous access is obtained with femoral or internal jugular dialysis catheter insertion as for intermittent hemodialysis and systemic anticoagulation is required.

CVVH is the renal replacement therapy of choice in intensive care units. It provides slow, controlled fluid and solute removal and hence reduces the risk of hemodynamic compromise or dialysis disequilibrium. The removal of immunomodulatory factors by the continuous circuit has a theoretical advantage in severe sepsis. It is, however, less efficient at solute removal. This has been addressed in some centers by adding a dialysis circuit to the conventional CVVH setup. This continuous venous–venous hemodiafiltration improves clearance and is considered by some to be the renal replacement therapy of choice in unstable, highly catabolic patients.

ACUTE PERITONEAL DIALYSIS

As described above, haemodialysis uses an artificial membrane as an interface between the blood and dialysate compartments and allows removal of solutes down a concentration gradient. In peritoneal dialysis (PD) the physiological principles are the same but in this instance the peritoneal membrane is used as an interface between the peritoneal capillary blood and a dialysate instilled into the peritoneal cavity via a peritoneal catheter. Solutes move across the peritoneal membrane according to their relative concentrations in each compartment and are then removed via drainage of the peritoneal dialysate. Ultrafiltration (net fluid removal) is achieved by establishing an osmotic gradient between the peritoneal capillary blood by adding dextrose or other osmotically active solutes to the dialysate.

PD can be used intermittently or continuously. Intermittent PD is usually administered for 24 h 2–3 times weekly and the dialysate exchange may be performed manually or via an automated cycling machine. Rapid (1–2 h) exchanges of 1.5–2 l dialysate bags are normally required to achieve adequacy. Continuous PD involving a daily regimen of exchanges of lower frequency (4–8 h) may be deployed manually or via an external cycler but this therapy is usually reserved for chronic maintenance dialysis where it continues to be widely used.

Acute PD was once part of the interventional armamentarium of the general physician when it was more widely available than other renal replacement techniques. Insertion of peritoneal catheters under regional anesthesia is, however, hazardous and has become something of a 'lost art'. Acute PD is also less efficient in terms of solute, particularly potassium removal and may be inadequate in catabolic patients while the osmotically driven ultrafiltration is similarly inefficient and difficult to regulate. The high volumes of peritoneal fluid instilled may embarrass diaphragmatic excursion and compound respiratory compromise in pulmonary edema while recent abdominal or cardiothoracic surgery is a contraindication. For all these reasons acute PD is rarely used in adult ARF and has been largely superseded by intermittent and continuous external dialysis and filtration circuits.

Acute PD does have some advantages in certain clinical situations where it may be considered. If there are difficulties in achieving vascular access it may be a more practical alternative and this has led to its widespread and continued use in pediatric nephrology. Bleeding diatheses or contraindications to anticoagulation are other indications. External blood circuits, regardless of ultrafiltration rates, still require rapid pump speeds and are more hemodynamically compromising. Acute PD may therefore be considered in hemodynamically unstable patients and in patients with severe cardiac failure or critical myocardial ischemia.

RECOVERY PHASE OF ACUTE RENAL FAILURE

Polyuria may occur on recovery from ARF of obstructive origin or due to ATN. The key consideration is maintaining hydration during this polyuric phase so as not to impede renal recovery. It is recommended to match output with oral fluid or normal saline with an extra 500–1000 ml/24 h to compensate for insensible losses while the creatinine is falling rapidly.

SPECIFIC CONDITIONS CAUSING ACUTE RENAL FAILURE

OBSTRUCTION

Urinary tract obstruction is a common cause of ARF. The specific conditions causing obstruction and their management are described elsewhere in this volume. In severe ARF (urea > 30 mmol/l, creatinine > 500 µmol) there is an increased risk of hemorrhage due to uremic platelet dysfunction and we recommend consideration of dialysis prior to invasive procedures such as stent or nephrostomy insertion. In pulmonary edema or when severe metabolic complications are present the patient should be similarly stabilized with dialysis prior to the resolution of anatomical obstruction. The prognosis for renal recovery after obstruction is dependent on the severity and duration of the obstruction.

HEPATORENAL SYNDROME

Hepatorenal syndrome ocurrs in fulminant hepatic failure from acute hepatitis or from decompensated chronic liver disease and is related to reduced renal perfusion via complex mechanisms. There is renal impairment with oliguria and very low urinary sodium (<10 mmol/l) and a bland urine sediment with no response to volume expansion. Treatment is supportive and prognosis ultimately depends on reversal of hepatic dysfunction, which sometimes can only be achieved with hepatic transplantation. The antidiuretic hormone analogs ornipressin and terlipressin, as well as N-acetylcysteine, misoprostol and octreotide have also been used with varying success.

GLOMERULONEPHRITIS AND RENAL VASCULITIS

Space does not permit a comprehensive review of these conditions. Glomerulonephritis should be considered in a presentation of nephritic or nephritic syndrome, when there is proteinuria or combined hematuria/proteinuria or when there is evidence of systemic inflammatory disease such as pulmonary hemorrhage, arthralgia, cutaneous vasculitis, neuropathy, sinusitis or fever. Red cell casts may be seen on urine microscopy. Involvement of a nephrologist and renal biopsy is mandatory. The biopsy may show glomerular crescents which are characteristic of a rapidly progressive glomerulonephritis. Diagnosis is further aided by measurement of antineutrophil cytoplasmic antibody (present in patients with Wegener's granulomatosis, Churg–Strauss syndrome and microscopic polyangiitis), antiglomerular basement antibody (Goodpasture's syndrome) and antinuclear antibody and complement (abnormal in systemic lupus erythmatosus). Other diagnoses are cryoglobulinemia and Henoch–Schönlein purpura. Immunosuppressive therapy including pulsed methylprednisolone, cyclophosphamide and plasma exchange are all used therapeutically in these conditions depending on classification and severity of renal involvement.

THROMBOTIC MICROANGIOPATHY

Thrombotic microangiopathy is characterized by microangiopathic hemolytic anemia, thrombocytopenia and variable renal and neurological complications. It may complicate malignant hypertension, scleroderma renal crisis and pregnancy or may present after a diarrheal illness associated with *Escherichia coli* infection. Many presentations are idiopathic. Fragments will be seen on the blood film with reduced haptoglobins and raised bilirubin and lactate dehydrogenase. Hematuria and proteinuria may be present. Fresh frozen plasma, prostacyclin and plasma exhange are commonly used treatments.

RHABDOMYOLYSIS

Rhabdomyolysis may complicate trauma, burns, hypothermia, hypernatremia and prolonged immobility. Creatine kinase is usually grossly elevated with dark (or black) urine testing positive for blood but without red cells on microscopy (myoglobinuria). Initial treatment is aggressive rehydration with normal saline. Some advocate urine alkalinization (pH >6.5) to improve myoglobin excretion, and 1.26% sodium bicarbonate may be given instead of normal saline for a period, however, urine alkalinization is often difficult to achieve. Hyperkalemia may be more severe than in other forms of ARF due to muscle release and this may expedite the need for dialysis.

MYELOMA

Myeloma may cause ARF through light-chain cast nephropathy (myeloma kidney), hypercalcemia, amyloid infiltration, acute interstitial nephritis and urate nephropathy. There may be a background history of anemia, bone pain, weight loss and infection. Diagnosis may be through detection of serum paraprotein, urine Bence Jones proteins, bone marrow biopsy or renal biopsy. Myeloma predisposes to ARF precipitated by NSAIDs, contrast media or diuretics. Treatment includes hydration, pulsed steroids and chemotherapy. Hypercalcemia may also be corrected with bisphosphonates and plasma exchange may be used to reduce light chain load acutely in myeloma kidney while the effects of chemotherapy are awaited.

ACUTE INTERSTITIAL NEPHRITIS

Tubulointerstitial inflammation may complicate drug therapy, infection or systemic disease including sarcoidosis, systemic lupus erythematosus and vasculitis. It may also be idiopathic. Eosinophilia, eosinophiluria, proteinuria or hematuria may be present, however, renal biopsy is required to establish the diagnosis. Any offending drugs should be withdrawn. Most renal physicians treat acute presentations with corticosteroids although there is no evidence base for this at present.

PREVENTION OF ACUTE RENAL FAILURE

Patients at particular risk of ARF are the elderly, diabetics, patients with diffuse arteriosclerosis or background renal disease and patients taking NSAIDs and ACE inhibitors. Some nephrotoxic insults such as dehydration, hemorrhage, sepsis and administration of nephrotoxic drugs or contrast media can be anticipated. It is therefore vital that risks of ARF in these situations are reduced with adequate hydration and close monitoring for development of incipient ARF. There is some evidence that *N*-acetylcysteine may be of benefit in contrast prophylaxis (600 mg twice daily for 48 h) but no other prophylactic agents are of proven worth. Adequate hydration and prompt treatment of intrinsic renal disease or obstruction are therefore of most importance in ARF prevention.

FURTHER READING

Agodoa L, Eknoyan G, Ingelfinger J et al. Assessment of structure and function in progressive renal disease. *Kidney Int Suppl* 1997; **63**: S144–S150.

Alkhunaizi AM, Schrier RW. Management of acute renal failure: New perspectives. *Am J Kidney Dis* 1996; **28**: 315–28.

Bellomo R, Ronco C. Indications and criteria for initiating renal replacement therapy in the intensive care unit. *Kidney Int Suppl* 1998; **66**: S106–S109.

Brady HR, Brenner BM, Lieberthal W. Acute renal failure. In: Brenner BM (ed). *Brenner and Rector's The Kidney*. Philadelphia: WB Saunders, 1996; 1200–52.

Bronson D. Preoperative evaluation and management before major non-cardiac surgery. In: Stoller J, Ahmad M, Longworth D (eds). *Intensive Review of Internal Medicine*, 2nd edn. Philadelphia: Lippincott Williams & Wilkins, 2000; 74–81.

Campese VM. Neurogenic factors and hypertension in renal disease. *Kidney Int* 2000; **57(Suppl 75)**: S2–S6.

Chertow GM, Lazarus JM, Christiansen CL et al. Preoperative renal risk stratification. *Circulation* 1997; **95**: 878–84.

Cosentino F. Drugs for the prevention and treatment of acute renal failure. *Cleve Clin J Med* 1995; **62**: 248–53.

Levey AS, Bosch JP, Lewis JB et al. A more accurate method to estimate glomerular filtration rate from serum creatinine: A new prediction equation. Modification of Diet in Renal Disease Study Group [See comments]. *Ann Intern Med* 1999; **130**: 461–70.

Walsh PC, Retik A et al. Etiology, pathogenesis and management of renal failure (Chapter 8). In: *Campbell's Urology* 8th edn. 2002.

4. Upper urinary tract obstruction

Marc E Laniado and Christopher RJ Woodhouse

PRESENTATION

Patients with upper urinary tract obstruction may be asymptomatic or present with pain, hematuria, renal failure and occasionally lower urinary tract symptoms. Significant factors relevant to the presentation of upper urinary tract obstruction as an emergency include the rate at which it develops, the cause of obstruction, the presence or absence of infection and an unobstructed contralateral system.

PAIN

Renal pain is felt in the ipsilateral costovertebral angle beneath the twelfth rib and lateral to the sacrospinalis (the renal angle). Pain may radiate around the umbilicus, or upper or lower abdomen. Pain due to acute obstruction is due to distension of the renal capsule whereas obstruction that develops insidiously, which is often due to extrinsic compression, may be painless. Often, patients with renal pain due to obstruction are restless unlike patients with pain because of peritonitis and gastrointestinal pain, which is constant, more severe anteriorly, and sometimes felt in the shoulder tip.

Steady pain in the kidney may also be caused by renal ischemia. Radicular pain has a similar distribution but is altered by movement and is not colicky. Ureteral distension and hyperperistalsis in the mid-ureter cause pain that may mimic appendicitis or diverticulitis. Lower ureteric pain produces frequency, urgency and suprapubic discomfort. Midline back pain and bilateral renal angle pain are seldom caused by upper urinary tract obstruction.

HEMATURIA

Total hematuria with wormlike clots if associated with flank pain suggests an upper urinary tract cause.

OTHER SYMPTOMS

Anuria occurs in the presence of either complete lower or upper urinary tract obstruction. Fevers and chills develop when obstruction is combined with infection.

In the context of acute obstruction, the history will obviously be short. However, there may well be a relevant past history. Ask questions about a history of urinary stones, cancer (prostate, bladder, cervical), tuberculosis, sickle cell hemoglobinopathies, renal transplantation, diabetes, pregnancy, liver cirrhosis and treatment with analgesics or protease inhibitors such as indinavir.

A recent history of surgery may indicate an iatrogenic cause for obstruction. There may have been previous treatment for urinary stones, prostate, bladder or cervical cancer.

EXAMINATION

Initial examination may be limited by the crippling pain of renal colic. It is often taught that the pain is similar to that of labor – only worse. Limited anecdotal experience suggests that this is true. It may be a kindness to give analgesia first and examine afterwards, accepting that an occasional case of Munchausen's syndrome may be missed.

Pyrexia suggests infection and tachycardia with shock raises the possibility of septicemia. Scars may indicate surgery for disorders possibly related to upper urinary tract obstruction. If obstruction has been present for sufficiently long then there may be signs of fluid overload. A patient may sit with the hip flexed secondary to a psoas abscess that has developed as a complication of obstruction, extravasation and infection.

Careful examination of the kidneys should be done, and occasionally a tense hydronephrosis or infected mass may be felt. Always examine the lower abdomen and pelvis. A pelvic mass may be felt rectally or on vaginal examination suggesting extrinsic compression of the ureter. The pelvic adnexa should be palpated. The prostate should be specifically examined. Occasionally, a stone may be felt in the ureter as it passes by the cervix.

Restricted spinal movements may indicate a musculoskeletal cause for pain. Local examination of the ribs may reveal a bone spur that could explain the pain. Hyperesthesia of the affected peripheral nerve should be ruled out.

INVESTIGATIONS

URINALYSIS

Blood may be present on urinalysis. False positives can occur due to menstrual contamination, dehydration and exercise. In a series of patients who underwent spiral computed tomography (CT) for acute loin, using the criterion of more than one red blood cell (RBC) per high-power field, reported sensitivity of 81% for detection of calculi.[1] However, 33% of those with stones had less than 5 RBC/HPF. With these figures, the presence or absence of microscopic hematuria is of little value in making a diagnosis of renal colic. Blood may also be present with infection and, of course, malignancy. Other positive findings such as glycosuria or proteinuria may prove to be of greater value than hematuria.

IMAGING

Since many years, the intravenous urogram (IVU) has been the standard initial investigation for cases of suspected upper tract obstruction. However, virtually identical information can be obtained from an ultrasound and plain abdominal radiograph (kidney/ureter/bladder – KUB). Pre- and post-contrast CT, especially with sagittal reconstruction surpasses both in the diagnostic information provided.

INTRAVENOUS UROGRAPHY

This is the most commonly used test to identify ureteric obstruction in patients presenting with renal colic. Relative contraindications include impaired renal function (creatinine clearance less than ~50 ml/min), pregnancy, treatment with metformin and allergy to contrast media. The contrast can be administered in the majority of patients before a serum creatinine is available unless there is anuria, diabetes, diastolic hypertension, or a personal or family history of renal disease. The contrast associated renal dysfunction is most likely in patients with impaired renal function, small vessel renal disease, diabetic nephropathy, congestive heart failure, hyperuricemia, proteinuria and when the contrast medium has already been given within 24 h (e.g. for other imaging). In such patients choose alternative investigations (spiral CT or KUB and ultrasound).

A KUB by itself identifies calculi in 45–59% when compared with spiral CT, retrograde ureterography and ureteroscopy. Furthermore, a KUB cannot identify non-calculous causes of obstruction.

Signs on the IVU that indicate acute obstruction include:

- an intense and delayed nephrogram (Figure 4.1a)
- delay in filling of the collecting system with contrast
- pelvicalyceal dilatation (Figure 4.1b)
- rupture of a fornix with urinary extravasation (Figure 4.1c)
- pyelovenous and pyelosinus backflow (seen as lines of contrast passing medially from the kidney).

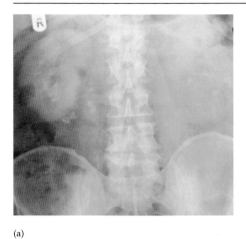

(a)

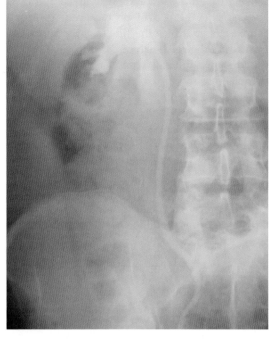

(c)

(b)

Figure 4.1

Intravenous urography. (a) Intense, delayed nephrogram, (b) pelvicalyceal dilation and (c) extravasation from a ruptured calyx.

An emergency IVU is often only a plain, 5-min and 20-min film. When delayed filling is seen, further films will be required. A rough estimate is six times the time required for contrast to fill the renal calyces. If the lower end of the ureter is poorly seen, a prone film may demonstrate the area better, as the middle and lower ureter becomes dependent and fills with contrast (Figure 4.2). There is some evidence to suggest that diclofenac can increase the apparent extent of obstruction and this must be borne in mind when interpreting imaging after ingestion of non-steroidal inflammatory drugs.[2]

An IVU is the preferred investigation when an 'anatomical road map' is required for percutaneous, endoureteral or surgical procedures,

or when a urothelial tumor is suspected. A spiral CT rather than an IVU is preferable when colic occurs in a diabetic patient in whom no stone has been detected on KUB or ultrasound and if papillary necrosis or a sloughed papilla is suspected. The advantages of the IVU include: it can be performed and interpreted with relatively little skill; it gives a rough estimate of renal function; and it can demonstrate a delay in renal excretion, which might indicate that endoluminal or percutaneous drainage is required.

ULTRASOUND

An ultrasound is an anatomical study and is used in circumstances in which an IVU is undesirable such as pregnancy, renal failure, or contrast allergy. It is observer dependent but is replacing IVU in centers with the necessary skills.

Important ultrasound findings are:

- Pelvicalyceal dilation: this indicates that obstruction might be present. If parenchymal thickness is preserved and the patient has renal colic then acute obstruction is likely. If parenchymal thickness is reduced, the obstruction is likely to be chronic.
- Asymmetry of 'ureteric jets': this is the urine pulsed into the bladder from the ureters, and is usually symmetrical unless obstruction is present. When a jet is absent from the ureter on the dilated side or there is significant asymmetry in jet frequency, hydronephrosis is likely to be obstructive. Continuous low flow from the ureter compared to the normal contralateral side may also be seen in obstruction. Ureteric jets are still present in pregnancy despite the physiological hydronephrosis that occurs. Their presence indicates that obstruction is unlikely. A unilaterally absent jet noted in the third trimester of pregnancy should not be interpreted as a sign of ureteral obstruction unless the finding persists in the contralateral decubitus position.

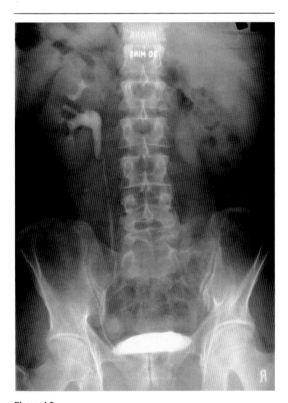

Figure 4.2

A prone intravenous urography (IVU) film demonstrating a distal vesicoureteric junction obstruction.

Other findings on ultrasound may be helpful. A hyperechoic lesion with an acoustic shadow may occur with stones or calcified necrotic papillae in the kidney, upper ureter or most distal ureter. Echoes within the collecting system may be due to infection and hemorrhage or a lesion of the urothelium, which can form clots and obstruct the ureter. Pelvic ultrasound can demonstrate extramural masses causing obstruction of the lower ureter. Transvaginal ultrasound may demonstrate stones in the distal ureter or other pelvic causes of non-calculous obstruction. However, an ultrasound is not able to demonstrate luminal or intraluminal non-calculous causes of obstruction, e.g. a transitional carcinoma.

The sensitivity of ultrasound for obstruction using dilatation as an indicator is reduced if:

- an ultrasound is performed before dilatation has occurred
- there is an intrarenal pelvis
- dehydration is present, or
- there is confusion between dilated calyces and cortical cysts.

The specificity of an ultrasound is lowered by:

- an extrarenal pelvis, which may be falsely interpreted as a dilated system
- vesicoureteric reflux and a high urine flow rate, which may give the appearance of a hydroureter or hydronephrosis.

Preferably, a spiral CT should follow an ultrasound that is inconsistent with the clinical scenario but an IVU or diuretic renogram may also help. An ultrasound can demonstrate ureteral stones in 19% compared with CT as a gold standard. Nevertheless, hydronephrosis due to obstruction may be present in 73% of those who have stones and this can be detected by ultrasound. In obstructive anuria, combined KUB and ultrasound are less sensitive than spiral CT for identifying calculous causes of obstruction

but similar for non-calculous causes. A spiral CT may be necessary to exclude stones and further determine the cause of obstruction. The specificity and positive predictive value for the diagnosis of a stone by ultrasound is very high making CT unnecessary for confirmation if a stone is seen on ultrasound.

In a patient with acute painful dilatation of a kidney, it is seldom difficult to make a diagnosis of obstruction. In doubtful cases isotope renography or measurement of the renal resistive index may be useful.[3]

COMPUTED TOMOGRAPHY

Unenhanced helical CT scans offer many advantages over the IVU in the diagnosis of loin pain and ureteric obstruction:

- Greater sensitivity for the detection of calculi especially those ≤2 mm in size.
- Information on extrinsic causes of ureteral obstruction and non-urological causes of flank pain (e.g. appendicitis, diverticulitis, bleeding aortic aneurysm and adnexal masses).
- Time saving (can be completed in one breath hold).

In the clinical presentation of renal colic, spiral CT has a sensitivity of 95% and specificity of 98%. Furthermore, in 27% of patients found not to have a stone a correct alternative diagnosis may be made by CT.[4]

The features of obstruction on CT are perinephric or periureteral fat stranding in association with hydronephrosis and hydroureter above the obstruction with normal ureter below (Figure 4.3). In the majority, ureteral dilation occurs 1–2 h after the pain develops but perinephric or periureteral stranding may not occur until after 8 h of pain.[5] Unilateral kidney enlargement is often present due to renal edema. Stranding of the perinephric fat may be present at the upper or lower poles only and should be compared with the contralateral kidney. Asymmetric stranding may be seen as a

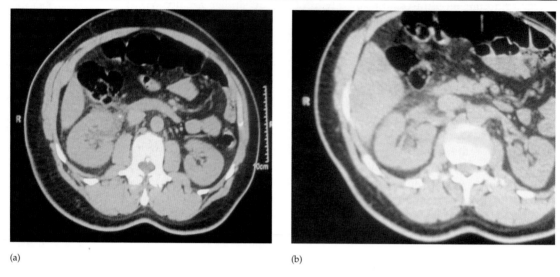

(a)

(b)

Figure 4.3

(a, b) Computed tomography scan demonstrating perinephric stranding with extra vasation.

loss of definition of the fat–kidney interface or as very fine linear stranding compared with the well-defined interface around the contralateral kidney. Collecting system dilatation is identified most easily at the upper and lower poles, which appear as round fluid-filled structures that partially obliterate the renal sinus fat compared with the contralateral kidney.

Spiral CT is not a functional study and so the relative grade of obstruction when compared with diuretic renography (see below) is more difficult to establish. In this respect, IVU may have an advantage. If the extent of obstruction might alter a treatment decision, a MAG-3 study may be needed, or if an anatomical road map of the ureter is required, an IVU is preferable, unless CT sagittal reconstruction is available.

CT can show all stones except matrix stones and protease inhibitor-related calculi (indinavir), but the features of obstruction are present even if the stones themselves are not seen. Stones in the ureter may be difficult to distinguish from phleboliths. Phleboliths are usually

surrounded by fat and so should have a black border on CT, whereas there is a thin circumferential rim – 'rim sign' – of soft tissue around a ureteric stone because of periureteral edema. The rim sign is highly specific (92–100%) for the presence of a stone, but rarely occurs without features of obstruction.[6] Furthermore, some ureteric stones will not show the rim sign. On CT, phleboliths may have a protruding gray tail and this is known as the 'comet-tail sign'. This is the soft tissue of the vessel within which the phlebolith lies. When the secondary features of obstruction are seen with an area of calcification, a stone is usually present even if the comet-tail sign is present or there is no rim sign.

Most importantly, the course of the ureter should be followed down from the kidney or up from the ureterovesical junction to determine if the calcification is in the ureter, confirming a stone (Figure 4.4a, b). Other calcifications that might occur and possibly cause confusion include calcified ovarian or uterine masses and calcified mesenteric lymph nodes. A gonadal vein can sometimes be confused with a dilated ureter and can be distinguished by following the superior course of the structure. In equivocal cases, image reformation in a curved frontal plane following the course of the ureter may demonstrate calcification within the ureter, or intravenous contrast can be used (Figure 4.4c). Therefore, there is a learning curve when using helical CT and this may preclude its use when expert interpretation is unavailable.

When the features of obstruction are present without a demonstrable area of calcification, the differential diagnosis includes a recently passed stone, urinary tract obstruction unrelated to stone disease (sloughed renal papilla/clot colic/stricture), matrix and protease inhibitor-related stones.

A CT scan is poor at determining the constitution of stones. Stones with a Hounsfield Unit density (HU divided by the maximum diameter of the stone) more than 76 HU/mm always contained calcium suggesting that alkalinization of urine to dissolve stones would be unsuccessful. Hounsfield units themselves are unhelpful. In some cases, further investigations are required following CT including plain radiography, retrograde urography, or nephrostography but mostly for treatment-related reasons.

NUCLEAR RENOGRAPHY

In the acute situation, diuretic renography is not commonly used, but may have a place after spiral CT to determine the degree of obstruction, the effect on function and the type or urgency of intervention required.

Commonly used agents for diuretic renography are mercaptoacetyltriglycine (^{99m}Tc-MAG-3), which is both filtered and secreted by the tubules, and diethylenetriaminepenta-acetic (^{99m}Tc-DTPA), which is filtered by the kidneys alone. The technique is important to obtain reliable results: the patient should be well hydrated and able to void efficiently or have a catheter in place. It should be possible to generate an adequate urinary flow rate and in patients with renal impairment, the dose of diuretic may need to be increased (Figure 4.5).

The effect of furosemide is maximal about 15 min after administration and the administration of furosemide 15 min before the renogram (F-15) reduces the number of equivocal responses. The result can be interpreted visually or by calculation of the clearance of the agent from the kidney ($T_{1/2}$). A $T_{1/2}$ of less than 10 min is considered normal, but greater than 20 min is abnormal.

MANAGEMENT

Although the management will always depend on the specific cause of obstruction, general principles include relief of obstruction to limit renal damage and prevention of infection. In the context of acute renal colic, intramural obstruction due to calculus is the most common cause, but the differential diagnosis includes sloughed renal papilla, blood clot, acute retroperitoneal pathology and accidental ureteric ligation.

Once obstruction has been diagnosed, the cause, the level of obstruction and the potential complications of not relieving the obstruction determine the management. When ureteric obstruction occurs in the late stages of malignancy, relieving obstruction may not always be appropriate. Otherwise, urgent indications to relieve obstruction are:

- obstruction of a single kidney or bilateral obstruction with deteriorating renal function
- infected urine (pyrexia >38.5 °C, rigors)
- uncontrollable pain
- deterioration in renal function
- high grade or complete obstruction that does not resolve quickly.

CALCULUS

The severe pain of ureteric colic demands early relief. Traditionally, intramuscular (IM) narcotics such as morphine or pethidine were used. Double-blind controlled trials have shown that there is no difference in immediate pain relief

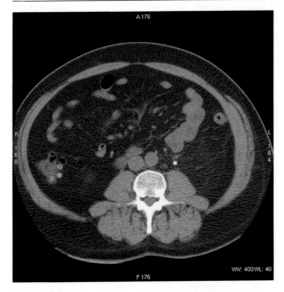

(a)

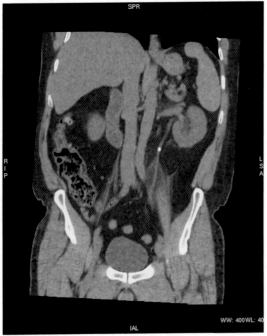

(b)

Figure 4.4

(a) A non-contrast CT scan showing a ureteric stone obstructing the left ureter. (b) The same scan reconstructed in the coronal plane demonstrating the exact level of the obstruction. (Courtesy of David Lloyd, University Hospital of Wales.)

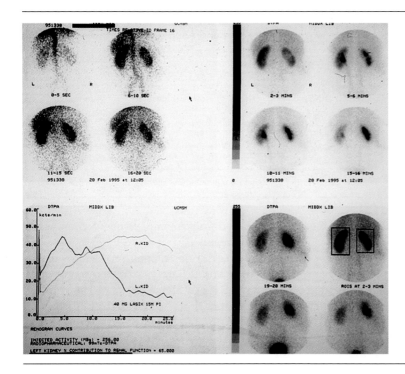

Figure 4.5

A Renal DTPA scan demonstrating right obstructive nephropathy. Upper left-hand panel: dynamic phase shows slightly reduced perfusion of the right kidney compared with left. Upper right-hand panel: progress of activity from the renal parenchyma into the pelvic-alyceal system from the right is slow and left is brisk. Lower right-hand panel: shows most of the activity from the left kidney has drained while the tracer is retained in the right kidney (kidney is more black). Lower left-hand panel: shows the time activity curve from the right kidney does not trend towards baseline. (Courtesy of Dr J Bomanji, UCL, London.)

between these and non-steroidal anti-inflammatory drugs (NSAIDs) such as diclofenac or ketorolac. The requirement for rescue analgesia is less with the NSAIDs than with narcotics.[7,8] The effect of the type of analgesia on spontaneous stone passage is seldom considered in the trials, but clinical experience suggests that it makes little difference. Diclofenac 100 mg IM or per rectum (in the UK) or ketorolac 60 mg IM (in the USA) is reasonable. Rectal diclofenac is particularly useful as it can be repeated at home. Rather surprisingly, two-thirds of patients with uncomplicated ureteric colic do not require a second dose of analgesia. Any further pain can usually be controlled with oral or rectal analgesia. After initial pain control and investigation in the emergency room, most patients can be discharged for outpatient follow-up.[9]

Factors determining whether stones will pass spontaneously include stone size and position. Prolonged symptoms and severe hydronephrosis are associated with less likelihood of spontaneous stone passage. The likelihood of the stone passing spontaneously is shown in Table 4.1.

In dogs with complete ureteral obstruction, irreversible loss of renal function does not occur before 2 weeks but can progress to complete loss of kidney function after 6 weeks. In man, there is little good evidence to determine how long obstruction can be allowed to persist without long-term damage. Although complete renal function may be regained following spontaneous passage of a calculus, it is possible that earlier rather than late intervention may recover more renal function.

Thus, if a spiral CT or ultrasound with KUB is performed for diagnosis, a diuretic renogram may be necessary if conservative management is planned for an extended period especially if there is no evidence of stone movement. In one study, patients had a MAG-3 renogram with furosemide immediately after spiral CT.[11] Several

Table 4.1 Percentage of spontaneous stone passage by size and position on computed tomography

Size (mm)	Position (%)				
	Proximal ureter	Mid-ureter	Distal ureter	Ureterovesical junction	All positions
1–4	47 (24–71)	80 (28–100)	77 (61–89)	92 (74–99)	75 (65–84)
5–7	63 (42–81)	0 (0–70)	71 (42–92)	50 (19–81)	60 (45–74)
>7	25 (7–52)	100 (16–100)	67 (9–99)	33 (1–91)	38 (19–59)
All sizes	48 (35–61)	60 (26–88)	75 (62–86)	79 (62–91)	77 (69–83)

Reproduced from Coll et al. *Am J Roetngenol* 2002; 178: 101–3[10] with permission from the *American Journal of Roentgenology*.

observations were made on the basis of the presence of obstruction diagnosed on MAG-3:

- Those who either never had obstruction or had experienced spontaneous decompression never required admission or emergency intervention.
- Those with complete or severe obstruction required admission and relief of obstruction to reduce pain or restore function.
- Those with mild obstruction could be managed by forced fluids, analgesics or, less frequently, elective surgery.

This study was a clinical experience rather than an investigation examining the prognostic or predictive value of diuretic renography in determining the type of intervention required.[11] Since patients without obstruction treated conservatively did not have a poor outcome, this study increases confidence in the safety of this course of management. Further studies are required to determine the place of combination CT and diuretic renography in the optimal management of acute obstruction.

For renal colic, clinical selection, KUB radiography, and even positive helical CT findings predict the extent of obstruction poorly (in one study, 35, 32, and 56% respectively[5]). An IVU shows the extent of drainage, which can act as a surrogate indicator of obstruction, and explains why IVU is still preferred by some urologists. If there is no obstruction, urgent intervention is not required unlike complete obstruction, when it is recommended.

Infection with obstruction can destroy a kidney within hours. Rarely, extravasation of urine through the ureter above the stone can result in a retroperitoneal and psoas abscess if infection occurs. Decompression of obstruction is essential in these cases either by nephrostomy or stenting (see below).

Thus, intervention is required if stones do not pass within 40 days, pain is uncontrollable, infection supervenes and, probably, if there is high-grade obstruction. If a smaller stone does not pass, the ureter is likely to be narrow and prior stenting of the ureter might be necessary to allow ureteric dilatation if intervention by ureteroscopy is planned.

Stones unlikely to pass spontaneously can be treated by extracorporeal shock wave lithotripsy (ESWL), rigid or flexible ureteroscopy with intracorporeal lithotripsy. Urgent ESWL without a JJ stent has a high success rate (80–90%) and requires fewer shocks than ESWL with a JJ stent. A stent in the ureter increases the intrapelvic pressure and reduces the peristaltic amplitude and rate. The success rate with large stones can be improved by pushing the stone in the renal pelvis with a ureteroscope before ESWL. Stones greater than 50 mm^2 area (product of the two maximum diameters) and in the proximal ureter have a higher likelihood of requiring more than one treatment with ESWL, and ureteroscopy or percutaneous nephrolithotomy may be the preferred choice of treatment by some patients.

Radiolucent stones on a plain radiograph and those with a Hounsfield unit density <74 HU on CT may be due to uric acid especially if a fasting urine pH is acidic. These stones can be dissolved by urine alkalinization with potassium citrate, and litmus paper can be used to test the extent of alkalinization achieved. Such stones may dissolve and not require additional interventional treatment.

Intensive medical treatment to increase the rate of spontaneous stone passage has infrequently been used, however, randomized controlled studies have shown that the combination of steroids, nifedipine and antibiotics can increase the rate of spontaneous stone passage and reduce the number of admissions to casualty.

PELVIURETERIC JUNCTION OBSTRUCTION

Obstruction of the pelviureteric junction (PUJ) may be accompanied by acute loin pain, usually precipitated by drinking a large volume of fluid in a short time (Dietl's crisis). The diagnosis and level of obstruction may be confirmed by an IVU (Figure 4.6) or spiral CT.

Rarely, the IVU appears completely normal in a patient with history of recurrent acute loin pain suggestive of PUJ obstruction. The pain is usually transient (lasting for 30–90 min) and by the time IVU is done the radio-graphic appearance is normal. It is then advisable to carry out IVU when the patient is in acute pain. The IVU in Figure 4.7 clearly demonstrates marked hydronephrosis during the acute episode while the appearance is normal looking during remissions. Such intermittent episodes of PUJ obstruction are usually due to the presence of an aberrant lower pole vessel.

In the presence of acute PUJ obstruction, insertion of an internal stent or nephrostomy is almost always associated with relief of pain and improvement in function. Decompression is essential if there is infection. The definitive treatment is pyeloplasty.

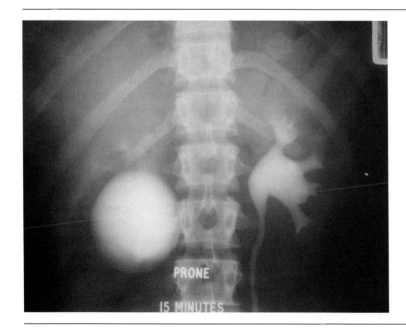

Figure 4.6

High-dose intravenous urography (IVU) demonstrating a significant anatomical narrowing of the pelvic-ureteric junction (PUJ). (Courtesy of Mr CRJ Woodhouse, UCL, London.)

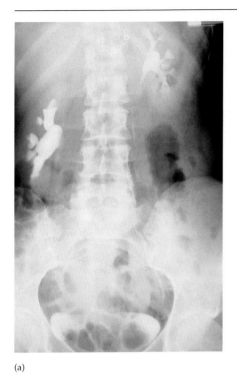

(a)

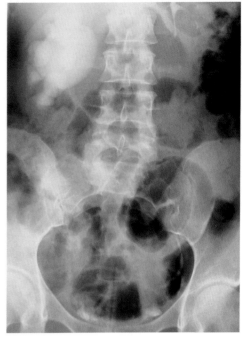

(b)

Figure 4.7

Intermittent PUJ obstruction. (a) Normal IVU in a patient with a history of intermittent right loin pain typical of PUJ obstruction taken during a pain-free period. (b) IVU of the same patient taken during acute pain demonstrating a typical appearance of an obstructed PUJ. (Courtesy of Mr F Mumtaz, Barnet and Chase Farm Hospital NHS Trust, London.)

PREGNANCY

Acute ureteric obstruction in pregnant women is most commonly due to ureteric calculi. Typical renal colic with microscopic or macroscopic hematuria is the most common presentation. Urinary tract infection may be present in a third of these patients.

DIAGNOSIS

Diagnosis is more difficult because of the physiological dilatation of the upper tracts that occurs in pregnancy by the second and third trimesters, which persists for up to 12 weeks after pregnancy. Dilatation seen on ultra sound beyond the 90th centile for gestation is strongly indicative of obstruction (Table 4.2).

Ultrasound should be the first investigation but has a sensitivity of between 35 and 95% and specificity of 90% for the identification of stones. Normally, the ureter is not dilated below the pelvic brim so a dilated infra-iliac ureter and high-grade hydronephrosis make obstruction likely. Distinction between a dilated ureter and the common iliac vein or an enlarged ovarian vein can be made by color Doppler. Asymmetric ureteric jets of urine indicate possible obstruction and it may be possible to show a stone at the ureterovesical junction on transvaginal ultrasound.

Table 4.2 Observed and adjusted percentiles of maximum calyceal diameter (mm)[a] of right and left kidneys by gestational age[b]

Gestational age (wk)	Observed percentiles				Adjusted[b] percentiles			
	Right			Left	Right			Left
	50th	75th	90th	90th	50th	75th	90th	90th
4–6	0.0	3.0	5.0	2.1	1.4	2.4	3.4	0.1
7–8	0.0	0.0	5.0	0.0	0.3	3.2	4.5	2.2
9–10	0.0	0.0	4.0	0.0	1.2	4.0	5.7	3.5
11–12	0.0	5.0	7.0	6.0	2.0	4.9	7.0	4.5
13–14	0.0	5.8	8.0	6.9	2.7	5.7	8.4	5.3
15–16	0.0	1.0	8.9	4.9	3.0	6.7	9.8	6.0
17–18	5.0	9.5	12.0	8.8	3.7	7.6	11.2	6.6
19–20	0.0	8.0	11.0	7.7	4.2	8.6	2.6	7.1
21–22	5.0	9.0	13.8	6.8	4.6	9.6	13.9	7.1
23–24	8.0	12.0	15.0	8.2	4.9	10.5	15.1	7.9
25–26	7.0	13.0	16.7	8.0	5.3	11.4	16.2	8.2
27–28	7.0	13.0	21.0	9.0	5.6	12.2	17.2	8.1
29–30	7.0	11.0	16.0	9.0	5.9	13.0	18.0	8.6
31–32	8.0	15.5	19.4	8.2	6.1	13.7	18.7	8.7
33–34	4.5	13.0	20.5	8.5	6.4	14.3	19.3	8.8
35–36	6.0	15.0	19.0	8.0	6.6	14.8	19.7	8.9
37–38	5.0	14.0	20.4	8.0	6.8	15.2	19.8	8.9
39–42	7.0	14.0	17.0	9.2	7.1	15.5	19.8	8.7

[a]Measurements are of the maximum diameter of the most dilated calyx of the kidney imaged in the longitudinal axis with the woman in the lateral position, normally hydrated, and after the bladder was emptied.
[b]Adjusted percentiles are those produced by curve fitting.
Reproduced from Faundes et al. *Am J Obstet Gynecol* 1998; **178**: 1082–6[12] with permission from Elsevier.

Radiation is most damaging in the first trimester and should be avoided. In the second trimester, the radiation dose below which no harmful effect occur is thought to be 5–15 rad (0.05–0.15 Gy) and a single radiograph gives 0.2 rad of exposure, which is less than 1% of the critical dose. Shielding of the asymptomatic side may further reduce the radiation exposure. Thus, a control film, 30-s nephrogram and 20-min film have minimal risk in the second and third trimester. The control film may be difficult to interpret if there is overlap with the fetal skeleton.

Magnetic resonance urography using T2-weighted fast spin echo sequences and diuresis enhancement distinguishes physiological dilatation from pathological causes. Stones cannot themselves be seen but appear as complete filling defects with a signal void at the level of obstruction. Perirenal fluid may surround the kidney.

TREATMENT

Almost two-thirds of women will pass calculi spontaneously with conservative treatment. In some, temporary measures to bypass the obstruction are required with definitive treatment usually reserved until after birth. Stents can be placed with a flexible cystoscope using ultrasound to monitor the position and locate the coil in the renal pelvis. These will need to be changed every 6–8 weeks because of the accelerated encrustation in pregnancy and should be placed preferably in the second or third trimester. Ultrasound-guided percutaneous nephrostomy may be needed in the first or second trimester or if a JJ stent is intolerable. Frequent urinary cultures are necessary because of the risk of infection.

In selected patients, especially those in early gestation, definitive treatment of the stone may be safer than repeated changes of ureteric stents. Flexible ureteroscopic access to the ureter may allow removal of stones with stone forceps or treatment with a laser, although it is technically demanding. Pneumatic lithotripsy of the stone with 7-Fr rigid ureteroscopes is also possible, but ultrasonic or extrahydraulic lithotripsy is contraindicated at any time during pregnancy.

SLOUGHED RENAL PAPILLA

Renal papillary necrosis may occur in patients with diabetes, pyelonephritis, urinary tract obstruction with urinary infection, analgesic abuse, sickle cell hemoglobinopathies, renal transplant rejection and liver cirrhosis. Patients present as if they have renal colic (Figure 4.8). If an IVU is performed, this may show signs of acute obstruction; medullary or papillary changes may be seen, such as irregular sinuses or medullary cavities, or an irregular calyx filled with contrast except centrally (seen as a ring sign) (Figure 4.9). Retained necrotic papillae may calcify and become echogenic on ultrasound resembling calculi. A helical CT may show signs of obstruction with either a non-calcified or calcified lesion. The diagnosis is made by the passage of necrotic tissue in the urine. They may pass spontaneously, but occasionally decompression will be required by a stent or nephrostomy if the obstruction persists. The sloughed papilla can be removed with a ureteroscope using a stone basket to trap the papilla. As infection is usually present, antibiotics are necessary.

BLOOD CLOT

Any cause of bleeding in the upper urinary tract may cause ureteric obstruction with consequent renal colic. A radiolucent filling defect may be seen on IVU. Often these will pass spontaneously, but occasionally decompression may be required. Further investigation for a tumor is required.

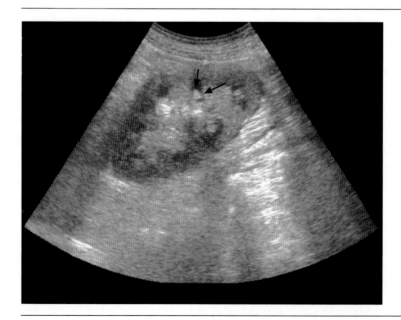

Figure 4.8

An ultrasound scan of the kidney suggestive of a papillary necrosis (sloughed papillae arrowed).

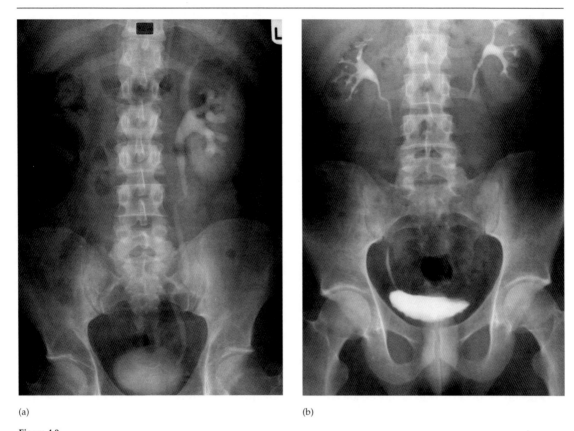

(a) (b)

Figure 4.9

(a) An IVU showing complete obstruction of the right kidney secondary to renal papillary necrosis. (b) A later IVU demonstrating complete relief of obstruction following the release of sloughed papillae.

MORE COMMON CAUSES OF CHRONIC OBSTRUCTION THAT MIGHT PRESENT ACUTELY

TUBO-OVARIAN ABSCESS AND INFLAMMATION

This cause of pelvic pain may be confused with renal colic. Pelvic inflammatory disease (PID) is possibly the most common cause of pelvic pain in the sexually active female. Specific features include dyspareunia, pelvic pain and tenderness, and cervical excitation. There may be symptoms of ureteric obstruction in acute cases. The most common pathogens are *Neisseria gonorrhoeae* and *Chlamydia trachomatis*.

Just under half may have associated ureteric dilatation at the level of the pelvic brim or just below. Ultrasound and spiral CT may demonstrate uni- or bilateral dilatation as well as a tubo-ovarian abscess. Conservative treatment is with oral ofloxacin 400 mg bd and metronidazole 500 mg tds for 14 days or intravenous cephalosporins with oral doxycycline 100 mg od. The abscess and ureteric dilatation resolves in 80%, but occasional surgical drainage is required.

APPENDICITIS

Acute obstruction of the ureter can occur in the presence of appendicitis, peritonitis, and an appendiceal abscess. An abdominal mass may be palpable. On a plain abdominal radiograph, a soft-tissue shadow obscuring the right psoas margin with most of the small bowel displaced to the left and a fecolith at the site of the appendix. If an IVU is performed, obstruction of the ureter may be seen. Confusion with renal colic from a stone is less likely if a spiral CT has been performed. Removal of the appendix relieves the hydronephrosis.

RETROPERITONEAL FIBROSIS

Patients may present with girdle-like pain and signs of chronic renal failure. Occasionally, the presentation may be similar to renal colic, but this is unusual. Imaging may show medial deviation of the mid-ureter on IVU and spiral CT, which will also show the retroperitoneal pathology surrounding the ureters and often the great vessels. Usually, stents will pass easily up the ureters but may not function for long because obstruction is by extrinsic compression and a nephrostomy may be required.

Abscesses can develop in the retroperitoneal space from either the kidney and ureter (e.g. infection of extravasated urine above a stone) or from inflammation of anterior structures such as appendix, diverticulae or bowel with Crohn's disease. A psoas abscess may develop which can obstruct or move the ureter medially. Patients may be pyrexial with a tender abdominal mass and the tenderness may extend to the iliac, groin or thigh areas. If a psoas abscess develops, patients sit with the hip flexed and find hip extension painful. On radiography, there may be air in the psoas and a scoliosis towards the side of the pain. Treatment consists of prompt drainage either through open surgery or percutaneous puncture.

GYNECOLOGICAL CAUSES OF OBSTRUCTION

Intraoperative ureteral injury

Intraoperative recognition of ureteral ligation can be treated by removal of the suture. If the ureter appears ischemic, excision of the ischemic area and ureteroureterostomy or ureteric reimplantation should be performed. Postoperative discovery may be prompted by pain, fever, drainage from the vagina or wound, nausea and vomiting, prolonged ileus, anuria and leukocytosis. An intravenous urogram will demonstrate the location of obstruction and help to identify a fistula. A ureteric stent should be passed retrogradely if possible and left for 6 weeks. If a stent cannot be passed, early ureteric reimplantation is required.

Endometriosis

Endometriosis is a rare cause of ureteric obstruction and less than a half of those affected have symptoms. The cyclical nature of symptoms such as loin pain, dysuria, urgency, urinary tract infection and hematuria, should make the diagnosis obvious. Extrinsic endometriosis of the adventitia or extraureteric tissue may cause the appearance of smooth strictures, but intrinsic endometriosis may appear as filling defects. Endourological biopsy can help make the diagnosis.

Uterine prolapse

By deforming the ureters and bladder, uterine prolapse may cause obstruction. Reduction of the prolapse usually alleviates obstruction and long-term treatment of the prolapse prevents further obstruction.

VASCULAR CAUSES

Aneurysms

Obstruction may occur in relation to aneurysms of the abdominal aorta or iliac artery. Post-aortobifemoral bypass, placement of the ureter behind the bypass can result in compression and fibrosis producing ureteric obstruction. Devascularization of the ureter can have similar consequences. Most patients present with flank pain between 2 weeks and 1 year after surgery. Diagnosis is by IVU or spiral CT and treatment by ureteric stenting or nephrostomy

Puerperal ovarian vein syndrome

This is also known as puerperal ovarian vein thrombophlebitis and occurs in 1 in 2000 pregnancies. Patients present with pain and fever 2 or more days after delivery. Examination of the adnexa may reveal a tender cord usually on the right and the diagnosis is best made by CT. Treatment is usually by antibiotics and anticoagulation.

GASTROINTESTINAL TRACT CAUSES

Diverticulitis

Diverticulitis itself can be confused with renal colic occasionally. Extension of the inflammatory process from a retroperitoneal perforation may result in a retroperitoneal abscess that can cause ureteric obstruction acutely.

Crohn's disease

Ureteral obstruction is usually slow in onset and occult developing after several months of bowel symptoms. Urinary symptoms are usually absent. Treatment of the bowel disease usually ameliorates obstruction.

MASS LESIONS

Retroperitoneal tumors

Primary retroperitoneal tumors can cause chronic obstruction and are rarely acute in presentation. Secondary peritoneal tumors may originate from the cervix, endometrium, prostate, bladder, ovary or other intra-abdominal structures. Such tumors tend to encase the ureter and may present with flank pain, sepsis, fever or acutely with renal failure. The diagnosis can be made by IVU or spiral CT, with the latter demonstrating the likely cause. There is a better prognosis for patients with carcinoma of the prostate, those previously untreated, and obstruction caused by direct extension of tumor arising from the pelvis in the absence of metastatic disease.

Lymphocele

Lymphoceles occur after renal transplantation, radical pelvic surgery and lymphadenectomy. Patients present with deteriorating renal function, lower abdominal pain, frequency, constipation, edema of the external genitalia and lower limbs. There may be a palpable mass on abdominal or pelvic examination. Spiral CT demonstrates a collection, deviation of the ureter medially and signs of obstruction if present. The aspirate from the collection will have potassium and creatinine levels similar to serum levels unlike the much higher levels characteristic of a urinoma. Unless renal failure is significantly acute, no urgent treatment may be necessary. Otherwise, retrograde ureteral catheterization or stent insertion will suffice until definitive treatment of the lymphocele.

MANAGEMENT OF OBSTRUCTION WITH INFECTION

Infection in an obstructed kidney is a life-threatening condition. Before the advent of nephrostomy and stents in the 1970s, patients commonly died. A randomized trial of retrograde ureteric stenting versus nephrostomy in patients with obstruction due to a stone showed that there was no important or significant difference in time to normalization of temperature, white cell count, discharge or complication rate by either technique.[13] In the patients (n = 42) in this study, the mean temperature was 38.7 °C, white cell count $15 \times 1000/mm^3$ and stone diameter 8 mm. Nephrostomies were cheaper, but they were more painful than retrograde stents. The choice is determined by the availability of interventional radiologists, surgeon preference and the potential need for percutaneous nephrolithotomy, ureteroscopy or extracorporeal shock wave lithotripsy (Table 4.3).

Patients should be resuscitated with fluid and antibiotics intravenously (gentamicin 5–7 mg/kg per day and amoxicillin 500 mg) before either intervention. After 5 days of antibiotics, an antegrade nephrostogram can be performed if a

---

Table 4.3 Advantages and disadvantages of percutaneous nephrostomy and retrograde stent

	Retrograde ureteric stent	Percutaneous nephrostomy
Advantages	• Internal drainage • No external collecting bag • Dilatation of the ureter facilitating future ureteroscopy	• Continuous monitoring of renal drainage • Better drainage (larger diameter tube) • Ability to flush the tube if it becomes blocked • More certain drainage than a JJ stent • Greater likelihood of lowering intrarenal pressure • May be better if a percutaneous approach is planned • Opportunity to perform Whitaker's test
Disadvantages	• Necessity for anesthesia • Risk of ureteric perforation • Less effective drainage (narrower tube) • Rise in intrapelvic pressure • May fail when due to extramural obstruction • Frequency, mild back discomfort	• Potential induction of sepsis • Back discomfort • Hemorrhage • Accidental tube displacement • Need for an external collecting bag • Need for an interventional radiologist

---

nephrostomy was inserted and the cause of obstruction identified.

PERCUTANEOUS ANTEGRADE NEPHROSTOMY TUBE

A 10–12-Fr catheter (locking loop-type catheter) is positioned in the renal pelvis by a radiologist or suitably trained urologist. The catheter is usually passed through a posterior lower pole calyx by the infracostal route to avoid empyema. An antegrade nephrostogram is not performed to avoid iatrogenic septicemia from pyelovenous or pyelosinus backflow of infected urine. Aspirated urine is sent for bacterial and fungal culture.

Antegrade percutaneous stenting is successful in 90% of cases. Reasons for failure include decompression of the collecting system secondary to rupture of a fornix, displacement and kinking of the tube. If there is no flow because the fluid is too viscous, the tube can be replaced with a larger lumen drain.

Retrograde stent insertion may be preferable if there is an uncorrected coagulopathy, no access to an interventional radiologist, or if it is likely the stone will be treated by ureteroscopy at a later date.

When obstruction occurs due to a steinstrasse, drainage of the kidney and relief of obstruction by a nephrostomy allows a dilated ureter to coapt thereby improving peristalsis and making stone passage more likely. In cases of a pyocalyx, the collecting system abscess is drained percutaneously. Similar to a pyonephrosis, a 10–12-Fr catheter is inserted below the twelfth rib and may need to be angled sharply to enter an upper calyx.

RETROGRADE URETERIC STENT

Retrograde stenting has been shown to be as effective as nephrostomy in treating patients with obstruction due to a stone and infection. A nephrostomy may be necessary if there is infection with obstruction due to a ureteral calculus greater than 15 mm in maximum diameter or steinstrasse, or because of pregnancy, urethral or ureteral stricture disease, ureteric reimplantation or urinary diversion. A single stent results in a rise in pressure in the renal collecting system, which lasts for at least 1 month and is reduced but not eliminated by a urethral catheter. Thus, in sick patients a nephrostomy may be preferable although one randomized trial indicated no difference in outcome between nephrostomy and retrograde in patients suitable for either.[13] Two ureteric stents may be preferable to allow pus to drain between the tubes as well as through them.

In general, ureteric stents almost always relieve obstruction caused by calculi or PUJ obstruction. Extrinsic compression is relieved by a stent in two thirds of patients. Significant predictors of failure of an internal stent to drain at 3 months include extrinsic compression, distal rather than proximal obstruction and severe hydronephrosis. In one study, the diameter of the stent inserted is probably not important in determining whether a stent will drain the kidney successfully. In gynecological malignancy, ureteric stents may fail and have been associated with fatal urosepis.[14] A stent may be ineffective if a tumor encases the ureter, which subsequently impairs muscle contraction and tissue distension that are required for peristalsis and the flow of urine around the stent.

Using wider stents, and changing them more frequently, may improve drainage down the ureter. Insertion of two stents has resulted in improved drainage in the presence of extrinsic obstruction.[15] Stiffer stents made of polyurethane are less compressible than those made of silicone and resist compression more effectively but have other disadvantages and so are not often used.

A retrograde stent may be necessary if the collecting system has decompressed for whatever reason making insertion of a percutaneous nephrostomy difficult.

RETROGRADE ACCESS TO THE URETER

Provided basic rules are followed, serious damage to the ureter can be avoided. Various techniques exist for situations where it is difficult to pass a guide wire or stent.

Patient selection
- Sterile urine (in the majority of circumstances).
- IV hydration.
- IV preoperative antibiotics (gentamicin and amoxicillin or gentamicin and cefuroxime, or third-generation cephalosporins).

- Availability of an image intensifier, a radiolucent operating table with an extension to allow adequate maneuvering of the image intensifier to view the kidneys.

Practical points: retrograde pyelography and guide wire insertion

Cystoscopy: use 30° lens in a 17/20/22-Fr rigid or 15-Fr flexible cystoscope. Perform a cystoscopy, visualize the ureteric orifice and then try to empty the bladder so that there is 100 ml or less of irrigation (this straightens and reduces the pressure on the intramural ureter).

Retrograde ureteropyelography: insert an open-tipped ureteric catheter (5-Fr Pollack) gently into ureteric orifice (Figure 4.10). Collect urine, if necessary, for cytology before the injection of a 1:1 mix of contrast and saline. Get an 'anatomic road map' of the ureter and attempt to demonstrate the pathology on the image intensifier.

Guide wire insertion: introduce an open-ended catheter (5-Fr Pollack) just into the ureteric orifice and then pass a guide wire (0.038" or 0.035" floppy-tipped polytetrafluoro ethylene (PTFE)-coated guide 'Bentson' wire) through and up the ureter past the pathology into the kidney. Alternatively, a hydrophilic-coated nitinol core wire may be used. These have a low coefficient of friction facilitating passage through resistant narrow segments of the ureter and are stiff, thus resisting kinking. If the catheter is not used, a submucosal flap at the ureteric orifice may result. If a guide wire will not pass easily, the following points may be of help:

- In men with a large prostate and J-hooked ureter, invert the cystoscope and retract the median lobe with the beak of the cystoscope to expose the ureteric orifice.
- Keep steady rather than intermittent intense pressure on the guide wire and it may slip past slowly.
- Advance the open-ended ureteric catheter over the wire within 1.5 cm of the end of the wire, which will stiffen and bring its fulcrum

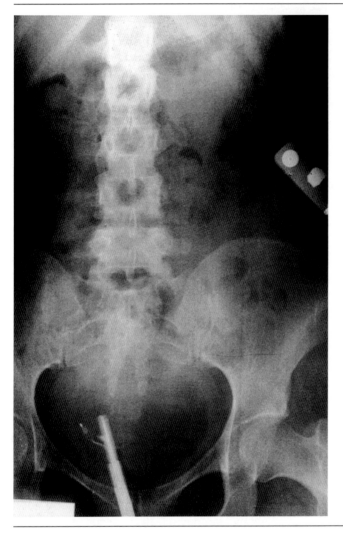

Figure 4.10

A ureteroscopic procedure to remove a distal ureteric stone using a dormia basket. (Courtesy of Mr CRJ Woodhouse, UCL, London.)

of bend closer to the end.

- Inject contrast, lidocaine jelly or a mixture (1:1) of both to act as lubricant.
- Change the floppy-tipped Bentson wire either to a hydrophilic superslippery (Glide) wire, a Sensor wire, or an angled Glide wire (Terumo, Japan; Microvasive, Boston Scientific Corporation).
- Place a guide wire under direct vision with a ureteroscope.
- Establish antegrade access, and pass a PTFE-coated or superslippery wire down to the

bladder. A flexible ureteroscope can also be passed antegradely to help insert a wire downwards. If this fails, a percutaneous nephrostomy can be left in place for 2 weeks after which a return to attempt ureteroscopy should be made in 2 weeks.

Tips for other problems:

Tortuous ureter: Bends in the upper ureter straighten on expiration, which can be controlled by the anesthetist, facilitating insertion of a guide wire or stent. Alternatively, insert a hollow 4-F or 7-F ureteral balloon-dilating catheter just distal to the problem area. Gently fill the balloon with contrast medium until there is just enough traction to grip the edges of the ureter when seen on the image intensifier. Pull down and straighten the ureter, and insert the guide wire through the internal lumen of the catheter beyond the tortuous area.

Perforation of the ureter: If a guide wire perforates the ureter, do not remove it but place another guide wire alongside. The first guide wire prevents the other wire from entering the perforation.

STENT INSERTION

- Have a guide wire in place.
- Pass the stent over the guide wire. Keep the cystoscope close to the ureteric orifice and the bladder reasonably empty to prevent the stent and wire buckling. Push the stent using the pusher up the guide wire slowly but steadily. The image intensifier can be used to monitor progress up the ureter. When the end of the stent is seen, which is usually marked in some way, remove the guide wire leaving 2 cm of stent visible from the ureteric orifice. Check the final position on the image intensifier.
- If a double J stent will not pass easily up the ureter, a ureteric catheter can sometimes be passed more easily and be left temporarily until ureteric dilatation occurs allowing easier passage of a stent. Alternatively, a percutaneous nephrostomy can be placed.

Choice of stent

Stent design should provide constant, unobstructed drainage and position. Stents of varying diameter have been constructed (4.7–18 Fr), but for the majority 7 Fr is ideal.

Lengths vary from 12 cm to 30 cm, but 24 cm will suit most adults. The length of stent required is best estimated by the height of the patient. Direct measurement can result in an overestimate of the required length because the redundant ureter is capable of significant shortening after stent insertion. In general, for a patient <178 cm (<5 ft 10 in) the stent length should be 22 cm; 178–193 cm (5 ft 10 in–6 ft 4 in) it should be 24 cm; and for >193 cm (>6 ft 4 in) it should be 26 cm.

For self-retaining stents, there is a coil at each end (double J). Some have a suture at the end, which can be left either completely out of the patient, or in the mid-urethra for easy removal with a flexible cystoscope.

A hydrophilic polymer usually lines the stent to allow smooth insertion and some need to be hydrated first. Silicone is a polymer with alternating silicone and oxygen atoms. It is thought to be non-irritating and resists encrustation but is very flexible sometimes making the insertion difficult and increasing the risk of stent migration.

Polyurethane, which contains repeating polyisocyanate and polyol units, is stiffer and resists compression more than silicone but may become brittle after extended use. Polyurethane can also cause ulceration of the ureter and more edema than silicone. C-flex is a silicone-modified thermoplastic elastomer, which is softer than polyurethane and has less shape memory. Percuflex is an olefinic block copolymer, which is stiff and has a low coefficient of friction. Percuflex stents are popular because they are easy to insert, have a high inner to outer diameter ratio, and enhanced retaining strength.

Single J stents are used to provide internal support to ureteral anastomoses created during various types of urinary diversion or to drain kidneys through the ureter into a catheter in the bladder. The proximal end stays in the renal pelvis while the distal open end is allowed to drain. These are not usually used in the setting of acute obstruction although they can be inserted with a flexible cystoscope.

INSERTION OF TWO URETERIC STENTS

In the cases of malignant extrinsic obstruction or obstruction with infection, two stents may be necessary. The following techniques can be used to insert these:

- A retrograde contrast study is performed. Two hydrophilic-coated 0.035″ flexitipped superslippery (Glide) wires are passed separately through a 21 Fr cystoscope with a double port bridge past the ureteral obstruction into the renal pelvis. A pair of 4.7-Fr double-J stents is inserted over each guide wire, and pushed simultaneously into the kidney. After placement of two stents the contrast material should drain promptly. The position of the stents can be confirmed on the image intensifier or by plain radiographs.
- Either spraying the stents with silicone or the injection of a mix of contrast/lidocaine jelly into the ureter can facilitate insertion of the stents. Stents can be changed later one after the other or simultaneously over a glide wire.

If two stents will not pass easily up the ureter, a superstiff guide wire (e.g. Amplatz, Boston Scientific) can be passed up the ureteric Pollack or Glide catheter, the catheter removed, and a dual-lumen catheter passed over the super-stiff wire. A retrograde pyelogram is performed through the second lumen and then a second super stiff wire passed through this lumen. The dual lumen catheter is removed leaving the two guide wires in the ureter. A 10-cm high-pressure balloon dilator is passed over the second wire and the entire length of the ureter dilated to 20 atm. After balloon dilatation, two 7 or 8-Fr ureteric catheters are passed simultaneously over the guide wires.

URETEROSCOPY

Circumstances in which ureteroscopy may be difficult include previous surgery on the ureter, prostate enlargement or a narrow ureter. Always have a guide wire ('safety' wire) in the ureter when performing ureteroscopy. Introduce the ureteroscope into the ureteral orifice alongside the safety guide wire, which is usually easier in females. If this fails, insert a second wire through the ureteroscope working channel ('working wire'), and 4–5 cm into the ureteric orifice. Invert the

ureteroscope to 180° so that the two wires splay the ureteric orifice open, and pass the ureteroscope through the opening. Ensure the bladder is almost empty to straighten and reduce the pressure on the intramural ureter. After entering the ureter, invert the ureteroscope so that it is now in the normal (0°) position and pass it up the ureter under direct vision without using force. In general, use the guide wire to straighten the ureter.

If it is not possible to insert the ureteroscope between two guide wires, either dilate the ureteric orifice or leave an indwelling JJ stent for 2 weeks. The latter is preferable if the entire ureter up to the pathology is narrow. Ureteric dilatation is necessary in less than 3% of ureteric orifices using 7.5–9.5 Fr ureteroscopes and is needed more commonly after pelvic or ureteral surgery, radiation, or extrinsic ureteral compression by tumor or fibrosis. Use serial Teflon dilators over a guide wire, or a balloon dilator (14–18 Fr, 10–20 atm).

Occasionally it is not possible to pass the ureteroscope over the pelvic brim as the ureter courses over the iliac vessels, in which case try the following:

- Apply pressure over the lower abdomen at the level of the pelvic brim to compress the iliac vessels and make the course of the ureter straighter.
- Elevate the loin.
- Insert the working wire along the ureter beside the safety wire and advance the ureteroscope under direct vision and radiographic control.
- Flexible ureteroscopy may be necessary if these measures fail, or insert a JJ stent to allow the ureter to dilate and then return in 1–2 weeks.

Give 20 mg of furosemide or more to generate a diuresis (to reduce the risk of pyelorenal reflux and infectious complications). Avoid excessive irrigation, which raises the pressure in the renal collecting system. Open the ports on the ureteroscope to allow drainage when movement up the ureter or visualization of pathology is not necessary. If there is only one channel, passing a catheter up the ureter will allow continuous drainage ameliorating the rise in pressure.

INSERTION OF A URETERIC CATHETER OR STENT WITH A FLEXIBLE CYSTOSCOPE

Male patients should be positioned supine and female patients in a frog leg position. Examine the flexible cystoscope to determine the relation between the lens and working port. After insertion of lubrication, introduce the flexible cystoscope into the bladder and identify the ureteric orifices. Keep the bladder as empty as possible. Insert a 0.035" Teflon-coated Bentson guide wire with a flexible tip into the ureteric orifice. By knowing the relation of the working port relative to the lens, it is possible to determine whether supination or pronation will align the working port with the trigone and ureteric orifice. If a Bentson wire cannot be passed, alternative guide wires as suggested above or a 0.035" or 0.038" hydrophilic angle-tip guide wire with a torque device can be helpful. If a superslippery wire is inserted, this will need to be replaced with a stiffer wire as kinking may occur. A 5-Fr open-ended ureteric catheter can be passed over the hydrophilic wire and the latter replaced with a Bentson PTFE wire so that a single J stent can be passed over this wire. Alternatively, the open-ended catheter can be left in place. This can be attached to a Foley catheter or passed down the end of a council tip catheter, which has an open end, to maintain a closed system. The position of the ureteric catheter or J stent can be confirmed with an image intensifier or plain radiograph.

STENT INSERTION THROUGH AN ILEAL CONDUIT

A gastroscope or flexible cystoscope can be used to facilitate stent insertion into the ureteric orifices of an ileal conduit. Retrograde stenting via the conduit is preferable but difficult without seeing the ureteric orifices and x-ray imaging alone may not be adequate. The flexible cystoscope has a small caliber, which makes it difficult to achieve an effective seal when used in an ileal conduit. Ileal conduits are readily distended by air with a gastroscope and the ureteric orifices can be seen easily. Guide wires can be passed under direct vision and their position confirmed with an image intensifier or plain radiographs.

CHANGE OF A BLOCKED STENT THROUGH A STENOSED ANASTOMOSIS BETWEEN AN ILEAL CONDUIT AND URETER

Perform a retrograde study of the ureter. Withdraw the stent so that 15 cm remain within the ureter proximal to the stenosed segment. Make a hole with an 18 gauge needle in the JJ stent, insert a 0.035" or 0.038" straight guide wire 5 mm through the hole into the lumen of the JJ stent, push the JJ stent back into the ureter such that the wire is passed through the stenosed segment. Advance an 5-Fr open-ended ureteric catheter over the guide wire and push it so that it withdraws the guide wire from the JJ stent allowing passage into the upper ureter into the kidney. Remove the blocked stent and pass a JJ stent up the guide wire into the ureter.

POSTOBSTRUCTIVE DIURESIS FOLLOWING RELIEF OF BILATERAL OBSTRUCTION

Diuresis may occur if there is bilateral ureteric obstruction or a single functional kidney is obstructed. Part of the diuresis is caused by impairment of concentrating ability or sodium reabsorption and the rest by retained urea, sodium and water that accumulate as a result of obstruction.

Patients most likely to have diuresis are those who are volume overloaded and with renal impairment. All patients should have their weight taken, a clinical estimate of volume status (postural blood pressure, jugular venous pressure) and their urine output measured. If the urine output is greater than 200 ml/h 2 h after relief of obstruction, it is helpful to know the type of diuresis. In the majority of cases, the diuresis is due to fluid overload and retained sodium. In this situation, fluid replacement is required when hypovolemia develops and the diuresis persists. Retained urea can produce an osmolar diuresis. If the urine is of low osmolality, then a pathological concentration defect is possible and supplemental fluid intake is necessary if the patient can manage until renal function stabilizes. If there is evidence of renal impairment, intravenous fluid supplementation is necessary with sodium-containing fluid. If the fractional excretion of sodium is increased, then a sodium wasting nephropathy may be present and copious sodium replacement is necessary until renal function recovers.

REFERENCES

1. Bove P, Kaplan D, Dalrymple N et al. Reexamining the value of hematuria testing in patients with acute flank pain. *J Urol* 1999; **162**: 685–7.
2. Kinn AC, Larsson SA, Nelson E, Jacobsson H. Diclofenac treatment prolongs renal transit time in acute ureteral obstruction: a renographic study. *Eur Urol* 2000; **37**: 334–8.
3. Shokeir AA, Abdulmaaboud M. Resistive index in renal colic: a prospective study. *BJU Int* 1999; **83**: 378–82.
4. Dalrymple NC, Verga M, Anderson KR et al. The value of unenhanced helical computerized tomography in the management of acute flank pain [See comments]. *J Urol* 1998; **159**: 735–40.
5. Varanelli MJ, Coll DM, Levine JA, Rosenfield AT, Smith RC. Relationship between duration of pain and secondary signs of obstruction of the urinary tract on unenhanced helical CT. *Am J Roentgenol* 2001; **177**: 325–30.
6. Heneghan JP, Dalrymple NC, Verga M, Rosenfield AT, Smith RC. Soft-tissue 'rim' sign in the diagnosis of ureteral calculi with use of unenhanced helical CT. *Radiology* 1997; **202**: 709–11.
7. Larkin GL, Peacock WF, Pearl SM, Blair GA, D'Amico F. Efficacy of ketorolac tromethamine versus merepidine in the ED treatment of acute renal colic. *Am J Emerg Med* 1999; **17**: 6–10.
8. Sandhu DP, Iacovou JW, Fletcher MS et al. A comparison of intramuscular ketorolac and pethidine in the alleviation of renal colic. *Br J Urol* 1994; **74**: 690–3.
9. Morris SB, Hampson SJ, Shearer RJ, Woodhouse CRJ. Should all patients with renal colic be admitted? *Ann Roy Coll Surg* 1995; **77**: 450–77.
10. Coll DM, Varanelli MJ, Smith RC. Relationship of spontaneous passage of ureteral calculi to stone size and location as revealed by unenhanced helical CT. *Am J Roentgenol* 2002; **178**: 101–3.
11. Sfakianakis GN, Cohen DJ, Braunstein RH. MAG3-F0 scintigraphy in decision making for emergency intervention in renal colic after helical CT positive for a urolith. *J Nucl Med* 2000; **41**: 1813–22.
12. Faundes A, Bricola-Filho M, Pinto ES, Joao L. Dilatation of the upper urinary tract during pregnancy: proposal of a curve of maximum caliceal diameter by gestational age. *Am J Obstet Gynecol* 1998; **178**: 1082–6.
13. Pearle MS, Lyle PH, Miller GL et al. Optimal method of urgent decompression of the collecting system for obstruction and infection due to ureteral calculi. *J Urol* 1998; **160**: 1260–4.
14. Feng MI, Bellman GC, Shapiro CE. Management of ureteral obstruction secondary to pelvic malignancies. *J Endourol* 1999; **13**: 521–4.
15. Rotariu P, Yohannes P, Alexianu M et al. Management of malignant extrinsic compression of the ureter by simultaneous placement of two ipsilateral stents. *J Endourol* 2001; **15**: 979–83.

FURTHER READING

Bird VG, Gomez-Marin O, Leveillee RJ et al. A comparison of unenhanced helical computerized tomography findings and renal obstruction determined by furosemide 99m technetium mercaptoacetyltriglycine diuretic scintirenography for patients with acute renal colic. *J Urol* 2002; **167**: 1597–603.

Borghi L, Meschi T, Amato F et al. Nifedipine and methylprednisolone in facilitating ureteral stone passage: a randomized, double-blind, placebo-controlled study. [See comments]. *J Urol*, 1994; **152**: 1095–8.

Clayman RV. Effectiveness of nifedipine and deflazacort in the management of distal ureter stones, *J Urol* 2002; **167**: 797–8.

Cooper JT, Stack GM, Cooper TP. Intensive medical management of ureteral calculi, *Urology* 2000; **56**: 575–8.

Cummings JM, Boullier JA, Izenberg SD, Kitchens DM, Kothandapani RV. Prediction of spontaneous ureteral calculous passage by an artificial neural network, *J Urol* 2000; **164**: 326–8.

Hamdy FC, Williams JL. Use of dexamethasone for ureteric obstruction in advanced prostate cancer: percutaneous nephrostomies can be avoided. *Br J Urol* 1995; **75**: 782–5.

Heidenreich A, Desgrandchamps F, Terrier F. Modern approach of diagnosis and management of acute flank pain: review of all imaging modalities. *Eur Urol* 2002; **41**: 351–62.

Liu JS, Hrebinko RL. The use of 2 ipsilateral stents for relief of ureteral obstruction from extrinsic compression. *J Urol* 1998; **159**: 179–81.

Motley G, Dalrymple N, Keesling C, Fischer J, Harmon W. Hounsfield unit density in the determination of urinary stone composition. *Urology* 2001; **58**: 170–3.

Pilcher JM, Patel U. Choosing the correct length of ureteric stent: a formula based on the patient's height compared with direct ureteric measurement. *Clin Radiol* 2002; **57**: 59–62.

Plata AL, Faerber GJ, Wolf JS Jr. Stent placement for the diagnosis of upper tract obstruction. *Tech Urol* 1999; **5**: 207–9.

Porpiglia F, Destefanis P, Fiori C, Fontana D. Effectiveness of nifedipine and deflazacort in the management of distal ureter stones. *Urology* 2000; **56**: 579–82.

Ruppert-Kohlmayr AJ, Stacher R, Preidler KW et al. [Active spiral computerized tomography in patients with acute flank pain–sense or nonsense?}. *Rofo Fortschr Geb Rontgenstr Neuen Bildgeb Verfahr* 1999; **170**: 168–73.

Shokeir AA, Abdulmaaboud M, Farage Y, Mutabagani H. Resistive index in renal colic: the effect of nonsteroidal anti-inflammatory drugs. *BJU Int* 1999; **84**: 249–51.

Shokeir AA, Mahran MR, Abdulmaaboud M. Renal colic in pregnant women: role of renal resistive index. *Urology* 2000; **55**: 344–7.

Shokeir AA, Shoma AM, Mosbah A. Noncontrast computed tomography in obstructive anuria: a prospective study. *Urology* 2002; **59**: 861–4.

Yossepowitch O, Lifshitz DA, Dekel Y et al. Predicting the success of retrograde stenting for managing ureteral obstruction. *J Urol* 2001; **166**: 1746–9.

5. Urinary retention and obstructive uropathy

Tim Nathan and Mark Emberton

Urinary retention is simply the inability to empty the bladder. This condition arises from bladder outflow obstruction, reduced bladder contractility or a combination of both. The inability to empty the bladder not only causes local symptoms but, in certain situations, which will be discussed in detail later, can result in profound effects on renal function due to the close hydrodynamic interaction between the lower and upper urinary tracts. Urinary retention can develop rapidly over a few hours, acute urinary retention (AUR), or develop more insidiously over months or years, chronic urinary retention (CUR) (Figure 5.1).

AUR is a common urological emergency, characterized by a sudden inability to micturate with painful distension of the bladder. It is the indication for surgery in 25–30% of men undergoing transurethral prostatectomy.[1] Painless AUR is rare and usually occurs secondary to a neurological pathology. In contrast, CUR is usually painless. Characteristically, patients with CUR continue to void, often with surprisingly minimal lower urinary tract symptoms. However, they have an ongoing inability to completely evacuate urine from the bladder, resulting in a large post-micturition residual volume. Diagnostic criteria for CUR in the literature arbitrarily specify that the residual volume has to be at least 300 ml, but patients with CUR can retain several liters without apparent distress. CUR does not usually present as an emergency except when it leads to complications of urinary stasis, such as urinary tract infection (UTI), pyelonephritis, bladder calculi, or renal failure. Some patients with chronic retention can subsequently develop painful retention. This has been referred to as acute on chronic urinary retention. In many instances it is difficult to distinguish this entity from AUR unless evidence of chronicity, such as obstruc-

tive uropathy, or prior documentation of significant residual volume, is present. However, when the residual volume is greater than 800 ml in a patient with painful retention, there is likely to have been a degree of chronic distension.

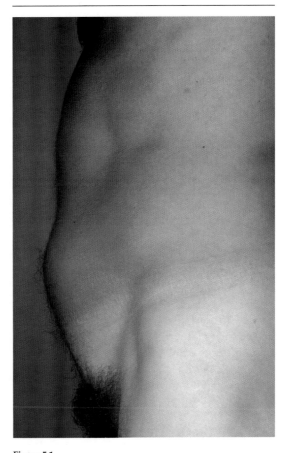

Figure 5.1

A large suprapubic swelling in a patient presenting with chronic urinary retention.

EPIDEMIOLOGY

The risk of AUR increases with age, and most cases occur in men over 60 years of age. A population-based, prospective study from Olmsted County, USA, found that the 5-year cumulative risk of AUR was six times greater in men in their seventies compared with those in their forties (10% vs. 1.6%).[2] It was calculated that a 60-year-old man would have a 23% probability of experiencing AUR if he were to reach the age of 80. AUR is uncommon in young men, women (male:female ratio 13:1)[3] and children. The epidemiology of CUR is less well documented but like AUR occurs mainly in elderly men.

AETIOLOGY AND PATHOGENESIS

Urinary retention occurs secondary to bladder outflow obstruction (BOO), impaired detrusor contractility, or a combination of both (Table 5.1). BOO can be due to a simple mechanical occlusion or a dynamic obstruction resulting from increased muscle tone. Impaired detrusor contractility may result from interruption of the sensory or motor innervation of the bladder wall, reflex detrusor inhibition, the influence of drugs or overdistension.

AUR and CUR have similar causes but why some develop acute painful retention whilst others develop more chronic forms is not well understood. Indeed many of the conditions which cause AUR are chronic. The etiology and pathogenesis of urinary retention will be discussed further but it must be borne in mind that the precise mechanisms involved are still poorly understood and the subject of much speculation.

ACUTE URINARY RETENTION

Table 5.2 lists the causes of AUR in men admitted to a teaching hospital during a 2-year period.[4] The increasing incidence of benign pro-

static hyperplasia (BPH) and impaired detrusor contractility, with age, accounts for the preponderance of AUR in elderly men. However, not all men with BPH develop urinary retention. The annual risk of AUR in men with symptomatic BPH has been estimated to be between 0.5 and 2.5%.[5] As mentioned above, the precise mechanisms leading to retention are unknown. Since a long time, prostatic infarction has been implicated as an important initiating event.[6] One study examining 200 prostatic adenomas removed by open enucleation, found prostatic infarcts in 85% of men with AUR, compared with 3% of men having surgery for symptoms alone.[7] However, other studies, albeit with smaller numbers of patients and based on examination of more limited tissue samples obtained at transurethral prostatectomy, have not shown such an association.[2,8] Factors which may predispose to prostatic infarction include an increased epithelial to stromal ratio,[8] hypotension during surgery, trauma and infection. Another mechanism in the pathogenesis of AUR, at least in some patients, may be stimulation of α-adrenergic activity (perhaps secondary to pain, bladder distension or prostatic infarction), resulting in elevated intraurethral pressures.[9] Modulation of the non-adrenergic, non-cholinergic nervous system has also been demonstrated in experimental animals in response to acute lower urinary tract obstruction,[9] but the role of such nerves in humans is uncertain.

Clinically, in approximately half the episodes of AUR associated with BPH, a triggering event may be identified such as surgery under anaesthesia, urethral instrumentation, ingestion of sympathomimetic, anticholinergic or opioid medication or other event. It is important to distinguish patients with precipitating factors, from those who develop spontaneous AUR, as they are less likely to eventually require prostatectomy (26 vs. 75%).[10] Surgery under general anesthesia appears to be a particularly important trigger, accounting for almost half of the cases in some populations.[2] Postoperative AUR

Table 5.1 Pathogenesis of urinary retention

Mechanism		Etiology
Bladder outflow obstruction	*Static obstruction*	• Benign prostatic hyperplasia • Prostate cancer • Constipation • Urethral/meatal stricture • Phymosis • Blood clot • Calculus • Foreign body • Pelvic mass • Hematocolpos due to imperforate hymen
	Dynamic obstruction	• Benign prostatic hyperplasia • Bladder neck dysynergia • Fowler's syndrome • Increased α-adrenergic activity in prostatic urethra due to pain or sympathomimetic medication
Impaired detrusor contractility	*Overdistension*	• Prolonged surgery under anesthesia without catheter • Excess fluid intake especially alcoholic beverages • Diuretic
	Drugs	• Anticholinergics • Opioids
	Derangement of sensory or motor innervation of bladder	• Frontal lobe lesion • Cauda equina/spinal cord compression from disk protrusion, hematoma, or spinal tumor/metastasis • Diabetic cystopathy • Herpes zoster or simplex affecting S2–4 dermatomes
	Reflex detrusor inhibition	• Painful anorectal stimuli, e.g. anal intercourse, anal fissures or hemorrhoidectomy

Table 5.2 Etiology of AUR in 310 men admitted to a teaching hospital[4]

Cause	Percentage
Benign prostatic hyperplasia	53.0
Constipation	7.5
Carcinoma of the prostate	7.0
Urethral stricture	3.5
Clot retention	3.0
Neurological disorders	2.0
Postoperative	2.0
Calculus	2.0
Drugs	2.0
Infection	2.0
Miscellaneous/unknown	16.0

commonly arises following a prolonged procedure during which the patient was not catheterized, leading to overdistension of the bladder. This may be exacerbated by any combination of opiate analgesia, anticholinergic medication, or high postoperative α-adrenergic activity. Urodynamic evidence of BOO is seldom found in those with postoperative AUR, and resumption of normal voiding occurs in the majority.[11]

The causes of AUR in women and children are listed in Table 5.3.[9] Women may develop AUR after surgery, secondary to cystitis, infravesical obstruction, insufficient detrusor function, obstetrical and gynecological conditions or hysterical reactions. In women in whom

---

Table 5.3 Causes of urinary retention in children and women[9]

	Cause
Children	• Cystitis • Postoperative • Voluntary overdistension • Congenital obstruction (anterior and posterior urethral valves, urethral polyp or atresia, ectopic ureterocele, hydrometrocolpos) • Acquired urethral obstruction (blood clot and/or tissue after surgery) • Neurogenic bladder • Trauma • Abscess (appendix, perirectal) • Tumors (sarcoma botryoides, teratoma) • Hypermagnesemia
Women	• Cystitis • Postoperative • Extrinsic compression, e.g. constipation, fibroids, ovarian cyst, gynecological tumors, retroverted impacted uterus (first trimester), pelvic prolapse, imperforate hymen leading to hematocolpos, Skene's gland abscess • Intrinsic urethral obstruction, e.g. meatal stenosis, urethral carcinoma, urethral diverticulum, urethral caruncle, Fowler's syndrome • Neurogenic, e.g. diabetes mellitus, demyelination, spinal cord compression • Psychogenic

---

a neurological or structural abnormality has been excluded, Fowler's syndrome should be considered.[12] The latter typically occurs in young women (usually in their twenties) and is characterized by abnormal electromyographic activity in the striated urinary sphincter causing a failure of relaxation which leads to urinary retention. There is strong association with polycystic ovarian disease suggesting an underlying hormonal etiology.

CHRONIC URINARY RETENTION AND OBSTRUCTIVE UROPATHY

CUR has been classified, on the basis of clinical presentation and urodynamic findings, into either low pressure CUR (LPCUR) or high pressure CUR (HPCUR),[13] although this distinction is not always clear cut.[14] LPCUR is so called, because the detrusor pressure during bladder filling remains low due to high bladder compliance. LPCUR does not cause hydronephrosis or compromise renal function. Two subsets of patients with LPCUR have been identified: those who void with a low flow rate and high detrusor pressure suggesting BOO; and those who void with a low flow rate and low detrusor pressure where impaired detrusor contractility is the underlying mechanism of retention. In contrast, HPCUR is characterized by raised detrusor pressures during all phases of the micturition cycle due to poor bladder compliance. Morphologically the HPCUR bladder is thick-walled and trabeculated, due to detrusor hypertrophy and marked collagen deposition. The reason why some develop such poor compliance in response to BOO, whilst others develop compliant bladders, and thus LPCUR, is not known.

The bladder spends 99.5% of its time in the storage (filling) phase. It is the high storage pressures, resulting from poor bladder compliance, that are thought to cause the hydronephrosis and obstructive nephropathy seen in HPCUR. Under conditions of normal hydration, the high intravesical pressures are not transmitted directly to the upper tracts due to the vesicoureteric valve mechanism. When urine production is stimulated, for example by fluid intake or a diuretic, the high upper tract urine flow combined with limited transport of urine across the vesicoureteric junction due to raised intravesical pressure, causes a rapid increase in renal pelvic pressure. This functional obstruction of the upper tracts, perhaps exacerbated by UTI, results in nephropathy (Figure 5.2).[15]

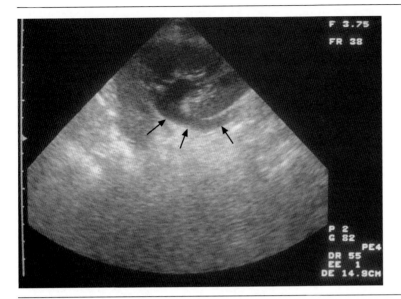

Figure 5.2

An ultrasound scan demonstrating hydroureteronephrosis in a patient with HPCUR.

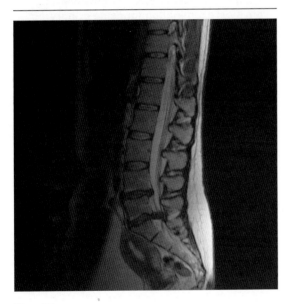

Figure 5.3

MRI of the spine showing a central disk prolapse in a patient presenting with painless urinary retention.

With progressive ureteric dilation, coaptive peristalsis is lost, and upper tract drainage becomes dependent on gravity. The hydrostatic pressure of 25 cmH$_2$O (18.4 mmHg), generated by the column of urine between the renal pelvis and bladder in the erect posture, becomes critical for upper tract drainage.[16] Thus, prolonged recumbency can lead to exacerbation of the renal impairment. With disease progression, even the nadir of detrusor pressure, which occurs at the end of micturition, may exceed 25 cmH$_2$O (18.4 mmHg). At this point a rapid deterioration in renal function ensues. Both glomerular and tubular functions are deranged. The glomerular filtration rate (GFR) is reduced leading to retention of urea and creatinine, and eventually severe uremia. Tubular dysfunction can result in a defective urinary concentrating mechanism, hyperkalemic acidosis and retention of salt and water. The latter manifests clinically as hypertension and congestive cardiac failure. If obstructive nephropathy is left untreated, progressive tubular atrophy due to apoptosis, interstitial fibrosis and glomerular sclerosis occur which can eventually lead to irreversible end-stage renal failure. Fortunately, patients usually present before this stage is reached and following relief of obstruction it is common to see some degree of recovery in renal function. This recovery occurs in two phases: an initial tubular phase followed by a glomerular phase.[17] The tubular phase is maximal in the first few days following relief of obstruction and lasts up to 2 weeks. It is characterized by diuresis and natriuresis accompanied by a fall in plasma creatinine. Although salt and water balance is restored, thus leading to rapid improvement of hypertension and congestive cardiac failure, approximately 10% of patients develop temporary 'overshoot' hypovolemia, necessitating intravenous saline infusion. Serum potassium levels usually fall during this diuretic phase but, occasionally, can rise due to the unresponsiveness of the distal tubule to aldosterone, which is physiologically suppressed during the obstructed state.[18] The secondary glomerular phase during which the GFR slowly recovers takes place between 2 weeks and 3 months after relief of obstruction.

CLINICAL FEATURES AND PATIENT ASSESSMENT

ACUTE URINARY RETENTION

A diagnosis of urinary retention can frequently be made based on the clinical history and examination without recourse to sophisticated diagnostic tests. AUR usually presents as a sudden inability to empty the bladder with marked urinary urgency and lower abdominal pain. Percussion and palpation of the lower abdomen will reveal a tense, distended, painful bladder. In obese and postlaparotomy patients, clinical detection of a distended bladder may be rendered more difficult. The patient's distress often necessitates immediate drainage of the bladder by catheterization (see below) before completing history taking and physical examination (Table 5.4). A large residual volume of urine drained after catheterization will confirm the diagnosis.

When a properly sited bladder catheter drains less than 300 ml, other diagnoses should be considered, particularly if the patient continues to be distressed. Conditions commonly misdiagnosed as urinary retention include intestinal obstruction, ascites, pelvic masses, aortic aneurysms and lower abdominal peritonitis.

Rarely, AUR is painless and suggests a neurological cause (see Table 5.1) which requires prompt evaluation. In addition to urinary symptoms, the patient may complain of bowel and/or sexual dysfunction. Neurological symptoms and signs will indicate the level of the lesion. Also, one should seek other clinical features suggestive of the underlying pathology, such as back pain and sciatica, which commonly occur in cauda equina syndrome (Figure 5.3).

Table 5.4 Important points in history and physical examination for acute urinary retention

History
- Previous history of lower urinary tract symptoms
- Presence of hematuria
- Presence of precipitating factors/events (see text and Tables 5.1–5.3)
- Past urological and gynecological history
- Drug history (opioids, anticholinergics, sympathomimetics)
- Neurological symptoms (sensory and motor disturbances, radicular pain, sexual/bowel dysfunction)
- Symptoms of uremia (malaise, lethargy, tiredness, shortness of breath on exertion, pruritus, anorexia, nausea and vomiting)

Examination
- Vital signs (pulse, blood pressure (BP), temperature)
- Hydration status (jugular venous pressure, postural BP changes, gallop rhythm, presence of pulmonary/peripheral edema)
- Signs of uremia (sallow complexion, fluid overload, Kussmaul's respiration, pericardial friction rub)
- Abdominal (palpation and percussion for bladder, exclude other causes of acute abdomen)
- External genitalia (meatal stenosis, phymosis, evidence of trauma or previous surgery)
- Digital rectal examination (anal tone, saddle sensation, prostate size, presence of malignancy, constipation)
- Per vagina (urethral pathology, pelvic masses, prolapse)

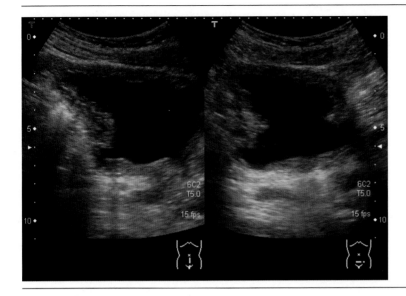

Figure 5.4

An ultrasound scan of the bladder demonstrating large amount of residual urine in a patient with LPCUR.

During digital rectal examination (DRE), sensory disturbance over the saddle area and reduced anal tone should raise the suspicion of a neurological cause. Urgent neurological or neurosurgical consultation may be required because delayed treatment can compromise eventual recovery.

CHRONIC URINARY RETENTION

The cardinal clinical features of HPCUR have been stated as enuresis, a tense painless bladder, hypertension and bilateral hydronephrosis.[13] However, patients with HPCUR often have minimal lower urinary tract symptoms. The symptom that typically causes the patient to seek medical attention is late-onset nocturnal enuresis, which is caused by a combination of the fall in urethral sphincter tone that normally occurs during sleep and the high intravesical storage pressures. This is often mistakenly referred to as overflow incontinence. Others with HPCUR present with symptoms of renal failure and the accompanying sodium and water retention. Hypertension and congestive cardiac failure occur in 50 and 20% of cases, respectively. Physical examination may reveal signs of uremia, fluid overload and a tense distended but painless bladder.

LPCUR often produces few symptoms and is usually an incidental finding during abdominal examination or ultrasound scanning (Figure 5.4). LPCUR cannot be considered a urological emergency, but it is important to differentiate this entity from HPCUR because LPCUR can be managed on an elective basis. The bladder, although distended, may be soft (non-tense) and difficult to feel. A normal serum creatinine level and absence of hydronephrosis on ultrasound scanning help to distinguish this condition from HPCUR.

INVESTIGATIONS

Urinary retention is readily diagnosed by history, physical examination and noting the residual volume after catheterization of the bladder. Additional investigations should be directed at identifying precipitating causes and the complications of urinary tract obstruction.

What are mandatory investigations in the emergency situation for a patient with uncomplicated urinary retention is open to debate. The authors recommend that urine dipstick and culture where indicated, and measurement of serum electrolytes, urea and creatinine, are the only baseline tests required. Other investigations should be directed by the clinical findings.

Serum prostate specific antigen (PSA) levels, should not be measured routinely in the acute setting as both AUR and urethral catheterization are known to elevate PSA. If a malignant prostate is suggested by DRE, PSA can be measured after an interval of 6 weeks. Occasionally, in those who are unwell with suspected extensive prostatic metastases requiring urgent treatment, early PSA testing may be justified.

An ultrasound scan to assess the upper tracts should be performed in the presence of a raised serum creatinine. Those with painless AUR require urgent imaging of the spine with magnetic resonance imaging (MRI) if there is clinical evidence of cauda equina syndrome or spinal cord impingement. Occasionally urodynamic investigations are required to distinguish HPCUR, LPCUR and neuropathic bladder disorders but this can be performed electively.

TREATMENT

Imediate treatment of painful urinary retention involves prompt bladder catheterization, which also is crucial in confirming the diagnosis (Figure 5.5). In those with painless retention, the presence of significant obstructive nephropathy (HPCUR), UTI or gross hematuria are also indications for urgent bladder catheterization (Figure 5.6). Local practice usually determines

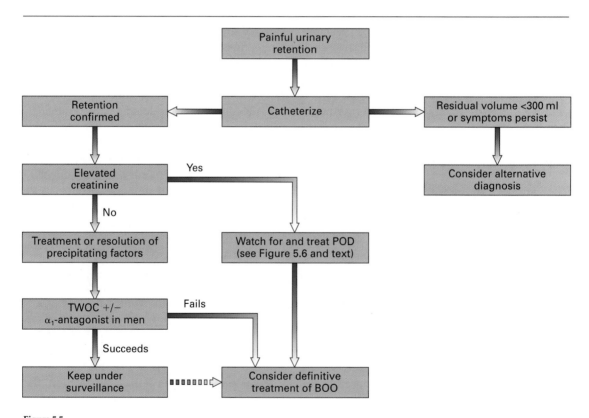

Figure 5.5

Management of painful urinary retention. POD, post obstructive diuresis; TWOC, trial without catheter; BOO, bladder outflow obstruction.

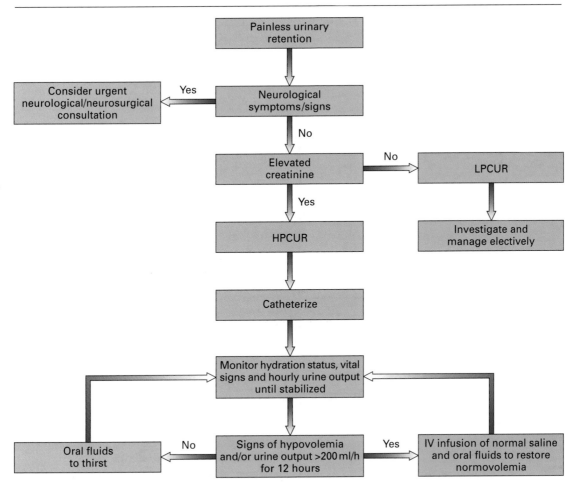

Figure 5.6

Management of painless urinary retention and postobstructive diuresis. HPCUR, High pressure chronic urinary retention; LPCUR, low pressure chronic urinary retention; IV, intravenous.

whether uncomplicated cases of AUR are admitted or sent home for later assessment in the urology outpatient department. The latter policy appears to be safe in the absence of concurrent uremia, sepsis, dehydration or other illness which would necessitate admission.[19] Those with painless retention and minimal derangement of renal function (LPCUR) do not need to be catheterized. Such patients can be investigated and managed electively.

BLADDER CATHETERIZATION

A summary of the techniques for urethral and suprapubic catheterization is provided in Tables 5.5 and 5.6. There is some debate among urologists regarding the optimal route of bladder catheterization. The urethral route is usually the most convenient as it is quick and usually straightforward. Also, it is more familiar to primary care and emergency room physicians and

---

Table 5.5 Technique of urethral catheterization

- Explain and discuss the procedure with the patient
- Place the patient in a comfortable supine position
- Prepare a trolley with all the required equipment
- Use an aseptic technique
- In men, inject 10–15 ml of water-soluble lubricant with local anesthetic into the urethra and massage it along. In women, apply lubricant directly to the catheter
- In men hold the penis under stretch perpendicular to the body
- Insert the catheter slowly and gently advance it along the urethra – avoid sudden or excessive use of force
- When the external sphincter is reached in men, stretch the penis parallel to the body and apply gentle, sustained pressure. Ask the patient to take slow deep breaths or strain as if passing urine to relax the sphincter
- Once the catheter is in the bladder inflate its balloon to the appropriate volume and attach drainage bag
- Record residual volume

Table 5.6 Technique of suprapubic catheterization

- Explain the procedure and obtain informed consent from the patient
- Correct any clotting defects
- Consider ultrasound guidance or urethral catheterization if there is a history of lower abdominal or pelvic surgery to avoid bowel injury
- Place the patient in a comfortable supine position
- Only proceed if the bladder is distended and easily palpable
- Prepare the trolley with the required equipment
- Prepare and drape the suprapubic area
- Select a point approximately 5 cm above the symphysis pubis in the midline
- Using 10 ml of 1% lignocaine (lidocaine) in a syringe and a 21-gauge $1\frac{1}{2}$ inch needle, insert the needle at right angles to the skin, anesthetizing the tissues as it is advanced
- When the needle has been fully inserted and all the local anesthetic expelled, withdraw the plunger
- If urine is aspirated, make a small incision in the skin, and insert the suprapubic catheter and obturator assembly according to the manufacturer's instructions
- If no urine is aspirated abandon the procedure

---

nursing staff, who are often the first to see the patient in painful retention. However, suprapubic catheters (SPCs) are recognized to have some important advantages particularly if prolonged catheterization is envisaged. SPCs are less likely to cause UTI or urethral strictures[20] and are less prone to interfere with sexual intercourse. Also a trial without catheter (TWOC) can be accomplished, simply by clamping the SPC, avoiding the discomfort of catheter removal and reinsertion if the patient fails to void. Complications of SPC insertion, such as catheter dislodgment, peritonitis secondary to bowel perforation or extravasation of infected urine, and tumor seeding in cases of bladder cancer, have been described.[9] For this reason, a previous history of transitional cell carcinoma of the bladder, or lower abdominal/pelvic surgery (which can cause intraperitoneal adhesions), are relative contraindications to SPC insertion. However, SPC is safe when performed by adequately trained personnel.[21] Although some would argue for routine use of SPC, the convenience of urethral catheterization usually outweighs any relative disadvantages in most instances. SPC does become necessary when urethral catheterization fails or is contraindicated, e.g. in the presence of a urethral stricture or urethral trauma (see below).

Clean intermittent self-catheterization (CISC) is an alternative to an indwelling urethral or SPC which, perhaps, should be more widely used. CISC is recognized to cause fewer complications than a catheter in situ for prolonged periods.[22] Also, patients can remain sexually active. However, CISC is a technique that requires a lot of patience, empathy and encouragement to teach, usually by a skilled dedicated nurse or continence advisor. For those presenting with acute painful retention out of hours, initially it is often more practical to insert an indwelling catheter. CISC can then be instituted at subsequent follow-up. There is evidence that this practice reduces the incidence of UTI and improves the chances of a return to spontaneous voiding.[23]

TYPES OF CATHETER

URETHRAL CATHETERS

The most commonly used type of indwelling urinary catheter is the self-retaining balloon catheter designed by Dr Frederick Foley in the 1920s. The basic two-way design has a channel for urine drainage and a smaller channel for inflation of the balloon (Figure 5.7b) Manufacturers now offer a wide variety of Foley catheters including three-way catheters that have a third channel for irrigation (Figure 5.7c). In-out catheters (e.g. LoFric, nelaton (Jacques)) are also available and are mainly used for measuring postmicturition residual volume, instillation of solutions into the bladder and CISC. Foley catheters are available in different sizes, balloon volumes and tip designs. Also catheters

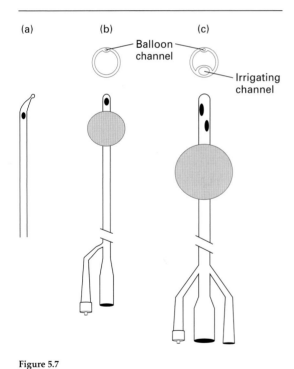

Figure 5.7

Common designs of urethral catheter in cross-sectional view. (a) Coude; (b) Standard two-way Foley; and (c) three-way Foley catheters.

are manufactured using a variety of materials. Factors governing catheter selection are discussed below.

Catheter size is usually expressed in Charrière (Ch), also known as French (Fr) gauge, which refers to the circumference of the catheter in millimeters. The diameter in millimeters is obtained simply by dividing the Ch (or Fr) gauge by π, e.g. a 16 Ch catheter would have a diameter of 5 mm. For a given diameter, a three-way catheter has a narrower channel for urine drainage than a two-way catheter due to the extra channel for irrigation (Figure 5.7c). In principle, the smallest size of catheter necessary to maintain adequate drainage should be used to minimize discomfort for the patient and reduce the risk of urethral complications. However, if the catheter is too small, it may be more difficult to insert in men due to kinking and coiling in the urethra, and more prone to blockage from debris or blood clots. In practice, in the presence of clear urine, a 14–16 Fr two-way Foley catheter should be considered in adults. Larger three-way catheters up to 22–24 Fr may be required for bladder lavage and irrigation in the presence of debris or hematuria.

Catheter balloons should be just large enough to hold the catheter tip securely in the bladder. A 5–10 ml balloon is ideal in most instances. Larger balloons (30–50 ml) are available usually on three-way irrigating catheters and are designed to be used after transurethral prostatectomy. Large balloons are more prone to cause bladder spasms and urinary leakage; also long-term use of large balloons may cause damage to the bladder neck. Catheter balloons should be filled to the manufacturer's stated volume. Otherwise the balloon may be misshapen resulting in catheter dislodgment and/or occlusion of the drainage holes.

Catheter tips vary in shape and the configuration of the drainage eyes. Straight tipped catheters will suffice in most instances. Catheters with curved tips (Coude and Tiemann, Figure 5.7a) have been designed to negotiate the S-shaped curve of the male bulbar urethra which may be exaggerated in the presence of prostatic enlargement. Most catheters have side eyes which can have a greater diameter than the lumen of the drainage channel, and allow more than one opening, thus reducing the chances of blockage.

Catheter material influences biocompatibility (Table 5.7) and mechanical properties such as stiffness. Latex Foley catheters are ubiquitous, fairly soft, relatively cheap and suitable for short periods of catheterization. With prolonged use, latex catheters are prone to encrustation and urethral irritation, sometimes resulting in stricture formation. Also latex catheters should be avoided in patients with a history of latex allergy.[24] The development of a variety of more inert biomaterials has permitted the manufacture of catheters suitable for long-term use (up to 12 weeks). These are generally more expensive than standard latex catheters, and should only be used when a prolonged period of catheterization is envisaged. Plastic catheters are stiff and may cause some patients urethral discomfort. Also, more care is needed during insertion to avoid urethral injury. However, this stiffness allows a thinner catheter wall, and thus a larger diameter internal drainage channel than an equivalently sized latex catheter. In addition the drainage channel lumen tends not to collapse when suction is applied. These features are particularly advantageous for three-way irrigating catheters, which may be required in patients with hematuria and clot retention.

Recent years have seen the development of reinforced latex and stiffer silicone three-way catheters, which combine the outer softness and comfort of these materials with adequate rigidity for bladder lavage.

SUPRAPUBIC CATHETERS

There are several types of SPC, some examples of which are illustrated in Figure 5.8. Narrow diameter pigtail (Bonnano) and malecot designs are easy to insert but are not suitable for long-term use due to a tendency to block, dislodge, become kinked or sometimes fracture below skin level. The internal fixation mechanisms of these catheters are weak and they need to be stitched to the skin, causing discomfort and predisposing to infection. The Lawrence Add-a-Cath trocar and peel away sheath allows suprapubic insertion of a standard Foley catheter which is securely retained by its balloon without the need for external fixation to the skin. It is ideal for inserting long-term Foley catheters suprapubically, where prolonged drainage is envisaged. Such catheters can be easily changed by nursing staff when a track has developed after 3 weeks.

DIFFICULT URETHRAL CATHETERIZATION

Difficulty in urethral catheterization is most often encountered in men, and occurs due to a variety of causes. In this situation, there is considerable potential to damage the urethra by

---

Table 5.7 Effect of catheter material or coating on duration of use

Duration of use	Catheter material
Short-term (1–14 days)	• Plain latex • Plastic (polyvinyl chloride)
Medium-term (2–4 weeks)	• Teflon (PTFE) or • Silicon elastomer coating applied to latex
Long-term (up to 12 weeks)	• All silicone • Hydrogel (latex encapsulated in a hydrophilic polymer coating)

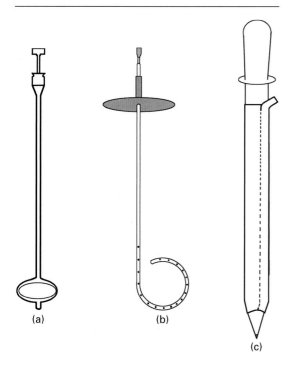

Figure 5.8

Common types of suprapubic catheter. (a) Malecot (Porges, UK); (b) Bonnano (Becton Dickinson, USA); and (c) Lawrence Add-a-Cath (Femcare Ltd., UK).

excessive use of force or injudicious use of urethral instrumentation. A urological history and examination, in conjunction with information gleaned from the initial failed attempt at catheterization will indicate the underlying problem. Retrograde urethrography or flexible cystoscopy, if available, may be helpful. The principles of successful catheterization are: gain the confidence of the patient; never to use excessive force; and only attempt maneuvers which one is experienced in. Insertion of a SPC will usually be the most appropriate course of action, if one is not expert in the use of urethral dilators, catheter introducers or urinary tract endoscopy.

Commonly, the S-shaped male bulbar urethra may impede the passage of a straight catheter,

particularly in the presence of prostatic enlargement with an elevated bladder neck. This situation can be aggravated by the tightening of the external sphincter that can result from patient anxiety and discomfort. Previous failed attempts at catheterization, especially if performed roughly and unsympathetically, will only make matters worse. Therefore, it is very important to relax the patient by adopting a reassuring manner and explaining how one intends to proceed. Intraurethral retention of lignocaine (lidocaine) gel for 15 min before attempting catheterization, by application of a penile clamp, can provide additional anesthesia. However, caution is advised if there is any urethral bleeding due to the risk of systemic absorption of lignocaine. The curved tip of a Coude catheter will often negotiate the bulb and prostate, where attempts with a straight catheter have failed. The use of curved catheter introducers is an alternative but is more likely to cause urethral damage, particularly in the hands of a novice.

Other causes of difficult catheterization in men include: anatomic variants, such as hypospadias, which may make identification of the external urethral meatus difficult for the unfamiliar; a narrowing or occlusion of the lower urinary tract due to phymosis, meatal stenosis, urethral strictures, postsurgical bladder neck contractures, tumors, or foreign body; a false passage, which is usually iatrogenic in origin; and traumatic disruption of the urethra. Narrowing of the lower urinary tract is a frequent cause of failed urethral catheterization. When a phymosis is encountered it can be dilated or a dorsal slit performed after administration of a local anesthetic ring block. A urethral stricture or other unpassable occlusion will usually require SPC in the emergency setting. Short strictures may be amenable to dilation, after administration of prophylactic antibiotics, intraurethral lignocaine and sedoanalgaesia, but this should only be performed after thorough endoscopic or radiological evaluation of the stricture to avoid excess urethral trauma.

Filiforms and follow-on gum–elastic bougies are particularly useful for dilating a tight stricture. The technique involves passage of multi filiforms (en fagot) until one enters the bladder. Follow on bougies attached to this filiform are then used to dilate the urethra. Long dense strictures may, however, require formal endourethrotomy under spinal or general anesthesia before a catheter can be inserted. A false passage can be bypassed by inserting a catheter over a guide wire directed into the bladder at flexible cystoscopy. An end hole will need to be created in the catheter to thread it over the guide wire.

Difficulty in catheterization of the female urethra is uncommon and usually occurs in the severely obese patient, where the external urethral meatus may be difficult to locate. Use of a vaginal speculum or an assistant to hold the labia apart is usually helpful. Also a finger in the vagina may be used to direct the catheter cephalad into the urethra. Occasionally, a structural abnormality of the introitus, such as labial fusion; or urethra, such as stenosis or iatrogenic false passage, may be encountered. As with men, unless one is experienced at urethral instrumentation, an SPC may be necessary.

POSTOBSTRUCTIVE DIURESIS

Following the relief of HPCUR, postobstructive diuresis (POD) and natriuresis occur in all cases, although this may only become clinically apparent when the diuresis is marked. The diuresis is beneficial in that it corrects the state of extracellular fluid overload. The majority (90%) of patients will self-regulate their fluid balance and stabilize with a marked improvement in plasma urea and creatinine levels within 1 week.[15] In approximately 10% of patients the diuresis is excessive and intravenous fluid replacement is required to prevent 'overshoot' hypovolemia. Occasionally (in <1%) the diuresis can be prolonged and life-threatening, due to severe tubular dysfunction. Thus, patients with POD need to be carefully monitored until they stabilize. In particular, assessment of hydration status and extracellular fluid volume should be done by measurement of daily weight, 4-hourly erect and supine blood pressure, and recording of jugular venous pressure and other signs of congestive cardiac failure. Urine output should also be monitored but is of secondary importance to the above. As discussed above, POD is self-limiting and clinically beneficial in 90% of cases. In this situation, strict intravenous fluid replacement of monitored urine output only serves to, unnecessarily, prolong the diuresis. Patients at risk of 'overshoot' hypovolemia, who do require intravenous fluid replacement, can be identified by a urine output which is consistently greater than 200 ml/h for the first 12 h after drainage of the initial residual urine. The aim of fluid replacement should be to achieve and maintain a normovolemic state based on above the clinical signs, rather than slavishly keeping up with the hourly urine output and estimated insensible losses.

Serum potassium levels should also be monitored carefully during POD. Usually the high potassium levels associated with obstructive uropathy will fall rapidly after catheterization. Occasionally, serum potassium levels may paradoxically rise during POD, due to a hyporesponsiveness of the distal nephron to aldosterone. This is a particular risk in patients who are taking a potassium-sparing diuretic or potassium supplements. Management of hyperkalemia is described in detail in Chapter 3.

Slow or intermittent bladder drainage was, at one stage, advocated for HPCUR to limit POD and prevent the hematuria that commonly occurs due to mucosal congestion after bladder decompression. However, this practice is no longer justified because it is now recognized that drainage of as little as 60 ml is accompanied by a large drop in intravesical pressure, resulting in the rapid onset of POD.[16] Intermittent clamping of the catheter may only serve to confuse patient monitoring. Postcatheterization hematuria should not cause concern as it is rarely severe and usually self-limiting.

TRIAL WITHOUT CATHETER

For patients presenting with a first episode of uncomplicated AUR it is reasonable to undertake a TWOC as some will resume spontaneous voiding. A TWOC is more likely to succeed where the obstruction has a largely dynamic component or there is a clearly identified precipitating factor which is reversible such as UTI, constipation, anesthesia, postsurgical pain, opiates, anticholinergic medication, etc. TWOC should not be done in those with associated obstructive nephropathy. Such patients have an absolute indication for deobstructing surgery.

The overall success rate of TWOC in men with AUR seen by urologists is only 23–28%.[9] Factors which predict failure of TWOC in men include, age over 75 years, drained residual volume >1000 ml, detrusor pressures <35 cmH$_2$O (25.7 mmHg), and absence of precipitating factors. Prolonging the duration of catheterization also seems to increase the chances of success, particularly in those with a residual volume over 1 liter.[25] Recently a randomized controlled trial has shown that administration of the α_1-antagonist, alfuzosin, prior to TWOC in men with benign prostatic obstruction can improve the success rate two-fold (55% vs 29% for placebo, $P = 0.03$).[26] After successful TWOC further urological follow-up is necessary because two-thirds will develop recurrent retention within the first year.[27] Those men who fail an initial TWOC or develop recurrent retention, usually require bladder outflow surgery.

FUTURE PROSPECTS

Progress is being made in the prevention and treatment of AUR in men. The 5α-reductase inhibitor finasteride, which causes modest reductions in prostatic volume by blocking the intraprostatic conversion of testosterone to the more active metabolite, dihydrotestosterone (DHT), has been shown in a randomized placebo controlled trial in men with sympto-matic BPH, to decrease the risk of AUR and surgery for BPH by 57 and 55%, respectively, over a 4-year period.[28] However, AUR and prostatic surgery were relatively infrequent occurrences in both the treatment and placebo groups, and the authors admitted that 15 men would have to be treated for 4 years to prevent one event. More recently, dutasteride, which inhibits both plasma and intraprostatic 5α-reductase activity, has shown a similar preventative effect to finasteride but possibly with a more rapid onset of action.[29] Because AUR is relatively infrequent and not life-threatening, a widespread program for prevention is not justified. Selective use of 5α-reductase inhibitors in men with known risk factors (moderate to severe lower urinary tract symptoms, large prostates, and poor flow rates) may be more appropriate. Also, there may be a role for secondary prevention in those who have had successful TWOC postretention, but this needs further study.

Alternatives to urethral catheterization are also under development. Temporary stents which hold open the bladder and prostatic urethra while still allowing the external sphincter to function are already available. At present such stents are more difficult to place than a urethral catheter, but this situation may change. If these devices could be inserted in primary care or the emergency room, hospital admission could be avoided. However, with time, these stents are still prone to displacement, infection and encrustation. Biodegradable stents are available but are still at an early stage of development. Temporary stenting of the prostate could in theory allow time for 5α-reductase inhibitors (or drugs, which may be available in the future, which can reduce the size of the prostatic adenoma) to work, thus avoiding the need for prostatectomy.

CONCLUSION

Urinary retention is a common, often distressing, urological emergency which usually occurs in elderly men. The diagnosis, in most cases, can be made on clinical findings without recourse to sophisticated investigations. Initial treatment simply involves bladder catheterization and management of associated complications. However, the immediacy of relief and the profoundness of gratitude expressed by a patient with painful retention after catheterization, are seldom encountered in other spheres of medical practice.

REFERENCES

1. Holtgrewe HL, Mebust WK, Dowd JB et al. Transurethral prostatectomy: practice aspects of the dominant operation in American urology. *J Urol* 1989; **141**: 248–53.
2. Jacobsen SJ, Jacobson DJ, Girman CJ et al. Natural history of prostatism: risk factors for acute urinary retention. *J Urology* 1997; **158**: 481–7.
3. Klarskov P, Andersen JT, Asmussen CF et al. Acute urinary retention in women: a prospective study of 18 consecutive cases. *Scand J Urol Nephrol* 1987; **21**: 29–31.
4. Murray K, Massey A, Feneley RC. Acute urinary retention – a urodynamic assessment. *Br J Urol* 1984; **56**: 468–73.
5. Roehrborn CG. The epidemiology of acute urinary retention in benign prostatic hyperplasia. *Rev Urol* 2001; **3**: 187–92.
6. Hubley JW, Thompson GJ. Infarction of the prostate and volumetric changes produced by the lesion. Report of three cases. *J Urol* 1940; **43**: 459–62.
7. Spiro LH, Labay G, Orkin LA. Prostatic infarction. Role in acute urinary retention. *Urology* 1974; **3**: 345–7.
8. Anjum I, Ahmed M, Azzopardi A, Mufti GR. Prostatic infarction/infection in acute urinary retention secondary to benign prostatic hyperplasia [Comment]. *J Urol* 1998; **160**: 792–3.
9. Choong S, Emberton M. Acute urinary retention. *BJU Int* 2000; **85**: 186–201.
10. Roehrborn CG, Bruskewitz R, Nickel GC et al. Urinary retention in patients with BPH treated with finasteride or placebo over 4 years. Characterization of patients and ultimate outcomes. The PLESS Study Group. *Eur Urol* 2000; **37**: 528–36.
11. Anderson JB, Grant JB. Postoperative retention of urine: a prospective urodynamic study [Comment]. *BMJ* 1991; **302**: 894–6.
12. Swinn MJ, Wiseman OJ, Lowe E, Fowler CJ. The cause and natural history of isolated urinary retention in young women [Erratum appears in *J Urol* 2002; **167**: 1805]. *J Urol* 2002; **167**: 151–6.
13. George NJ, O'Reilly PH, Barnard RJ, Blacklock NJ. High pressure chronic retention. *BMJ (Clin Res Ed)* 1983; **286**: 1780–3.
14. Styles RA, Ramsden PD, Neal DE. Chronic retention of urine. The relationship between upper tract dilatation and bladder pressure. *Br J Urol* 1986; **58**: 647–51.
15. Jones DA, George NJ. Interactive obstructive uropathy in man [Review]. [63 refs]. *Br J Urol* 1992; **69**: 337–45.
16. George NJ, O'Reilly PH, Barnard RJ, Blacklock NJ. Practical management of patients with dilated upper tracts and chronic retention of urine. *Br J Urol* 1984; **56**: 9–12.
17. Jones DA, George NJ, O'Reilly PH, Barnard RJ. The biphasic nature of renal functional recovery following relief of chronic obstructive uropathy. *Br J Urol* 1988; **61**: 192–7.
18. Jones DA, George NJ, O'Reilly PH. Postobstructive renal function. *Semin Urol* 1987; **5**: 176–90.
19. Pickard R, Emberton M, Neal DE. The management of men with acute urinary retention. National Prostatectomy Audit Steering Group. *Br J Urol* 1998; **81**: 712–20.
20. Horgan AF, Prasad B, Waldron DJ, O'Sullivan DC. Acute urinary retention. Comparison of suprapubic and urethral catheterisation. *Br J Urol* 1992; **70**: 149–51.
21. Abrams PH, Shah PJ, Gaches CG, Ashken MH, Green NA. Role of suprapubic catheterization in retention of urine. *J R Soc Med* 1980; **73**: 845–8.
22. Lapides J, Diokno AC, Silber SJ, Lowe BS. Clean, intermittent self-catheterization in the treatment of urinary tract disease. *J Urol* 1972; **107**: 458–61.
23. Patel MI, Watts W, Grant A. The optimal form of urinary drainage after acute retention of urine. *BJU Int* 2001; **88**: 26–9.
24. Young AE, Macnaughton PD, Gaylard DG, Weatherly C. A case of latex anaphylaxis. *Br J Hosp Med* 1994; **52**: 599–600.
25. Djavan B, Shariat S, Omar M, Roehrborn CG, Marberger M. Does prolonged catheter drainage improve the chances of recovering voluntary voiding after acute retention of urine (AUR)? *Eur Urol* 1998; **33 (Suppl 1)**: 110.
26. McNeill SA, Daruwala PD, Mitchell ID, Shearer MG, Hargreave TB. Sustained-release alfuzosin and trial without catheter after acute urinary retention: a prospective, placebo-controlled [Comment]. *BJU Int* 1999; **84**: 622–7.
27. Hastie KJ, Dickinson AJ, Ahmad R, Moisey CU. Acute retention of urine: is trial without catheter justified? *J R Coll Surg Edinb* 1990; **35**: 225–7.
28. McConnell JD, Bruskewitz R, Walsh P et al. The effect of finasteride on the risk of acute urinary retention and the need for surgical treatment among men with benign prostatic hyperplasia. Finasteride Long-Term Efficacy and Safety Study Group [Comment]. *New Engl J Med* 1998; **338**: 557–63.
29. Roehrborn CG, Boyle P, Nickel JC, Hoefner K, Andriole G. Efficacy and safety of a dual inhibitor of 5-alpha-reductase types 1 and 2 (dutasteride) in men with benign prostatic hyperplasia. *Urology* 2002; **60**: 434–41.

6. Upper urinary tract trauma

Michael J Metro and Jack W McAninch

Approximately ten percent of patients sustaining abdominal trauma have an injury of the genitourinary tract. Upper tract trauma comprises injuries to the kidney, renal pelvis, and ureter.

RENAL INJURY

The kidney is the most commonly injured genitourinary organ, with renal trauma present in approximately 5% of all abdominal trauma.[1,2] Staging of renal injuries consists of clinical, radiologic and, occasionally, surgical information, the combined use of which has improved the capacity for detection, classification and appropriate treatment. Advances in the imaging and subsequent staging of renal trauma, along with improvements in treatment strategies, have decreased the need for surgical intervention and increased renal preservation.[3,4] The goals of treatment include accurate staging, maximal preservation of renal function and minimal complications.

CLASSIFICATION OF RENAL INJURIES

Traditionally, renal trauma has been classified by mechanism, either blunt or penetrating. Overall, 80–90% of renal injuries result from blunt trauma, occurring most commonly in falls, motor vehicle accidents and assaults.[4] The majority of blunt renal injuries are minor and are managed conservatively. At our institution, only 2.5% of blunt renal injuries have required exploration and surgical repair.[2,5] Penetrating renal injuries, often the result of gunshot and stab wounds, require operative intervention more commonly because of the frequency of severe damage and associated intra-abdominal injuries.[6]

Accurate determination of the grade of renal injury is a key factor in deciding the mode of management.[7] The Organ Injury Scaling Committee of the American Association for the Surgery of Trauma has classified traumatic renal injuries into five grades (Figure 6.1).[8]

INDICATIONS FOR RENAL IMAGING

The indications for renal imaging have been well described.[4,10] Computed tomography (CT) with and without contrast has replaced intravenous pyelography to become the technique of choice in suspected renal trauma. In all large series, hematuria has been the most common sign: its presence suggests potential injury, although its degree does not correlate with the severity of injury.[4,10] It is imperative that the first catheterized or voided urine specimen be obtained for examination, as hematuria may clear upon subsequent voiding or within hours after catheterization. On the basis of our experience, we follow the criteria below and assess patients radiographically in the presence of the following:

- penetrating trauma to the flank or abdomen, regardless of degree of hematuria
- blunt trauma in adults with either gross hematuria or microhematuria and shock (defined as systolic blood pressure 90 mmHg or below at any time after injury)
- deceleration injuries
- major associated intra-abdominal injuries and microhematuria
- flank or abdominal trauma in all pediatric patients with any degree of hematuria.

Before a renal injury can be selected for non-operative management, it must be radiographically imaged and accurately staged (Figure 6.2). An incompletely staged renal injury requires

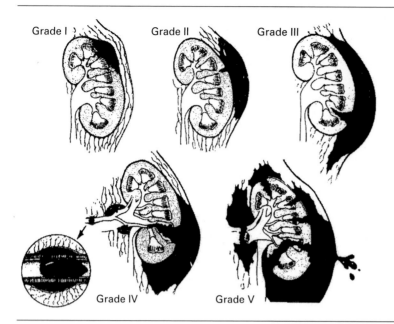

Figure 6.1

Grades of renal trauma, based on the American Association for the Surgery of Trauma's Organ Injury Severity Score for the Kidney. (Reprinted from Miller KS, McAninch JW. In: *Traumatic and Reconstructive Urology.* Philadelphia: WB Saunders, 1996; 89–94[9] with permission from Elsevier.)

surgical exploration. The widespread use of CT and the accumulated experience with the non-operative management of high-grade renal injuries have led to decreased rates of renal exploration.

INDICATIONS FOR SURGICAL EXPLORATION

The indications for renal exploration fall into two categories: absolute and relative.

ABSOLUTE INDICATIONS

Persistent renal bleeding constitutes an absolute indication for renal exploration. The intraoperative finding of an expanding, pulsatile or uncontained retroperitoneal hematoma indicates persistent bleeding, usually owing to major parenchymal or vascular injury. In these cases, exploration with reconstruction at the time of initial exploration is mandatory.[11]

If adequately staged, many major renal injuries can be managed expectantly. Expectant management is not necessarily non-operative management: it is a period of close observation (and sometimes repeat radiographic study), which determines when the injury might need surgical intervention. This being said, however, Grade V injuries will require intervention owing to their severity – either pedicle avulsion or extensive parenchymal destruction.

RELATIVE INDICATIONS

Both blunt and penetrating trauma can produce large areas of non-viable tissue, which is often best managed by early surgical debridement. When injuries with significant devitalized parenchyma are managed expectantly, short-term complications such as persistent urinary extravasation and abscess formation occur more commonly, as can long-term morbidity, such as hypertension. This was demonstrated by Husmann and Morris,[12] who showed that major renal lacerations associated with devitalized fragments constituting more than 25% of the unit resulted in an 80% rate of complications, including perinephric abscess, infected urinoma and delayed hemorrhage, requiring open surgi-

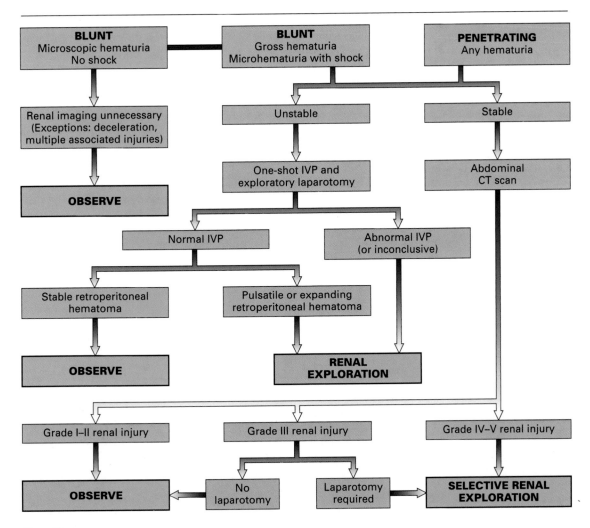

Figure 6.2

Algorithm for treatment of patients with renal trauma. IVP, intravenous pyelogram (Reprinted with permission from Meng MV et al. *World J Urol* 1999; **17**: 71–7.[1])

cal management. When immediate exploration and renal repair were performed in similar patients with associated pancreatic or bowel injuries, morbidity was reduced to 23%.[13] On the basis of this knowledge, grades III and IV injuries with significant devitalized fragments and concomitant intraperitoneal organ injuries should prompt immediate surgical repair.

In our experience, patients with a large, non-viable fragment and urinary extravasation or retroperitoneal hemorrhage, even without significant intraperitoneal injury, may also benefit from early renal exploration. The intervention is usually partial nephrectomy, which minimizes potential post-traumatic complications.

Urinary extravasation

Urinary extravasation alone does not necessitate surgical intervention, but commonly reflects a major renal injury (Grade IV) from a laceration of the renal pelvis, a parenchymal laceration into the collecting system, or an avulsion of the ureteropelvic junction (UPJ). Blunt trauma can lead to rupture of a renal fornix and significant urinary extravasation without an associated parenchymal injury.[14] When the degree of extravasation is small and the mechanism is blunt injury, most instances of urinary extravasation will resolve spontaneously (Figure 6.3). Larger degrees of extravasation may still subside without intervention, but serial CT scans are indicated for monitoring owing to the greater risks of complication and lower rates of spontaneous resolution. Intervention is indicated in persistent leakage, significant urinoma formation, or sepsis development. Recent literature has shown a >75% spontaneous resolution

rate of urinary extravasation associated with Grade IV renal injuries. With persistent extravasation, percutaneous or endoscopic methods have been effective in most cases.[15,16] Glenski and Husmann[15] reported 47 patients with major renal lacerations and urinary extravasation: 15% required endoscopic stenting for persistent leakage and only 9% of these required further intervention (exploration).

Immediate exploration is indicated in suspected UPJ avulsion. Although these injuries are rare, they rarely heal spontaneously. They are suggested by the non-visualization of the ipsilateral ureter on CT or intravenous urography (IVU) and by the presence of significant contrast extravasation both medially and perirenally. They occur more commonly in children who suffer trauma associated with rapid deceleration.[17]

Gunshot wounds to the kidney have the propensity for significant tissue damage from

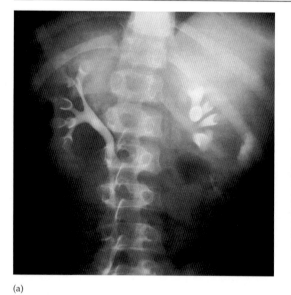
(a)

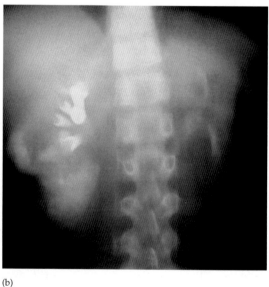
(b)

Figure 6.3

(a) IVU following a blunt renal trauma demonstrating a renal pelvis injury as indicated by extravasation of the contrast. (b) Tomogram indicating a renal injury to the calyx of the lower pole.

the 'blast effect' of the projectile's temporary and permanent cavities. (High-velocity missiles or close-range shotgun blasts are particularly devastating.) The risk of delayed complications is likewise increased. With urinary extravasation from gunshot wounds, the threshold for exploration should be lower than that for stab wounds or blunt trauma.[6]

INCOMPLETE STAGING

Imaging and accurate staging can obviate renal exploration in many cases. When imaging criteria are met,[4,10] we radiographically stage renal injury by CT when possible. Often, however, the instability of associated injuries will make complete staging impossible, and a more aggressive approach is warranted. An intraoperative 'single-shot' high-dose IVU should be obtained. A bolus of 2 ml/kg of intravenous contrast is injected and a single film is exposed at 10 min.[18] Any abnormality or incomplete evaluation warrants renal exploration. Thus, in a patient with unstaged blunt renal trauma, a retroperitoneal hematoma, and equivocal findings on 'single-shot' IVU, exploration would be

indicated. In addition, all patients with penetrating renal trauma with retroperitoneal hematoma who have not had adequate preoperative staging should undergo exploration and repair. This approach has resulted in a high rate of renal salvage and has not increased the rate of unnecessary nephrectomy.[19]

VASCULAR INJURY

With renovascular injury, prompt diagnosis and immediate operative repair are mandatory for renal preservation. The detection of renal pedicle injuries, however, is frequently delayed because associated life-threatening injuries take precedence. Over 50% of trauma victims with renal vascular injuries present in shock, and the mortality ranges from 10 to 50% (Figure 6.4).[20]

Renal pedicle injuries more commonly occur in pediatric patients with blunt trauma owing to the greater absorptive force of the child's kidney, which is proportionately larger than the adult's with lesser perinephric fat and degree of musculoskeletal development. The inelastic intima of the artery can be disrupted during deceleration injuries, which can lead to throm-

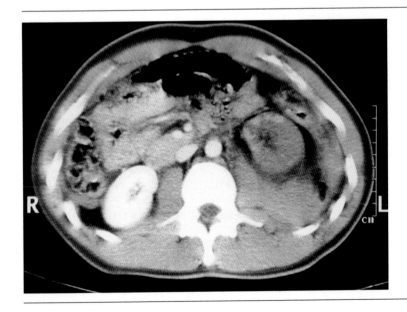

Figure 6.4

A CT scan showing a complete absence of contrast in the left kidney as a result of complete avulsion of the renal pedicle.

bosis of a segmental or main renal artery with consequent parenchymal ischemia or infarction. Main renal artery injuries have the lowest rate of repair and salvage.[21] Surgical repair undertaken within 12 h has the greatest chance of salvage; nevertheless, revascularization has demonstrated only a modest 10–30% overall success rate in multiple reports.[21–24] Even with early intervention (within 5 h), Cass et al[21] found significantly reduced function in the few kidneys appropriate for vascular repair. Complications of attempted repair included increased operative time in critically ill patients, hypertension and delayed nephrectomy. Thus, renal preservation is best attempted within 12 h of the initial injury, in cases of bilateral injury, or in injury to solitary renal units. Patients in whom the injury appears to be incomplete or perfusion seems intact intraoperatively can also be considered for reconstruction.

When the diagnosis of renal artery thrombosis is delayed or repair is not otherwise indicated, nephrectomy should be performed at exploration for associated injuries. When exploration is not needed, isolated renal artery thrombosis can be safely observed, with the kidney allowed to atrophy slowly over time. Complications of bleeding, infection, and hypertension requiring nephrectomy are rare.[25]

RENAL EXPLORATION

EARLY VASCULAR CONTROL

To ensure good renal salvage rates, certain principles regarding renal exposure should be followed. As nephron preservation is the primary goal, and as uncontrolled hemorrhage is often the cause of total nephrectomy, we perform preliminary proximal vascular control in all cases of renal trauma.[26]

Exposure of the renal vasculature
Proximal vascular control was initially described by Scott and Selzman.[27] A transabdominal midline incision from the xiphoid to the pubic symphysis provides the best access to the abdominal viscera and vasculature. The transverse colon is lifted from the abdomen and placed on the chest under moist laparotomy sponges. The root of the small bowel mesentery and the underlying retroperitoneum are exposed by lifting the bowel up and to the right. A vertical incision is made over the aorta superior to the superior mesenteric artery and into the retroperitoneum, and this is extended upwards to the ligament of Treitz. Often, the aorta is difficult to palpate because of retroperitoneal hematoma. In these cases, the inferior mesenteric vein is used as a guide for the incision, which is made just medial to it, and the dissection is carried down to the anterior surface of the aorta (Figure 6.5).

Upon identification of the aorta, dissection is continued superiorly until the left renal vein is identified crossing the aorta. This is the key landmark for the identification of the remaining renal vessels (Figure 6.6). Loops are placed around the individual vessels, which are left unoccluded unless heavy bleeding that cannot be controlled by direct manual compression of the renal parenchyma is encountered. The artery is first occluded and, if bleeding persists, the vein is clamped to reduce back-bleeding. Warm ischemia time should be less than 30 min if possible.[29] In our experience, occlusion of the renal vessels was required in only 17% of cases, but there is no reliable method to identify these before exploration. On average, it takes only 12 min to isolate the renal vessels.

Once vascular control has been achieved, the colon is reflected medially and the retroperitoneal hematoma is evacuated after Gerota's fascia has been incised laterally (Figure 6.7). The entire kidney must be well exposed to examine the renal pelvis, parenchyma, and vessels fully.

PRINCIPLES OF RECONSTRUCTION

The first step in reconstruction involves adequate debridement: all non-viable tissue should be sharply excised and removed. Preservation of one-third of one kidney provides sufficient

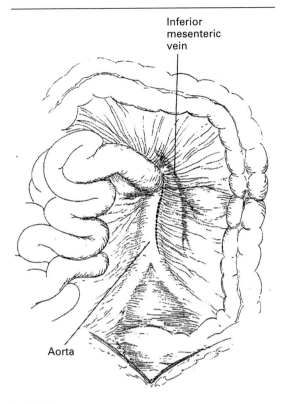

Figure 6.5

Surgical approach to the renal vessels and kidney. The retroperitoneal incision is made over the aorta medial to the inferior mesenteric vein. (Reprinted with permission from McAninch JW. In: *Stewart's Operative Urology*, 2nd edn. Baltimore: Williams & Wilkins, 1989; 234–9.[28])

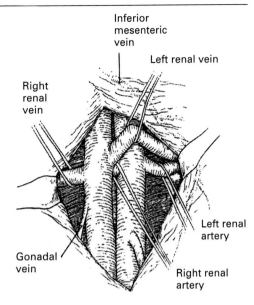

Figure 6.6

Anatomic relationships of the renal vessels. (Reprinted with permission from McAninch JW. In: *Stewart's Operative Urology*, 2nd edn. Baltimore: Williams & Wilkins, 1989; 234–9.[28])

renal function to avoid dialysis. The renal capsule should be preserved if at all possible, as it makes eventual closure more successful. Parenchymal vessels should be suture ligated with 4/0 chromic sutures. Persistent, smaller venous bleeding will usually stop after the parenchymal defect is closed.

Lacerations in the collecting system should be closed in a watertight fashion with running 4–0 chromic suture. Careful injection of dilute methylene blue into the renal pelvis after gentle occlusion of the proximal ureter can aid identification of injuries and confirm adequate closure of the collecting system. Additional drainage by internal stent or nephrostomy tube is not routinely required.

After reconstruction, the defect should ideally be covered with renal capsule by reapproximation of the parenchymal edges. This is done with interrupted 3/0 Vicryl sutures tied over gelfoam bolsters. This improves hemostasis and reduces the risk of urinary extravasation. We place titanium surgical clips on the sutures to aid identification of the suture line on postoperative CT scans. If the renal defect is significant, it can be packed with a hemostatic agent such as Avitene (microfibrillar collagen hemostat; Bard, Murray Hill, NJ, USA) or Tissel (fibrin glue; Baxter Deerfield, IL, USA) or with perinephric fat (Figure 6.8).

In rare cases, a devitalized polar segment will require partial nephrectomy with amputation and closure of the collecting system. Omentum is a good choice to cover the polar defect if renal capsule is not available. In all renorrhaphies, a 2.5 cm (1″) Penrose drain is left dependently to

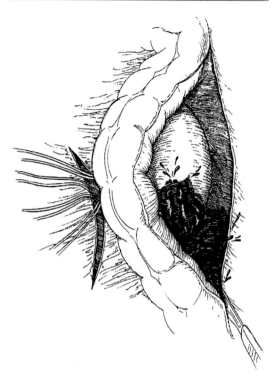

Figure 6.7

The retroperitoneal incision lateral to the colon, exposing the kidney. (Reprinted with permission from McAninch JW. In: *Stewart's Operative Urology*. Baltimore: Williams & Wilkins, 1989; 234–9.[28])

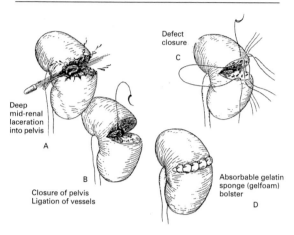

Figure 6.8

Technique of renorrhaphy after midpole Grade IV injury. (Reprinted with permission from: McAninch JW. In: *Stewart's Operative Urology*. Baltimore: Williams & Wilkins; 1989; 234–9.[28])

allow drainage of the retroperitoneum. A suction drain should not be used, as it can promote urinary leakage from the repaired collecting system. Vicryl mesh can be placed around the kidney to stabilize the renorrhaphy repair or when large or multiple parenchymal defects are difficult to cover.

URETERAL AND RENAL PELVIC TRAUMA

Ureteral and renal pelvic injuries are uncommon, accounting for less than 1% of all urological trauma.[30] Ureteral injuries may result from external trauma, but iatrogenic injuries are more common. During abdominal surgery, the ureter is vulnerable because of its inconspicuous location adjacent to the iliac vessels, colon, and uterus. In addition, various abdominal diseases can affect the normal ureteral course, causing it to deviate and making it more difficult to identify. This chapter focuses only on injuries from external trauma.

When ureteral and renal pelvic injuries result from external trauma, the mechanism is usually penetrating, and multiple organ injuries are frequently associated. Ureteral injuries from blunt trauma are rare. They usually occur in children and involve disruption at the level of the UPJ. At San Francisco General Hospital, the majority (86%) are confined to the renal pelvis or upper ureter.

DIAGNOSIS

Although hematuria of some degree is usually present, it may be absent in up to 31% of patients.[31] Findings on IVU may be negative in patients with ureteral injury, and a high index of suspicion is essential for early diagnosis.

RADIOGRAPHIC DETECTION

With the widespread use of CT in patients with multiple injuries, ureteral injuries are now being identified predominately with this imaging modality. Extravasation of contrast is the sine qua non of the diagnosis, but radiographic findings may be vague, including decreased calyceal excretion, mild hydronephrosis, and ureteral dilation or deviation. Alternatively, if CT has not been done, a single- or multiple-shot IVU after 2 ml/kg of contrast can be obtained intra-operatively. If the results are inconclusive, retrograde ureterography can be performed, but this is usually impractical in the trauma setting.

INTRAOPERATIVE DETECTION

Direct visual inspection is the most reliable means of assessing ureteral integrity. Urinary extravasation and ureteral discoloration or bruising are indicative of ureteral trauma. Intravenous or direct collecting system injection of indigo carmine or methylene blue may aid intraoperative recognition. Because high-velocity missiles can lead to a delayed blast injury to the ureter, this must be considered during intraoperative inspection of a gunshot wound, and prophylactic measures such as stenting of contused ureters should be considered.

CLASSIFICATION

The classification of ureteral injuries is based on the system of the Organ Injury Scaling Committee of the American Association for the Surgery of Trauma (Table 6.1).[32]

MANAGEMENT

Selection of appropriate surgical management depends on the patient's condition, promptness in injury recognition, and location and grade of injury. In a stable patient in whom the ureteral injury is identified immediately, prompt surgical repair is the preferred option.

TECHNIQUES OF RECONSTRUCTION

General principles of ureteral reconstruction include careful debridement, creation of a watertight tension-free anastomosis, isolation of the anastomosis from associated injuries, and adequate ureteral and retroperitoneal drainage. Management decisions must take into account the blood supply of the ureter, which is a freely anastomosing network arising from multiple vessels. The blood supply of the upper ureter derives mainly from the renal arteries; of the midportion from the aorta and iliac arteries; and of the lower portion from the superior vesical, vaginal, middle hemorrhoidal and uterine arteries. Ureteral dissection should be performed with great care to preserve its vasculature.

Grade I injuries should be managed, at the very least, with internal ureteral stenting. If the segment appears to have compromised blood supply or viability, it should be resected and primary repair with a ureteroureterostomy performed over a ureteral stent. This is done with

Table 6.1 Classification of ureteral injuries		
Grade I	Hematoma	Contusion without devascularization
Grade II	Laceration	<50% transection
Grade III	Laceration	>50% transection
Grade IV	Laceration	Complete transection, <2 cm devascularization
Grade V	Laceration	Avulsion with >2 cm devascularization

Based on the system of the Organ Injury Scaling Committee of the American Association for the Surgery of Trauma; data from reference 32.

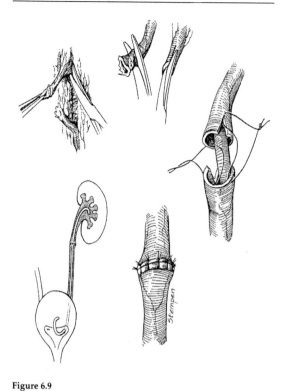

Figure 6.9

Ureteroureterostomy. (Reprinted with permission from Presti JC Jr, Carroll PR. In: *Perspectives in Colon and Rectal Surgery*. St. Louis: Quality Medical Publishers, 1988; 98–106.[33])

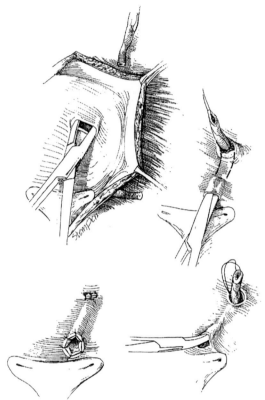

Figure 6.10

Ureteral reimplantation: the injured ureter is brought through a new opening in the bladder wall, and a submucosal tunnel is created; the completed repair shows a widely patent neohiatus. (Reprinted with permission from Presti JC Jr, Carroll PR. In: *Perspectives in Colon and Rectal Surgery*. St. Louis: Quality Medical Publishers, 1988; 98–106.[33])

fine 5/0 absorbable suture such as Dexon or Vicryl in an interrupted fashion (Figure 6.9). Grades II and III injuries can be closed primarily over a stent, or they can be managed by debridement, excision and ureteroureterostomy. Stents used during ureteral repair should be maintained for 4–6 weeks. Grades IV and V injuries require more mobilization to facilitate resection of the damaged ureter and allow tension-free ureteroureterostomy.

DISTAL URETERAL INJURIES

Injuries to the distal third of the ureter, below the iliac vessels, are best managed by submucosal bladder reimplantation. This is done with a combined intravesical and extravesical approach, bringing the ureter through the posterior bladder wall just medial to the original hiatus. A submucosal tunnel is created and the distal ureter is then spatulated and secured to the bladder wall with interrupted 5/0 absorbable sutures. A ureteral stent is generally used, and the bladder is closed in two layers (Figure 6.10).

Psoas hitch

Injuries involving the entire lower third of the ureter are best managed by a psoas hitch in conjunction with ureteral reimplantation. This ensures tension-free anastomosis. The proximal ureteral end is debrided and a traction suture is placed distally to facilitate handling. The bladder is mobilized away from its peritoneal reflection and the contralateral superficial lateral pedicle is ligated to facilitate mobilization. An oblique anterior cystotomy is made, perpendicular to the involved ureter. With the index and middle fingers, the bladder dome is guided over the ipsilateral iliac vessels toward the psoas tendon and anchored to this with three interrupted sutures. Care is taken to avoid entrapping the genitofemoral nerve. The ureter is then reimplanted, as described above, and the bladder wall is closed in two layers, leaving a suprapubic tube for drainage (Figure 6.11).

Boari flap

Very rarely, injuries that involve the entire lower two-thirds of the ureter require more extensive mobilization of the bladder to effect reimplantation with no tension. A boari flap uses an anterior bladder wall flap to bridge ureteral defects up to 15 cm long. The bladder is mobilized as described above, and a full-thickness U-shaped incision is made in its anterior wall. The width of the flap should be approximately three to four times the ureteral diameter, maintaining a wider base to ensure an adequate blood supply. The flap is raised toward the involved ureter, and the bladder wall is hitched to the psoas tendon. The ureter is reimplanted submucosally into the flap, which is then closed in a tubularized configuration (Figure 6.12). Bladder closure is then completed as described. If additional length is needed, a reverse nephropexy can add an extra 3–4 cm. This is preformed by mobilizing the kidney away from Gerota's fascia and fixing the renal capsule caudally to the underlying retroperitoneal muscles.

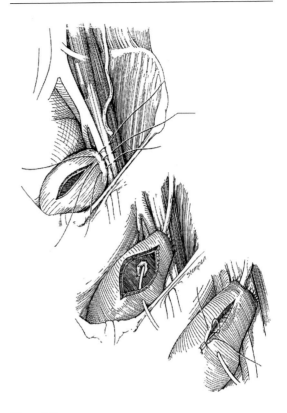

Figure 6.11

Psoas hitch. Top: an oblique anterior cystotomy is made perpendicular to the injured ureter. Middle: the bladder is guided toward the psoas tendon. Bottom: completed psoas hitch with reimplanted ureter. (Reprinted with permission from Presti JC Jr, Carroll PR. In: *Perspectives in Colon and Rectal Surgery*. St. Louis: Quality Medical Publishers, 1988; 98–106.[33])

Transureteroureterostomy

Injuries involving the distal half of the ureter, with insufficient bladder capacity or severe pelvic scarring that would make a bladder flap a poor option, can be managed with transureteroureterostomy. The posterior peritoneum is incised, exposing both ureters. The diseased ureter is brought through a retroperitoneal window carefully and should be brought across to the recipient ureter above the inferior mesenteric artery to avoid any angulation. A longitudinal ureterotomy is made in the recipient

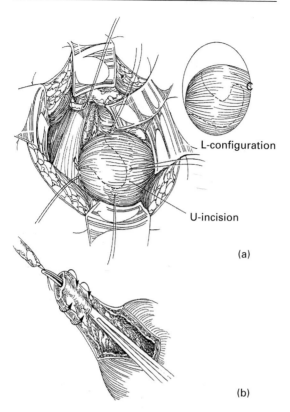

L-configuration

U-incision

(a)

(b)

Figure 6.12

Anterior bladder wall (boari) flap: (a) a U-incision is made on the anterior bladder wall (inset shows the alternative L-configuration, which can add additional length); (b) the ureter is reimplanted into the flap, which is then fashioned as a tube. (Reprinted from Armenakas NA. *Atlas Urol Clin North Am* 1998; **6**: 71–84[34] with permission from Elsevier.)

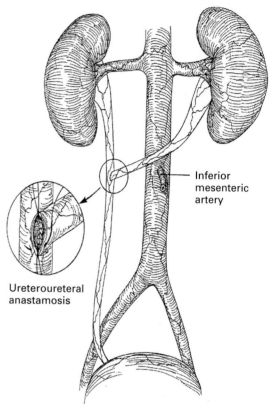

Inferior mesenteric artery

Ureteroureteral anastamosis

Figure 6.13

Transureteroureterostomy. (Reprinted from Armenakas NA. *Atlas Urol Clin North Am* 1998; **6**: 71–84[34] with permission from Elsevier.)

ureter and an end-to-side anastomosis is created with fine absorbable suture. The repair should be stented with a double-J ureteral catheter across the anastomosis (Figure 6.13). The procedure should be used selectively as it can potentially jeopardize the integrity of the normal ureter.

In all traumatic repairs of the ureter and kidney, a retroperitoneal drain should be placed at the site of reconstruction to limit urinoma formation. A passive drain such as a Penrose is preferable as suction drains can prolong leakage by exerting negative pressure on the suture line.[34]

CONCLUSIONS

Our treatment guidelines and algorithms for the management of upper tract trauma are based on over 25 years' experience in treating renal and ureteral injuries at San Francisco General Hospital, along with the accumulated knowledge of other trauma centers.

Our experience with renal trauma has validated our approach and reconstructive techniques. Renal exploration is necessary in only 2% of all blunt injuries and in 57% of penetrating injuries. Of the penetrating injuries, 42% of renal stab wounds required exploration and repair while 76% of gunshot wounds required reconstruction.[35] The principles of early vascular control have yielded a high rate of renal salvage, with only 11% of renal explorations requiring nephrectomy. We have yet to lose a kidney consequent to exploration.

The key to the successful management of ureteral and renal pelvic injuries is early recognition. Indeed, delay in diagnosis is the most common factor in morbidity. Because the clinical and radiographic evaluations are often indeterminate, maintaining a high index of suspicion is paramount in making the diagnosis promptly. Successful surgical management requires familiarity with the broad reconstructive armamentarium outlined here and meticulous attention to the specific details of each procedure.

REFERENCES

1. Meng MV, Brandes SB, McAninch JW. Renal trauma: indications and techniques for surgical exploration. *World J Urol* 1991; **17:** 71–7.

2. McAninch JW, Carroll PR, Klosterman PW, Dixon CM, Greenblatt MN. Renal reconstruction after injury. *J Urol* 1991; **145:** 932–8.

3. McAninch JW, Carroll PR. Renal trauma: kidney preservation through improved vascular control – a refined approach. *J Trauma* 1982; **22:** 285–90.

4. Miller KS, McAninch JW. Radiographic assessment of renal trauma: our 15 year experience. *J Urol* 1995; **154:** 352–5.

5. Nash PA, Bruce JE, McAninch JW. Nephrectomy for traumatic renal injuries. *J Urol* 1995; **153:** 609–11.

6. McAninch JW, Carroll PR, Armenakas N, Lee P. Renal gunshot wounds: methods of salvage and reconstruction. *J Trauma* 1993; **35:** 279–83.

7. Brandes SB, McAninch JW. Reconstructive surgery for trauma of the upper urinary tract. *Urol Clin North Am* 1999; **26:** 183–99.

8. Moore EE, Shackford SR, Pachter HL et al. Organ injury scaling: spleen, liver, and kidney. *J Trauma* 1989; **29:** 1664–6.

9. Miller KS, McAninch JW. Indications for radiographic assessment in suspected renal trauma. In: McAninch JW (ed.) *Traumatic and Reconstructive Urology.* Philadelphia: WB Saunders, 1996; 89–94.

10. Nicolaisen GS, McAninch JW, Marshall GA, Bluth RF, Carroll PR. Renal trauma: re-evaluation of indications for radiographic assessment. *J Urol* 1985; **133:** 183–7.

11. Holcroft JW, Trunkey DD, Minagi H, Korobkin MT, Lim RC. Renal trauma and retroperitoneal hematomas: indications for exploration. *J Trauma* 1975; **15:** 1045–52.

12. Husmann DA, Morris JS. Attempted non-operative management of blunt renal lacerations extending through the corticomedullary junction: the short-term and long-term sequelae. *J Urol* 1990; **143:** 682–4.

13. Husmann DA, Gilling PJ, Perry MO, Morris JS, Boone TB. Major renal lacerations with a devitalized fragment following blunt abdominal trauma: a comparison between nonoperative (expectant) versus surgical management. *J Urol* 1993; **150:** 1774–7.

14. Borirakchanyavat S, Nash PA, McAninch JA. Renal forniceal rupture following blunt abdominal trauma. *J Urol* 1995; **153:** 315A.

15. Glenski WJ, Husmann DA. Non-surgical management of major renal lacerations associated with urinary extravasation. *J Urol* 1995; **153:** 315A.

16. Matthews L, Smith EM, Spirnak JP. Nonoperative management of major blunt renal lacerations with urinary extravasation. *J Urol* 1997; 157: 2056–8.

17. Townsend M, DeFalco AJ. Absence of ureteral opacification below ureteral disruption: a sentinel CT finding. *AJR Am J Roentgenol* 1995; **164:** 253–4.

18. Morey AF, McAninch JW, Tiller BK, Duckett CP, Carroll PR. Single shot intraoperative excretory urography for the immediate management or renal trauma. *J Urol* 1999; **161:** 1088–92.

19. McAninch JW, Carroll PR, Klosterman PW, Dixon CM, Greenblatt MN. Renal reconstruction after injury. *J Urol* 1991; 145: 932–7.

20. Carroll PR, Klosterman PW, McAninch JW. Surgical management of renal trauma: analysis of risk factors, technique and outcome. *J Trauma* 1988; **28:** 1071–7.

21. Cass AS, Burbick M, Luxenberg M, Gleich P, Smith C. Renal pedicle injury in patients with multiple injuries. *J Trauma* 1985; **25:** 892–6.

22. Cass AS. Renovascular injuries from external trauma. *Urol Clin North Am* 1989; **16:** 213–20.

23. Clark DE, Georgitis JW, Ray FS. Renal artery injuries caused by blunt trauma. *Surgery* 1981; **90:** 87–96.

24. Maggio AJ, Brosman, S. Renal artery trauma. *Urology* 1978; **11:** 125–30.

25. Peterson NE. Complications of renal trauma. *Urol Clin North Am* 1989; **16:** 221–36.

26. Carroll PR, Klosterman PW, McAninch JW. Early vascular control for renal trauma: a critical review. *J Urol* 1989; **141:** 826–9.

27. Scott RF, Selzman HM. Complications of nephrectomy: review of 450 patients and a description of a modification of the transperitoneal approach. *J Urol* 1966; 95: 307–12.

28. McAninch JW. Surgery for renal trauma. In: Novack AC, Pontes ES, Streem SB (eds). *Stewart's Operative Urology.* Baltimore: Williams & Wilkins, 1989; 234–9.

29. Carroll PR, McAninch JW, Wong A, Wolf JS Jr, Newton C. Outcome after temporary vascular occlusion for the management of renal trauma. J Urol 1994; **151:** 1171–3.

30. Presti JC, Carroll PR. Ureteral and renal pelvic trauma: diagnosis and management. In: McAninch JW (ed.). *Traumatic and*

Reconstructive Urology. Philadelphia: WB Saunders; 1996; 171.

31. Presti JC, Carroll PR, McAninch JW. Ureteral and renal pelvic injuries from external violence: diagnosis and management. *J Trauma* 1989; **29:** 370.

32. Moore EE, Cogvill TH, Jurkovich GJ et al. Organ injury scaling III: Chest wall, abdominal vasculature, ureter, bladder and urethra. *J Trauma* 1992; **33:** 337–9.

33. Presti JC Jr, Carroll PR. Intraoperative management of the injured ureter. In: Schrock TR (ed.). *Perspectives in Colon and Rectal Surgery*. St Louis: Quality Medical Publishers, 1988; 99–106.

34. Armenakas NA. Ureteral trauma: surgical repair. *Atlas Urol Clin North Am* 1998; **6:** 71–84.

35. McAninch JW, Carroll PR. Renal exploration after trauma: indications and reconstructive techniques. In: McAninch JW (ed.) Traumatic and Reconstructive Urology Philadelphia: WB Saunders, 1996; 105.

7. Lower urinary tract trauma

Kiaran J O'Malley and Anthony R Mundy

External trauma to the pelvis can cause devastating injury to the lower urinary tract. Management of such injuries is often controversial and challenging, and may have a major bearing in preventing lifelong complications and morbidity. This chapter discusses the mechanisms by which major bladder and urethral injuries occur and describes the initial diagnostic and imaging techniques. Then the various management options for these injuries are discussed and the rationale for our unit's (Institute of Urology, London) preferred strategies are outlined.

BLADDER TRAUMA

Injuries to the bladder may occur following blunt or penetrating trauma, may arise spontaneously, or on occasion may develop after urologic, surgical, or self-instrumentation. Bladder injuries after blunt or penetrating trauma are rare and constitute only 2% of abdominal injuries requiring surgery. This low figure owes much to the fact that in adults, the empty bladder lies in a protected position within the bony pelvis. Moreover, when the bladder is injured, it often occurs in association with other severe injuries. The successful management of bladder trauma relies on clinical suspicion and early diagnosis followed by prompt therapeutic intervention.

MECHANISMS OF INJURY

With bladder filling the fundus distends slightly in the lateral direction and the dome rises easily into the abdominal cavity as its covering of peritoneum is pushed anteriorly. In children, however, the bladder is an abdominal organ and only reaches its adult pelvic position after puberty. The difference between the anatomic relationships of adult and child bladders is reflected in the different distribution of the types of bladder injury with a higher incidence of intraperitoneal injuries seen in children.

Extraperitoneal bladder rupture rarely occurs in the absence of a pelvic fracture. In such circumstances the normal protective effect of the pelvic ring is lost and the shearing force of the fracture may tear the bladder from its ligamentous attachments. Less frequently, a bony spicule from the site of fracture may lacerate the bladder. In Corriere's experience,[1,2] less than 40% of bladder lacerations occur in the area of the pelvic fracture and in the majority of patients there is no clear relationship between the fracture and the site of extravasation. This suggests that the usual manner for extraperitoneal bladder rupture may be a bursting type of injury similar to the intraperitoneal bladder injury or a tearing of the bladder wall as described. Extraperitoneal bladder injury in the absence of pelvic girdle disruption usually involves patients with a history of pelvic surgery. It is believed that the dome is fixed in these cases thereby making the lateral bladder wall the weakest and most susceptible area to injury (Figure 7.1).

Intraperitoneal bladder rupture is usually an injury of violent deceleration – the absence of such extreme circumstances should lead one to consider pre-existing disease of the bladder. These injuries are understood to occur when there is a sudden increase in pressure in a full bladder leading to rupture of the dome. The dome is the least supported wall of the full bladder having its muscle fibers widely separated and offering the least resistance to a sudden change in intravesical pressure, as shown by Oliver and Taguchi.[3] This may also explain why spontaneous bladder ruptures most frequently

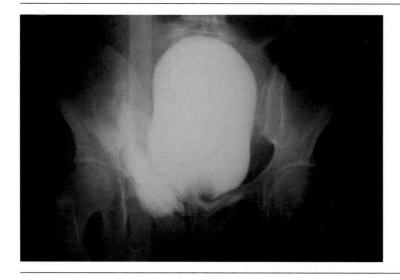

Figure 7.1

Cystogram showing typical pattern of contrast extravasation following an extraperitoneal bladder perforation associated with pelvic trauma.

occur at the dome and are intraperitoneal. A further possible cause of an intraperitoneal bladder perforation is a high fracture of the pelvic ring causing a bony fragment to separate off and lacerate the dome.

Overall, bladder rupture is due to blunt trauma in 85% of cases, and 89% are in association with a pelvic fracture injury. However, between 5 and 10% of all pelvic fractures only will also have a rupture of the bladder. The remaining 15% are due to a variety of penetrating injuries (surgical misadventure, external violence, or an internal migration of drains, stents or prostheses). Penetrating injuries can involve the bladder irrespective of its level of distension and there is rarely any doubt what the mechanism of injury is.

Sandler et al[4] described a classification for bladder injuries based on the radiological findings and patterns of extravasation but it plays little if any role in the clinical management of these patients. A more practical and simpler classification of bladder ruptures would be *intraperitoneal*, *extraperitoneal*, or *combined* injuries. Peters reviewed some of the more recent major series and found 34% of injuries to be intraperitoneal, 58% to be extraperitoneal,

and 8% to be combined bladder injuries.[5] Not surprisingly, urethral injury is the most commonly reported urological injury in association with bladder rupture; it is present in 10–20% of cases. Similarly, 15–30% of traumatic posterior urethral disruptions also have a bladder rupture – the importance of performing a complete evaluation of the lower urinary tract in these patients is obvious.

DIAGNOSIS AND IMAGING

The major prerequisite for the diagnosis of a bladder rupture is to recognize the history or precipitating events likely to have caused such an injury. Evaluate the patient for symptoms and signs for this diagnosis. Classic findings consistent with a bladder rupture include suprapubic pain and tenderness, difficulty or failure to void and hematuria. All patients with a ruptured bladder will have hematuria and this will be macroscopic in 95%. Signs of peritoneal irritation may be observed after intraperitoneal bladder injuries. In patients with pelvic fracture injuries, the external urethral meatus in men and the vaginal introitus in women should be specifically examined for blood.

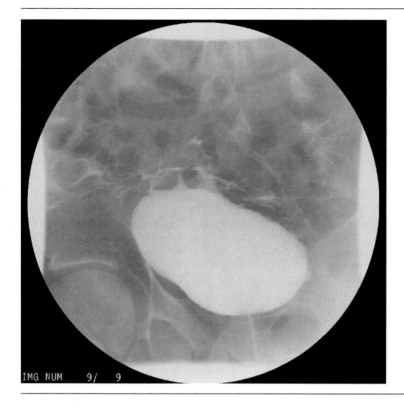

IMG NUM   9/   9

Figure 7.2

Cystogram demonstrating contrast extravasation amongst bowel loops after intraperitoneal rupture of the bladder.

If bladder injury is suspected based on clinical impression, cystography should be performed immediately unless life-threatening injuries mandate prompt surgical exploration (Figures 7.2 and 7.3). Even then, a cystogram may be obtained in the operating theater unless laparotomy is planned regardless of the cystogram findings. In a stable patient either standard or computed tomograph (CT) cystography can be performed but the choice is largely dictated by the clinical situation and the availability of CT facilities. If CT is being done to assess for intra-abdominal injuries, CT cystography can easily be accomplished at the same time by instilling 350 ml of diluted (3–5%) contrast material. If on the other hand retrograde urethrography is to be performed initially, then conventional cystography should follow on and is just as reliable a method of establishing the diagnosis as CT.

A five-film retrograde cystogram can be performed as follows:

1. Remove 250 ml from a half liter bag of normal saline and replace it with water-soluble contrast medium.
2. Obtain a plain anterioposterior (AP) radiograph of the pelvis (film 1).
3. Perform retrograde urethrography, if indicated, following the technique described later in this chapter.
4. Insert a 14-Fr Foley catheter and record the residual volume of urine, if any.
5. Connect the 50% contrast in the saline bag to the urethral catheter and instill 100 ml of contrast and apply a clamp to the catheter.
6. Hang the half liter bag of 50% contrast on a drip stand at 75–100 cm above the pelvis.
7. Take a repeat AP pelvic radiograph after

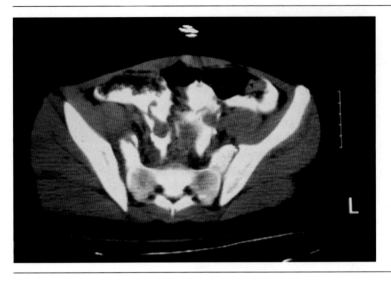

Figure 7.3

Computed tomography (CT) cystography illustrating an intraperitoneal perforation of the bladder.

100 ml of contrast (film 2) – gross extravasation will be evident at this point.

8. Unclamp the catheter and instill a minimum of 400 ml of contrast in adults.
9. Take a repeat AP pelvic radiograph, plus a lateral radiograph, after 400 ml of contrast (films 3 and 4).
10. Place the half liter bag on the floor and empty the bladder.
11. Take a repeat AP pelvic radiograph after bladder emptied (film 5) – small perforations may be obscured when the bladder is full.

If a bladder contraction occurs during filling as heralded by leakage of contrast solution around the catheter, or reflux back up the drip chamber, no further contrast needs to be instilled. In children, 60 ml and an additional 30 ml per year of age up to a maximum of 400 ml should be instilled.

The accuracy of cystography for the diagnosis of bladder rupture has been reported to range from 85–100%. False-negatives are a well recognized hazard and careful attention to proper technique is essential to achieve a high degree of accuracy. The post-drainage film is important,

and even more so when a lateral film cannot be obtained because of intense pain in patients with pelvic fractures. If a bladder rupture is indeed diagnosed, leave the catheter in!

MANAGEMENT

EXTRAPERITONEAL INJURIES OF THE BLADDER

It has been shown that extraperitoneal bladder rupture can be effectively managed by urethral catheter drainage for 10–14 days if the injury is only to the bladder. Repeat cystography should be performed at this timepoint and 85% of ruptures should be healed. If extravasation is still present, catheter drainage for another week should see almost all uncomplicated extraperitoneal leaks sealed. Clearly, if the patient has a concomitant urethral injury precluding urethral catheterization, a suprapubic catheter needs to be placed followed by cystography to define the extent of the injury.

However, if a laparotomy is being performed for associated injuries, the bladder should be formally repaired simultaneously. This is done by opening the dome of the bladder and repairing the rupture intravesically with a single continuous absorbable 3/0 suture. Any foreign material encountered (such as bone fragments), should be removed but extensive debridement should be resisted as it merely makes the defect larger. The pelvic hematoma associated with the bladder should be left undisturbed as further hemorrhage may ensue. A large catheter should be left in place for 10–14 days – failure of the catheter to provide adequate drainage (e.g. clots, persistent extravasation) may culminate in an open surgical repair.

Inspect the bladder neck, distal ureters, prostate, rectum and vagina for injuries. If present, these should be immediately repaired to prevent the development of fistulas, pelvic abscess, incontinence or bladder neck stenosis. Tissue interposition is required where concomitant vaginal or rectal injuries are identified. These injuries are more frequently encountered in children.

INTRAPERITONEAL INJURIES OF THE BLADDER

Intraperitoneal rupture of the bladder, usually due to a bursting-type effect, can result in several large rents in the bladder. They should all undergo open exploration and formal repair urgently. They cannot be as accurately defined by cystogram and are associated with a significant risk of peritonitis and metabolic complications within 24 h. A midline incision should be made to allow a complete evaluation of all the abdominal viscera. The bladder should be opened by extending the laceration in the dome and allowing a complete assessment of the bladder. The remaining pelvic organs should be inspected for injuries as described previously. A two-layered repair is performed as the bladder is closed on its abdominal and vesical surfaces with continuous absorbable 3/0 suture material. A 22-Fr urethral catheter is adequate for drainage if good hemostasis has been accomplished.

PENETRATING INJURIES TO THE BLADDER

All penetrating injuries of the bladder should be explored and repaired as an emergency. A midline incision is required as there is a high risk that other organs may have been injured; ureteric injuries have been identified in 29% of penetrating bladder injuries by Rober et al.[6] Clear urine should be observed emerging from each ureteric orifice. If not, ureteric catheters should be passed to determine if either ureter has been injured. Bladder closure and drainage is performed as described earlier.

Laparoscopic surgery is believed to entail a two to ten-fold greater risk of bladder injury than conventional open surgery. Cardinal signs of bladder injury during laparoscopy are clear fluid in the operative field, gas in the urinary bag or a visible laceration. Intravesical instillation of methylene blue through the catheter can confirm the presence and site of the injury. Laparoscopic repair may be undertaken if the injury is small and favorably located, and if the requisite expertise is readily available.

URETHRAL TRAUMA

Urethral injuries resulting from trauma can be some of the most devastating and complex injuries of the urinary system. Urethral trauma can be categorized into anterior and posterior injuries, and complete and partial ruptures. There are a number of other classifications but these do not alter the management.

The early management of urethral injury is critical in preventing lifelong morbidity and minimizing the major debilitating complications of impotence, incontinence and stricture formation. However, it cannot be overemphasized that initially the other injuries are usually far more important than the injury to the urethra, and that fractures of the pelvis can be associated with significant blood loss.

ANTERIOR URETHRAL INJURY

The incidence of *major* anterior urethral injury is relatively low compared to that of the posterior urethra and it occurs more often as an isolated event. Overall, anterior urethral injuries are less serious and their management is less demanding and controversial.

MECHANISM OF INJURY

The great majority of anterior urethral injuries are due to instrumentation, usually iatrogenic but occasionally self-inflicted, and result in minor contusions only. Disruptions of the anterior urethra are caused by blunt trauma, classically the straddle-type injury from a fall onto the perineum, and also by penetrating trauma, e.g. gunshot or stab wounds (Figure 7.4).

Any patient who presents with a history of falling astride forcefully against a blunt object such as a bicycle frame or a fence should be evaluated for a potential anterior urethral injury. A blow or kick to the perineum can cause a similar injury. The mechanism of injury is compression of the bulbar urethra between the blunt object and the underside of the symphysis pubis. In some cases, straddle injuries may be mild enough that patients may not seek medical attention initially and present many years later with a symptomatic bulbar urethral stricture with a remote history of trauma.

Penile fractures are associated with a ruptured urethra in 15–20% of cases. Typically, these patients will report having heard a cracking sound during intercourse followed by sharp pain, rapid detumescence, penile swelling and extensive bruising. Hematuria or inability to void after such an event suggests urethral involvement.

DIAGNOSIS AND IMAGING

The presence of an anterior urethral injury can usually be suspected from the clinical history. Trauma patients who present with blood at the meatus, or inability to void should have a retrograde urethrogram. Hematuria and dysuria should also raise suspicion for a urethral injury. A case can be made for routine urethrography in all patients with penile fractures.

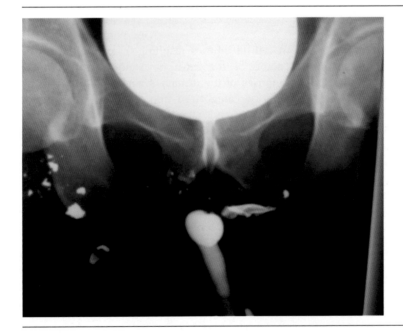

Figure 7.4

Penetrating injury to the urethra resulting following a gunshot.

Key points of retrograde urethrography for any urethral injury are as follows:

1. Plain radiograph of the pelvis will show fractures.
2. The patient should be placed in the oblique position during the study to prevent a false foreshortening of the urethra in the antero-posterior axis.
3. 14-Fr Foley catheter is inserted just inside the meatus and the balloon is inflated with 1–2 ml of saline to secure it.
4. 50 ml of non-diluted, water soluble contrast is prepared in a syringe and is injected under pressure with fluoroscopic screening with the penis under stretch.
5. A sufficient volume of contrast must be injected in order to distend the urethra as underfilling the urethra may fail to reveal an injury.
6. Extravasation, loss of urethral continuity, and the presence/absence of contrast in the bladder should be identified.

Retrograde urethrography allows definition of the extent of injury in patients with anterior urethral injury. Patients with a clinical presentation indicative of an injury but with a normal retrograde study are diagnosed as having a contusion. The presence of contrast extravasation with some contrast reaching the bladder indicates a partial disruption, whereas contrast extravasation without contrast reaching the proximal urethra or bladder indicates complete disruption.

These days many, perhaps the majority of cases, are in the Accident and Emergency room before they have had the time to develop blood at the meatus. The diagnosis is then made from failure to pass a catheter. It is important to remember that being able to pass a catheter does not exclude a partial rupture so the surgeon must be alert to the potential problems if the catheter is removed within a few days.

The presence and extent of a hematoma provide information about the status of several anatomic planes. Patients with urinary extravasation secondary to an injury in which Buck's fascia is intact present with a hematoma in a sleeve distribution limited to the shaft. In contrast, patients in whom Buck's fascia has been breached can present with a 'butterfly' hematoma in the perineum extending into the scrotum.

MANAGEMENT

It is likely that in a severely injured patient a catheter will have been inserted during initial resuscitation by the trauma team. Enormous importance has been placed recently on not catheterizing a patient urethrally if there is the likelihood of a urethral injury, as it has been suggested that this may convert a partial tear to one that is complete. In the senior author's opinion, it is extremely unlikely that gentle passage of a urethral catheter will do any additional damage to that caused by the original insult. In addition, in urethral surgery considerable force is required to divide the urethra, making it difficult to accept that a gentle attempt at the passage of a urethral catheter could do a similar job.

Initial management of patients with anterior urethral injuries should be to provide adequate drainage of urine and to minimize potential complications such as stricture formation, fistula, and/or infection. Ideally, when called to see a stable patient with blood at the external urethral meatus or other signs and symptoms suggestive of a urethral injury, a retrograde urethrogram should be performed as a urethral injury can then be confirmed or excluded. In an unstable patient an attempt to pass a catheter can be made, but if any resistance is encountered a suprapubic catheter should be placed and a retrograde study performed when appropriate.

Further management of anterior urethral rupture depends on its type. Partial tears are managed with a suprapubic or urethral catheter, and repeat retrograde urethrograms performed at 2-weekly intervals until healing is demonstrated.

Any residual stricture can usually be managed with direct visual urethrotomy.

Blunt trauma resulting in complete disruption of the anterior urethra warrants suprapubic catheterization followed by anastomotic or patch urethroplasty at 3–6 months. Excellent long-term results can be anticipated. Blunt trauma due to deceleration can result in associated injuries and significant spongiosal and soft-tissue damage that may render primary repair difficult.

A primary repair may be indicated in certain circumstances; urethral injury in association with a penile fracture should be repaired primarily to minimize the potential of developing chordee and/or painful erections, and sharp penetrating injuries with an almost surgical laceration should also undergo early reconstruction. Patients selected for primary repair should ideally have no signs of hemodynamic instability, no major associated injuries, and focal urethral defects of 2 cm or less.

POSTERIOR URETHRAL INJURY

Posterior urethral injuries are not common and take a low priority in the management of patients with pelvic fracture injuries as these individuals almost always have multiple injuries with more serious consequences. Most patients are best treated by a suprapubic catheter for 3 months and then an end-to-end anastomotic urethroplasty in those who have developed urethral occlusions. There is a role for delayed primary repair and for endourological management in selected patients, but their exact roles have yet to be defined.

MECHANISM OF INJURY

Posterior injuries are caused by fractures of the pelvis in 90% of cases, and 5–10% of pelvic fractures have an associated urethral injury. Orthopedic surgeons consider three types of pelvic fracture – (i) anteroposterior compression injuries; (ii) lateral compression injuries; and (iii) vertical shear injuries. Most fractures of the first and second type affect the anterior pelvic ring and are stable as far as the fracture is concerned. Vertical shear injuries are more commonly the result of a fall from great height and are the worst because they are the most unstable. Instability is produced by posterior bony or ligamentous injuries around the sacroiliac joint in addition to anterior bony disruption, allowing one side of the pelvis to move separately from the other. This produces the so-called Malgaigne's fracture. In unstable injuries, immediate external fixation and subsequent internal fixation are routinely used to control the bleeding from the fracture, to immobilize the fracture and to reduce pain and facilitate mobilization, and many orthopedic surgeons fix stable injuries for similar reasons.

A ruptured urethra occurs in 5–10% of patients and is said to be a shearing injury through the membranous urethra. In the senior author's experience the injury more closely resembles an avulsion injury rather than a shearing injury and very often represents injury to the membranous urethra from the proximal bulbar urethra rather than through the membranous urethra itself.[7] Typically a ruptured urethra occurs with a 'butterfly' fracture of the pubic symphysis and the related pubic rami, with or without sacroiliac joint disruption, or otherwise with a Malgaigne's fracture.

It is said that about 66% of posterior urethral injuries are complete ruptures and the remainder are incomplete, generally on the basis of the radiological appearance. Our feeling is that true incidence of complete ruptures is probably higher.

A ruptured bladder occurs in 5–10% of pelvic fracture injuries and in about one-third of those with urethral injuries. In 85% of cases it is an extraperitoneal bladder injury. In the majority of instances the ruptured bladder is attributed to a bursting or shearing injury. Impotence occurs in 10–20% of pelvic fracture injuries and in about half of those with urethral injuries. The site of injury to the neurovascular structures responsible for erection can be closely related to the fracture sites.

DIAGNOSIS AND IMAGING

The diagnosis of a posterior urethral disruption should always be considered in pelvic fracture injuries. When the urethra is ruptured there is blood at the external urethral meatus in the vast majority of cases. Some investigators have reported over 90% in their series and therefore when there is no blood at the meatus a ruptured urethra is unlikely.

In the absence of blood at the meatus clearly one should proceed with urethral catheterization in the usual manner. In the presence of blood at the meatus a gentle attempt at passing a catheter urethrally is a perfectly reasonable option for reasons detailed earlier but only on the proviso that the surgeon is alert to the possibility of complications following catheter removal within a few days. If this proves difficult or fails to produce more than a few drops of blood or blood-stained urine, then radiological assessment with urethrography should follow (Figure 7.5). Whatever the abnormality, a suprapubic catheter should be placed, with ultrasound guidance if necessary.

It is commonly said that inability to feel the prostate in its normal location is suggestive of a distraction injury, but the circumstances of physical examination in these patients usually makes assessment very difficult. The finding of blood on the examining finger heralds the possibility of a rectal injury.

MANAGEMENT

The ruptured posterior urethra in association with a pelvic fracture results in not so much a stricture in most patients as a distraction defect (Figures 7.6 and 7.7). There is no continuity of the urethra, the lumen is (usually) completely obliterated and there is simply a block of fibrous tissue between the ends of the urethra.

There is considerable controversy about the immediate management of pelvic fracture injuries of the posterior urethra. The options include primary realignment, primary repair, delayed primary repair a few days later, delayed primary realignment a few days later, and suprapubic catheterization and repair 3 months or so later.

Early surgery for ruptured posterior urethra

The traditional treatment in these patients involves so-called 'railroading'. This used to be achieved by an open surgical procedure but currently it is more commonly performed endoscopically by a variety of endourological maneuvers. Probably the most common technique is to pass a flexible cystoscope through the suprapubic tract, a rigid cystoscope up the urethra and then a guide wire between them so a catheter can be passed over the wire. This is said to reduce the stricture rate and to facilitate subsequent surgery, however stricture rates of over 70% are reported.

Open railroading has been associated with a higher incidence of complications such as impotence, incontinence, infection and bleeding, but

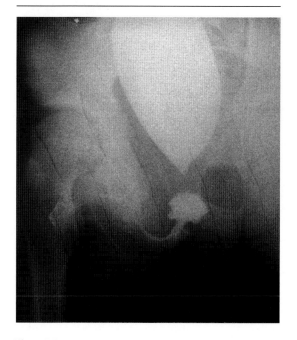

Figure 7.5

An ascending urethrocystogram indicating a ruptured bulbar urethra. (Courtesy of Mr CRJ Woodhouse, UCL, London.)

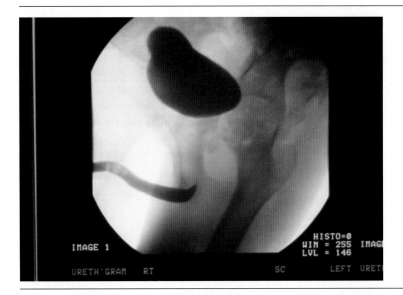

Figure 7.6

Ascending and descending urethrography showing a posterior urethral distraction injury defect and pelvic fracture.

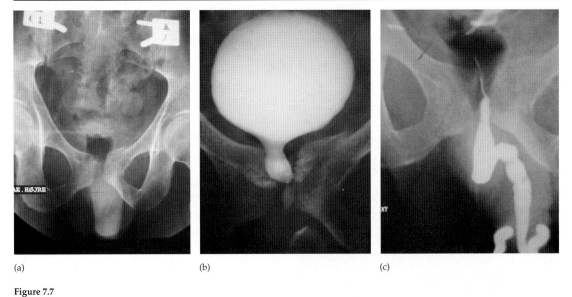

(a)   (b)   (c)

Figure 7.7

Posterior urethral distraction injury: (a) Plain film showing fracture, (b) descending urethrogram illustrating complete disruption, (c) ascending urethrogram that demonstrates the distal extent of the injury – the epithelial-lined tract seen to track superiorly should not be confused for the urethral lumen.

this may simply have reflected the selection of patients undergoing this procedure. It also makes urethroplasty more difficult because of vertical extension of the inflammatory fibrotic process both up and down the urethra on either side of the injury. This more than offsets the theoretical advantage of realignment. Primary repair by end-to-end anastomosis has only been attempted anecdotally to our knowledge but it may be considered when it is the only injury (apart from the pelvic fracture) in a fit, healthy patient with a proven complete rupture.

Delayed primary repair and realignment for ruptured posterior urethra

Delayed primary repair has been reported for the distracted 'pie-in-the-sky' bladder. Several other reconstructive surgeons have attempted delayed primary repair, and not just for the markedly distracted bladder, although again these are only anecdotal reports. It is generally agreed that even just evacuating the hematoma

– a few days after the injury when it would not immediately recur – seems to be valuable in improving the long-term outcome of urethral injury, irrespective of the possible benefit of urethral repair. Evacuation of the hematoma can be achieved by the percutaneous placement of one or two drains under radiological guidance. Evacuating the hematoma may also reduce stretching of the neurovascular bundles and therefore improve the rate of impotence associated with fractured pelvis.

Before either open or endoscopic realignment is considered it is important that one confirms that the urethra is indeed ruptured. Dramatic though the 'pie-in-the-sky' bladder is, the urethra may actually just be stretched through the pelvic hematoma rather than ruptured (Figures 7.8 and 7.9). This may be another indication that the nature of the injury represents more of an avulsion than a shear and another indication, perhaps, that evacuating the pelvic hematoma might be worthwhile in its own right.

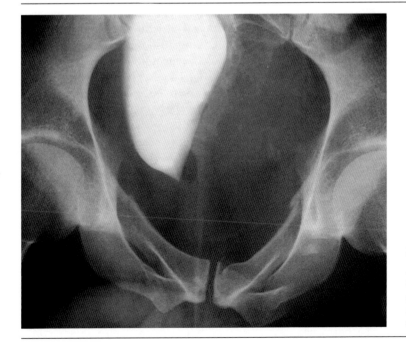

Figure 7.8

A cystogram demonstrating a 'pie-in-the-sky' typical of a ruptured membranous urethra in a patient with a fractured renal pelvis. (Courtesy of Mr CRJ Woodhouse, UCL, London.)

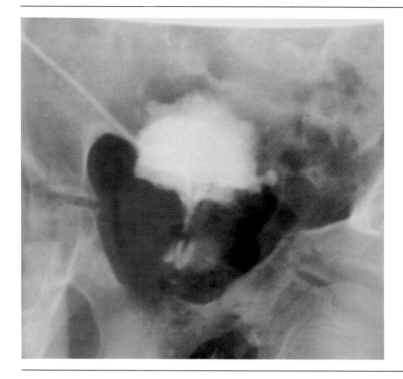

Figure 7.9

The 'pie-in-the-sky' bladder lifted dramatically out of the pelvis by the pelvic fracture hematomata.

Delayed surgery for ruptured posterior urethra

The gold standard of treatment remains suprapubic catheterization for 3 months and end-to-end bulboprostatic anastomosis at that stage. This is performed transperineally in the vast majority of cases using a 'progression approach'. The progression approach capitalizes on the elastic lengthening inherent in the urethra and then on the ability to straighten out the natural perineal curve of the urethra by a series of maneuvers, thereby reducing the gap between the two ends to allow a tension-free anastomosis. These maneuvers include crural separation, inferior pubectomy and re-routing of the urethra to bridge the gap. By following these steps end-to-end repair is almost always possible irrespective of the length of the stricture (Figure 7.10).

Certainly, suprapubic catheterization and delayed urethroplasty cause the least harm in the early stage of management, and in practice produce a 10-year stricture-free survival of at least 90%. It is against this standard that all other methods of managing these injuries must be judged.

COMPLICATIONS

The complications of such surgery, other than failure manifest by re-stricturing, are generally the complications of the original injury, i.e. urgency and stress incontinence with a full bladder because of damage to the urethral sphincter mechanism, and impotence caused by damage to the neurovascular bundles as they run along the inferior pubic rami.

Impotence

The incidence of impotence after pelvic fracture has been variably reported from 2.6 to 75%. When urethral injury is present the incidence is about 42%; without urethral injury it is 5%. In a

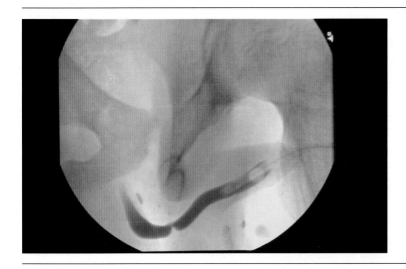

Figure 7.10

Classic appearance of a bulbar stricture presenting 4 months after a fall astride a wall in an 8-year-old boy.

review of 15 series, the incidence of impotence after suprapubic indwelling catheterization as initial management was 22.5%, and after railroading it was 42%. This may be a reflection of the severity of injury in the two groups of patients rather than a reflection of the nature of the initial management. More severely injured patients are more likely to have a laparotomy and, therefore, to undergo railroading and are also more likely to be rendered impotent by their injury.

The vast majority of patients, 80–85%, are said to be impotent because of vascular damage and a minority because of neurogenic damage. Nobody has ever really quantified the psychogenic component and its influence. Reasonable success with intracavernosal agents suggests a much higher incidence of neurogenic damage.

Occasionally impotence is the result of surgery but some authorities contest this. The neurovascular bundles are at their most vulnerable as they course laterally alongside the membranous urethra to run into the penile hilum. Thus the dissection associated with an inferior pubectomy is particularly liable to damage these structures. A detailed history of erectile activity and nocturnal penile tumescence studies should both be obtained prior to reconstruction. Patients with abnormal tumescence studies should undergo Doppler assessment of the penile arteries.

Incontinence

It is said that the urethral sphincter mechanism is either overtly destroyed or essentially nonfunctional after a pelvic fracture injury in the vast majority of cases and continence thereafter is dependent on bladder neck function. Thus, if the bladder neck is normal and the bladder itself is stable the patient will be continent, although a degree of stress incontinence and urgency may be present, especially in the case of a full bladder, particularly during the first few months after urethroplasty. Notably however, recent work suggests that at least half of our patients with pelvic fracture distraction injuries *have* evidence of sphincter activity after reconstruction.[7] In addition, some patients may also develop bladder neck fibrosis as a long-term complication of pelvic fracture injury (Figure 7.11).

Some patients may have voiding difficulty due to an acontractile bladder, presumably as a result of damage to the pelvic plexus as another consequence of the pelvic fracture. These patients are continent but require self-catheterization to void.

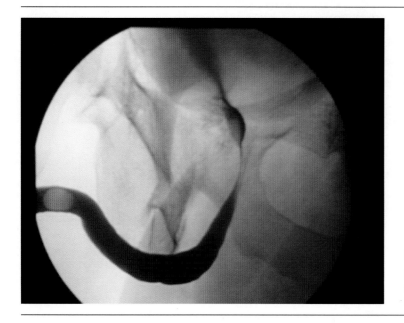

Figure 7.11

Normal appearance of the external sphincter mechanism in a patient with bladder neck stenosis.

RUPTURED URETHRA IN FEMALES

This is supposedly rare but large series of pelvic fractures have shown an incidence of about 5%, many of which are overlooked or misdiagnosed.[8] The general view is that urethral injuries in females are more commonly a longitudinal tear from the bladder through the bladder neck and into the sphincter mechanism (Figure 7.12).

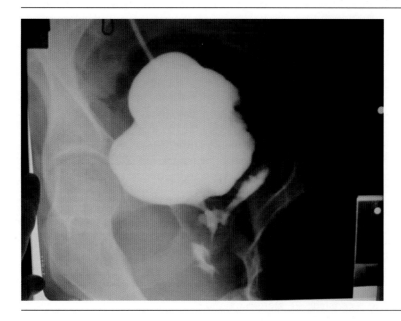

Figure 7.12

Female urethral disruption injury.

Direct repair should be performed at the same time as bladder repair. Vaginal bleeding is usually the way such injuries present and long-term management is more an incontinence problem than a structural one.

PELVIC FRACTURE INJURIES IN CHILDREN

In children the bladder neck and prostate are injured more commonly than in adults. Not only do these children suffer from strictures, but the impotence rate is nearly twice the rate found in adults and 25% of these children suffer from incontinence, whereas this is rare in adults. Both impotence and incontinence, may not be manifest until after puberty; thus, the prognosis should always be guarded until after puberty. See also Chapter 11 on Pediatric Urological Trauma.

REFERENCES

1. Corriere JN Jr, Sandler CM. Management of extraperitoneal bladder rupture. *Urol Clin North Am* 1989; **26:** 49–60.
2. Corriere JN Jr, Sandler CM. Bladder rupture from external trauma: diagnosis and management. *World J Urol* 1999; **17:** 84–9.
3. Oliver JA, Taguchi Y. Rupture of the full bladder. J Urol 1982; **128:** 25–6.
4. Sandler CM, Hall JT, Rodriguez MB et al. Bladder injury in blunt pelvic trauma. *Radiology* 1986; **158:** 633–8.
5. Peters PC. Intraperitoneal rupture of the bladder. *Urol Clin North Am* 1989; **16:** 279–82.
6. Rober PE, Smith JB, Pierce JM. Gunshot injuries of the ureter. J Urol 1990; **30:** 83–6.
7. Andrich DE, Mundy AR. The nature of urethral injury in cases of pelvic fracture urethral trauma. *J Urol* 2001; **165:** 1492–5.
8. Venn SN, Greenwell TJ, Mundy AR. Pelvic fracture injuries of the female urethra. *BJU Int* 1999; **83:** 626–30.

FURTHER READING

Andrich DE, Mundy AR. Urethral strictures and their surgical treatment. *BJU Int* 2000; **86:** 571–80.

Hernandez J, Morey AF. Anterior urethral injury. *World J Urol* 1999; **17:** 96–100.

McAninch JW (ed.). *Traumatic and Reconstructive Urology*. Philadelphia: WB Saunders, 1996.

McAninch JW, Santucci RA. Genitourinary trauma. In: Walsh PC, Retik AB, Vaughan ED, Wein AJ (eds). *Campbell's Urology*, 8th edn. Philadelphia: WB Saunders, 2002.

Morey AF, Hernandez J, McAninch JW. Reconstructive surgery for trauma of the lower urinary tract. *Urol Clin North Am* 2002; **26:** 49–60.

Mundy AR. Results and complications of urethroplasty and its future. *Br J Urol* 1999; **71:** 322–5.

Mundy AR. Pelvic fracture injuries of the posterior urethra. *World J Urol* 1999; **17:** 90–5.

Palmer JK, Benson GS, Corriere JN Jr. Diagnosis and initial management of urological injuries associated with 200 consecutive pelvic fractures. *J Urol* 1983; **130:** 712–14.

Pierce JM Jr. Disruptions of the anterior urethra. *Urol Clin North Am* 1989; **16:** 329–34.

Webster GD, Mathes GL, Selli C. Prostatomembranous urethral injuries: a review of the literature and a rational approach to their management. *J Urol* 1983; **130:** 898–902.

8. Adult urinary tract infections

Gregory J Malone and David L Nicol

Urinary tract infection (UTI) is a common problem in the general community, being the most frequent bacterial infection. Most simple UTIs are diagnosed and treated by primary care physicians. Urologists, however, are frequently involved in the management of moderate and severe uncomplicated, and, essentially all, complicated UTIs. Uncomplicated pyelonephritis, as an example, accounts for approximately 25% of all UTI-related admissions for inpatient treatment. Complicated UTIs secondary to urinary tract catheterization, urolithiasis, obstructive uropathy, instrumentation, diabetes mellitus, pregnancy, immunosuppression and congenital or secondary variations of urinary tract anatomy such as prune belly syndrome, ileal conduits and bladder augmentation are further diagnoses requiring inpatient treatment. A working knowledge of the basic pathophysiology and the diagnostic and treatment principles of management of UTIs is important for every urologist to acquire and maintain. This chapter aims to provide a practical overview of the management of important UTIs that *present as emergencies* to both junior and senior urology trainees caring for the adult population.

DEFINITIONS

Bacteriuria is the presence of bacteria in the urine from upper and lower urinary tract sources. It can occur in the presence or absence of both pyuria and symptoms. A **urinary tract infection** (UTI) occurs when a microbial agent, usually bacterial, invades and colonizes the urinary tract. In the immunocompetent host this infection results in an inflammatory mediated response. This response will manifest as local and/or systemic signs and symptoms, the elucidation of which will allow a diagnosis of UTI to be made.

UTIs can be classified as either uncomplicated (simple) or complicated. **Uncomplicated** UTIs are those infections in a structurally and functionally normal urinary tract, when the patient is not pregnant, and when there is no history of recent antimicrobial use. Examples of simple UTIs include most isolated or recurrent lower UTIs and acute pyelonephritis in female patients. **Complicated** UTIs are those that occur in a structurally and/or functionally abnormal urinary tract, for example where urolithiasis causes obstructive uropathy and in those patients with a neuropathic bladder.

INCIDENCE

UTIs are diagnosed far more frequently in female patients, when compared with male patients (~30:1). The exception to this is in young children where UTIs are more common in males, up to approximately 6 months of age. Furthermore, in female patients, the incidence of UTIs increases with advancing age. Approximately 1% of girls 5–15 years of age will have bacteriuria. This increases to 5% in early adulthood. Overall, up to 30% of all females aged between 20 and 40 years will experience an acute bacterial UTI requiring treatment. The risk of a UTI increases with complicating upper and lower urinary tract pathology. Approximately 20% of women and 10% of men over 70 years of age will have bacteriuria upon culture of their urine.

PATHOGENESIS

UTIs arise, most commonly, from the ascending route whereby bacteria enter the bladder via the urethra. Large bowel commensal organisms colonizing the perineum, the perianal region, and the prepuce in the male are the most common sources. Other routes of infection, which are far less common, include the hematogenous and lymphatic pathways, and the spread of bacteria from adjacent organs.

RISK FACTORS FOR URINARY TRACT INFECTION

Host factors predisposing to UTIs include urinary stasis, local trauma, abnormal urinary tract anatomy and function, diabetes mellitus, immunosuppression, debility, poor hygiene and aging. Factors specific to females include deficient estrogen status and short urethral length. Mechanical and other factors mediate the ability of the enterobacteria to colonize, invade and damage the urinary tract. In women, risk factors include sexual intercourse, especially with a new partner, unusually vigorous intercourse, delayed postcoital micturition, history of previous UTIs, and the use of spermicide and contraceptive diaphragms. Elderly patients have an increased incidence of asymptomatic bacteriuria and UTI due to reduced urogenital estrogen, reduced nutritional status, an inability to maintain body homeostasis, poorer bowel function, increased comorbidities and a greater incidence of dysfunctional voiding.

Foreign bodies entering the urinary tract and breaching natural defense mechanisms may also contribute to an increased risk of UTI. These include external urinary drainage devices such as indwelling urethral catheters, suprapubic catheters and nephrostomy drainage tubes. Dysfunctional voiding in the male, with high voiding pressures and grossly elevated residual volumes may predispose to UTIs. Furthermore, augmentation or substitution of the lower urinary tract with bowel segments substantially increases the risk of developing a UTI.

DIABETES MELLITUS

Diabetes mellitus is an important predisposing condition for UTI. It is a common multisystem disease with potentially serious effects on urinary tract anatomy and function. Complications which can arise in a subset of diabetic patients include diabetic nephropathy, papillary necrosis, renal artery stenosis, and diabetic cystopathy. Bacteriuria is twice as common in glycosuric and diabetic patients when compared with the non-diabetic population. Diabetic patients also have a higher incidence of complicated upper and lower UTIs, such as renal and perinephric abscesses, emphysematous pyelonephritis, emphysematous cystitis, xanthogranulomatous pyelonephritis and fungal infections. Diabetes has a strong association with Fournier's gangrene, a life-threatening synergistic infection. Furthermore, morbidity and potential mortality is greater in diabetic patients with UTIs. Investigation of diabetic patients is further compounded by the added risk of contrast nephropathy, especially in those patients with reduced renal function, dehydration, sepsis or treat with metformin. Finally, it is essential that the treating urologist be aware that the clinical condition of the diabetic patient may deteriorate rapidly and response may be suboptimal with more conservative treatment strategies.

COMMON ORGANISMS

Commensal organisms in the large bowel are the usual source of UTIs, with aerobic Gram-negative rods the most common bacteria isolated. The type of pathogenic organism and antibiotic sensitivity will often vary according to whether the infection is community or hospital acquired. Community-acquired infections most commonly result from *Escherichia coli* (80%). Other enterobacteria, such as *Proteus mirabilis* and *Klebsiella* spp., are also frequent pathogens. Gram-positive organisms common to community-acquired UTIs include *Enterococcus faecalis* and *Staphylococcus saprophyticus*. Nosocomial infections are typically the result of *E. coli* (50%), *Pseudomonas aeruginosa*, *Klebsiella* spp., *Enterobacter* spp., *Citrobacter*, *Serratia marcescens*, *Providencia stuartii* and *S. epidermidis*, and are often more resistant to frequently prescribed antibiotics.

Less common causative organisms can produce UTIs in the presence of a grossly abnormal urinary tract, immunosuppression or a foreign body. These include fungi such as *Candida albicans*, *Mycoplasma* species including *Ureaplasma urealyticum*, and viral organisms such as Adenovirus in immunosuppressed bone marrow transplant recipients. Urethral infections result from *Chlamydia trachomatis*, *Neisseria gonorrhoeae*, *U. urealyticum*, and occasionally *Gardnerella vaginalis*.

Indwelling urinary catheters are the most common source of nosocomial infections and Gram-negative bacteremia in the hospital environment. There is an approximately 1–2% risk of infection with a single catheter passage, highlighting the importance of meticulous aseptic catheter insertion technique. The risk of acquired infection is directly related to the duration of catheterization, with the risk of bacteriuria increasing by approximately 10% per day postinsertion in women and approximately 3–4% per day in men. The source of this infection is – via the catheter, the periurethral region, the drainage bag, or connector disruption with contamination. Catheterization for less than 5 days should be aimed for in the hospital environment as bacteriuria from short-term catheterization usually clears quickly. Long-term catheterization results in bacteriuria by providing a breach in the natural defense mechanisms and also provides a direct reservoir for bacteria due to adherence to the catheter surface. Upon removal of a long-term catheter, clearance of bacteriuria may be improved by administering a short course of antimicrobials.

INTERACTION BETWEEN THE HOST AND BACTERIA

To produce a UTI the inoculated organism must adhere, multiply, colonize and finally, invade the urinary tract. At each of these steps in the progression towards a urinary tract infection, the interaction between the host and the infecting organism will determine whether an infection ensues, or whether the process is aborted prior to an infection being established. Host and bacterial factors, including the size of the bacterial inoculum, determine the susceptibility of each patient to a potential UTI. The similar clonality of urine and fecal isolates of *E. coli*, highlight the dominance of particular strains causing cystitis in the rectal flora of those patients with recurrent bacteriuria.

BACTERIAL FACTORS (FIGURE 8.1)

Bacterial adherence to uroepithelial cells is reliant upon bacterial pili. These are surface adhesion molecules (adhesins) that allow the organism to attach to the urothelium. The type 1 pilus and the P pilus, present on *E. coli*, have been most investigated and reported. Type 1 or mannose-sensitive pili cause hemagglutination and, furthermore, allow the bacteria to bind to the uromucoid of uroepithelial cells, the intestinal mucosa and urethral catheters, thereby allowing colonization. P pili (mannose-negative) bind to the P blood group antigen found on uroepithelial cell surfaces. The P pilus facilitates ascent of the *E. coli* in the anatomically normal urinary tract, resulting in the dominance of this organism in pyelonephritis. Both type 1 and P pili are antigenic sites targeted by host humoral immunity to prevent binding. Other pili important in bacterial adherence and host immune modulation include x-adhesins and the 075X fimbria.

Additional bacterial virulence factors in UTIs include hemolysins, bacterial enzymes such as collagenases and elastases, and inducible iron

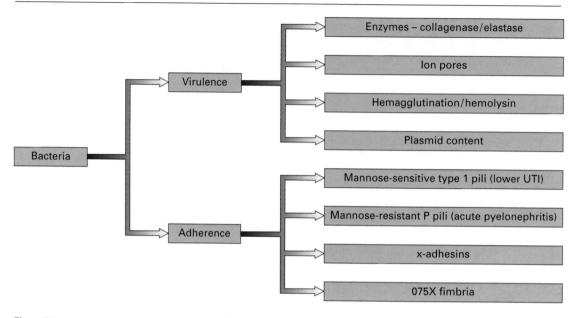

Figure 8.1

Bacterial factors that influence the host–bacteria interaction in urinary tract infection (UTI).

channels. These factors are more prevalent in bacteria isolated from the urinary tract than those isolated from the colon. Colony establishment and growth is an energy-dependent process and this requires suitable environmental conditions within the host to be effective. These conditions include a suitable urine pH and temperature, and nutritive support.

HOST DEFENSE (FIGURE 8.2)

Multiple mechanisms are involved in host defense and prevention of an established UTI in both female and male patients. Estrogen status in females is an important natural defense mechanism in the prevention of bacterial adherence. Estrogen augments proliferation and regular shedding of introital and vaginal epithelium. Furthermore, estrogen results in the accumulation of glycogen and growth of lactobacilli with

acidification of the local environment, thus preventing colonization by uropathogens such as *E. coli*. Factors specific to male defense mechanisms include long urethral length, urine flow with its clearing effect, and prostatic secretions, including zinc-containing substances.

Cell surface antigen status is another important natural defense mechanism. Antigens which appear to be important include Lewis antigens, P group antigens and to a lesser extent ABO blood group status. Lewis antigen positive patients have a lower risk of bacterial binding to uroepithelial, vaginal and other mucosal cells. P group antigen expression is extremely common in the community giving the P pili expressing bacteria a natural selection advantage and subsequently an increased infection risk.

Multiple factors in urine can be inhibitory to bacterial infection. Low urine osmolality in

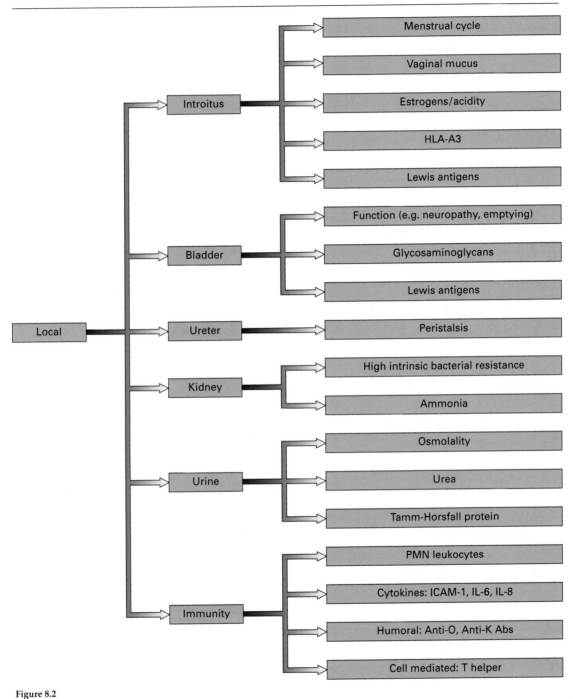

Figure 8.2

Local host defense factors that govern host susceptibility in urinary tract infection. HLA, human leukocyte antigen; PMN, polymorpho nuclear; ICAM, intercellular adhesion molecule; IL, interleukin.

association with dilute urine can prevent bacterial growth. Also, the polymorphonuclear (PMN) leukocytes naturally found in urine destroy bacteria. Other substances found in urine that are inhibitory to bacteria include urea, organic acids, Tamm-Horsfall protein and certain oligosaccharides. Tamm-Horsfall protein appears to act via a direct effect on bacterial binding plus host immune modulation.

Natural immunity to UTIs is an important defense mechanism. The PMN leukocyte response is usually triggered once infection occurs with local release of cytokines. Humoral immunity is induced with the production of anti-O and anti-K antibodies. The primary response is the production of IgM with delayed IgG elevation. IgA is thought to play an ill-defined roll. Cellular immunity with an increase in T-helper cells and subsequent production of cytokines amplifies this host response.

Table 8.1 Principles of management of acute severe urinary tract infections

Acute management
- Establish diagnosis
  - Clinical
    - History, examination, observations
    - Dipstick analysis +/−
  - Microbiological assessment
  - Radiological assessment
- Treatment of infection
  - Local – antibiotic therapy
  - Systemic – modification of physiological response/Gram-negative sepsis
- Upper tract management
  - Conservative
  - Urinary tract drainage – antegrade/retrograde

Definitive management
- Endoscopic antegrade/retrograde procedures
- Open procedure/nephrectomy

Ongoing management and follow-up
- Risk factor modification

PRINCIPLES OF MANAGEMENT (TABLE 8.1)

DIAGNOSTIC MODALITIES

Appropriate treatment of all UTIs requires accurate categorization of the disease process and exclusion of all complicating factors. This includes determination of infection site, contributing anatomical variation, complexity of the infection, and the likelihood of recurrence. Investigations commonly performed in the acute work-up of a patient with suspected UTI include dipstick analysis, urine culture, hematology and radiological studies. These investigations are also of value in the follow-up of patients after definitive therapy has been undertaken.

REAGENT STRIPS

Standard reagent testing strips include nitrite dipstick to detect bacteriuria, and leukocyte esterase estimation to detect pyuria. The nitrite test is only positive for coagulase-splitting bacteria. The sensitivity of nitrite analysis ranges between 27 and 70% with a specificity of 85–94%. The leukocyte test is reported to be accurate to 10–12 leukocytes/high-power field (HPF) of centrifuged urine. Leukocyte esterase reagent strip sensitivity is between 55 and 85%, with a specificity of 60–94%. When combined, the sensitivity of nitrite testing in addition to leukocyte esterase detection has a false-negative rate of approximately 20%, which is inadequate for the accurate assessment of most UTIs.

For the young female patient presenting with an isolated simple UTI to a primary care physician, the use of this diagnostic method may be justified. However, if an accurate midstream urine culture is not obtained then an opportunity is lost for any subsequent bacterial assessment and tailored antimicrobial prescribing. Standard reagent strips should ideally only be used as screening aids in the initial diagnostic work-up of patients with a clinical diagnosis of UTI, until urine culture and antimicrobial sensitivity results are available. The sole use of reagent strip testing in the definitive management of serious and recurrent UTIs, where specific urine cultures with appropriate antibiotic sensitivities are required, is inadequate.

URINE CULTURE

The accepted gold standard for diagnosing a UTI is a positive culture with pyuria, from an uncontaminated or clean-catch specimen of urine. The role of this laboratory-based urine analysis is to obtain a quantitative bacterial measurement, identify the infective organism, and classify drug sensitivities for subsequent treatment. Various methods are used to obtain urine for subsequent laboratory processing. Midstream urine is the most commonly employed technique for collecting uncontaminated urine. This technique requires the patient to collect the middle portion of a single void in a sterile container. The fresh specimen must be processed within 60 min of collection or refrigerated (4 °C) immediately upon collection if processing is to be delayed. The length of delay should be as short as possible, and no longer than 24 hours from the time of collection. To diagnose a UTI (Table 8.2) the urine culture must grow >100 000 colony-forming units (CFUs) of a single isolate per milliliter of urine. However, up to 30% of women with symptomatic UTIs will grow between 100 and 10 000 CFUs/ml, and if symptoms are consistent with a UTI then this may be considered adequate evidence to initiate antibiotic therapy. A common cause for these reduced colony counts is excessive hydration.

The most accurate method of assessing the white and red cell counts in a urine specimen is with a hemocytometer reading performed on unspun urine, however for convenience, most laboratories will examine the centrifuged urine sediment microscopically. The specimen should demonstrate pyuria (>10 white cells/mm^3 of urine), with minimal introital contamination (<10 epithelial cells/mm^3 of urine) on microscopy, to be considered an adequate sample on which clinical management decisions can be based. Other techniques used to obtain uncontaminated urine for subsequent microscopy and culture include suprapubic aspiration and urethral catheterization with subsequent urine collection. Both these methods reduce the risk of contamination. Using these techniques, >100 CFU/ml of urine, without evidence of contamination, will be adequate for diagnosing a UTI in symptomatic patients.

In isolation, the presence of pyuria correlates poorly with the definitive diagnosis of a UTI. Confounding the diagnosis of UTI further is the finding of sterile pyuria. This is a negative urine culture in the presence of pyuria. The differential diagnosis of sterile pyuria includes a previously treated UTI, urolithiasis, urinary tract tumors, pregnancy, foreign bodies such as a ureteric stent, tuberculosis and other atypical organisms, and spurious causes such as vaginal contamination.

URINARY TRACT IMAGING

The aim of urinary tract imaging (Table 8.3), in those patients with infection is to diagnose underlying conditions requiring additional treatment – to allow adequate urinary drainage, avoid deterioration in renal function and clinical status, and prevent recurrence of infection. Generally, plain radiography with a KUB (kidney, ureter, bladder) radiograph plus a urinary tract ultrasound scan is a sufficient first-line investigation to screen for significant pathology. If abnormalities are identified then subsequent imaging should be tailored to the clinical situation. In most cases intravenous urography (IVU) or computed tomography (CT) imaging are the most appropriate second-line investigations. CT scans, however, are generally superior to renal

---

Table 8.2 Midstream urine criteria for urinary tract infections

>100 000	CFUs/ml – single isolate
>10	white cells/mm^3 of urine
<10	epithelial cells/mm^3 of urine

Table 8.3 Imaging modalities used in the investigation of urinary tract infections

- Plain abdominal radiograph (KUB)
- Ultrasonography
- Intravenous urography
- Computed tomography
- Nuclear medicine renography (MAG3/DTPA/DMSA)
- Magnetic resonance imaging (MRI/MRU)
- Antegrade or retrograde urography

---

ultrasonography and IVU for the evaluation and management of adult patients with acute renal infection. Both unenhanced and contrast-enhanced CT, at varying excretory phases, are excellent imaging modalities. CT offers advantages in distinguishing degree and type of involvement of the renal parenchyma, a more accurate diagnosis of acute abscesses, and rapid identification of obstructing pathology such as urolithiasis. In those patients with poor renal function or contrast allergies, and evidence of urinary tract obstruction, magnetic resonance urography, nuclear medicine renography and retrograde urography may be more appropriate. Generally however, these investigations are uncommon in the acute setting, with antegrade imaging via nephrostomy or retrograde urography via cystoscopic catheter insertion performed after a decision to intervene has been made.

In adult female patients diagnosed with an isolated episode of simple acute bacterial cystitis, imaging is generally not necessary. Concerning details in the patient's history, such as hematuria and loin pain, may necessitate imaging in infrequent cases. Those patients presenting with acute pyelonephritis should generally have a urinary tract ultrasound (in combination with a KUB radiograph) during their management – as a screening modality – to exclude any complicating pathology. Because uncomplicated UTIs in men are not common, diagnostic evaluation with ultrasound scans and plain abdominal radiographs should also be undertaken in order to identify complicating pathology within the urinary tract. Other investigations required in these patients include uroflowmetry, residual volume estimation and possibly flexible cysto-urethroscopy in selected cases.

Table 8.4 Aims of management of urinary tract infections (UTIs)

- Relieve symptoms
- Eradicate bacterial infection
- Exclude complicated UTIs
- Prevent urinary tract damage
- Prevent recurrent UTIs

ANTIBIOTIC THERAPY

Antimicrobial agents are the mainstay of therapy in UTIs (Table 8.4) and should follow basic principles. Many different antibiotics are used in the treatment of both community and nosocomial UTIs. The ideal antibiotic should achieve high renal tissue and urine levels, be bactericidal, and have a broad spectrum of activity. The major drugs suitable for the treatment of UTIs are listed in Table 8.5. The more frequent prescribing of certain drugs in the management of UTIs relates to drug efficacy as well as cost. The commonly prescribed drugs include gentamicin, ciprofloxacin, trimethoprim/sulfamethoxazole, amoxicillin and the cephalosporins. Atypical organisms such as the chlamydiae and mycoplasmas will require tailored antibiotic prescribing with the tetracyclines and erythromycin. *Trichomonas vaginalis* infections should be treated with metronidazole.

Table 8.5 Antibiotics used in the management of urinary tract infections

- **Aminoglycosides** (gentamicin/tobramicin)
- **Fluoroquinolones** (ciprofloxacin/norfloxacin)
- **Trimethoprim/sulfamethoxazole**
- **Aminopenicillins** (amoxicillin/ampicillin), alone or in combination with **clavulanic acid**
- **Cephalosporins** (cephalexin, cephalothin, ceftriaxone)
- **Carboxypenicillins** (carbenicillin/ticarcillin)
- **Uredopenicillins** (mezlocillin/piperacillin)
- **Monobactams** (aztreonam)
- **Carbapenems** (imipenem)

Gentamicin is generally the most suitable antimicrobial for the treatment of serious UTIs as it fulfills many of the necessary requirements including bactericidal activity. Gentamicin in combination with β-lactams and vancomycin has the added advantage of synergistic activity. These drugs in combination increase the diffusion of gentamicin across bacterial cell membranes thereby improving efficacy. Furthermore, gentamicin exhibits a post-antibiotic effect with a large once daily dose producing bacteriostasis several hours after dosage, despite low concentrations.

Bacterial *antibiotic resistance* can arise after the initiation of antibiotic therapy and is becoming an increasing problem in managing both simple and complicated UTIs. Resistance usually results through one of three mechanisms. First, natural resistance occurs with the absence of any drug-sensitive strains prior to the initiation of therapy. Second, the selection of resistant mutants can occur in up to 10% of infections, whereby the original bacterial strain is replaced by a resistant strain, usually within 48 h of antibiotic treatment. These mutations can be of bacterial transport molecules and molecules aiding the binding of antibiotics to bacterial proteins, for example the 30S ribosomal subunit binding to gentamicin. Finally, plasmid-mediated resistance (R-factor) is the most important mechanism of bacterial resistance, and is due to the transfer of multidrug resistance (MDR) genes leading to the production of 'killer' enzymes. With the increasing prevalence of antibiotic-resistant strains of bacteria, including *E. coli*, it is important to obtain periodic advice from regional clinical microbiologists/infectious diseases physician if empiric treatment of UTIs is contemplated.

The dosage regimen for uncomplicated cystitis and pyelonephritis is relatively well defined through clinical trials and is outlined in the appropriate sections that follow. The choice of antimicrobials, and adjustments in dosage and length of treatment will be influenced by coexisting conditions such as pregnancy, diabetes mellitus, anatomical variation, urolithiasis, neuropathy, renal impairment, hepatic impairment, immunosuppression and age (pediatric cases are not discussed in this chapter).

GRAM-NEGATIVE SEPSIS AND THE PHYSIOLOGICAL RESPONSE

Gram-negative sepsis (GNS) is a potentially fatal complication of UTIs, and infections from other sources with Gram-negative pathogens. This process generally starts as localized infection that becomes systemic in a patient whose condition is compromised by underlying medical and surgical comorbidities. GNS is a **systemic inflammatory response syndrome** (SIRS) caused by the host's natural, although at times exuberant, physiological response to an infectious agent. This process originates at a local cellular and biochemical level, and is manifest at a systemic (or clinical) level (Table 8.6). The infectious agents in GNS are the Gram-negative organisms (e.g. *E. coli*, *Klebsiella* spp., *Enterobacter* spp., *Serratia* spp., *Pseudomonas aeruginosa*, and *Proteus mirabilis*). The lipid-A component of the lipopolysaccharide (endotoxin) in the Gram-negative cell wall is responsible for most of the toxicity in GNS as it generates a florid host-mediated response.

Table 8.6 Clinical features of Gram-negative sepsis

• Hypotension	Systolic blood pressure <90 mmHg
• Hyperthermia / Hypothermia	>37/<36 °C
• Tachycardia	>100 beats per min
• Tachypnoea	respiratory rate >20 per min/$Paco_2$ <32 mmHg
• Leukocytosis / Leukopenia	>12 000/<4000 mm^3
• Possible multiorgan failure	

The initial event in GNS is the localized host reaction to the infectious process, i.e. an acute inflammatory response, neutrophil and macrophage infiltration and initiation of the complement and coagulation cascades. This confined process evolves into a systemic response due to poor control of the local infection, or a massive bacterial load with the release of bacterial products (cell wall components/endotoxins) from the pathogens either at localized sites or within the circulation. The bacterial endotoxemia induces cellular processes in the host, resulting in the release of endogenous mediators that subsequently act on various biochemical and cellular pathways. Tumor necrosis factor (TNF), interleukin (IL)-1, IL-6 and IL-8 are the principal mediators with their release resulting in further cascading effects. Clinical signs of sepsis, such as fever, tachycardia and hypotension are directly related to host cytokine levels. Complement activation, with elevation in production of C3a and C5a of the membrane attack complex, leads to local tissue damage. Numerous other mediators are involved in GNS including catecholamines, histamine, kinins, prostaglandins, leukotrienes, endorphins, and the platelet activating factor. These factors in concert serve to amplify the cytotoxic and inflammatory response producing oxygen free radicals, lysosomal and granular enzyme release, plus a procoagulant state with possible disseminated intravascular coagulation (DIC) with a clotting factor consumption coagulopathy.

The clinical outcome in GNS (Figure 8.3) results from multiple system failure combining to overwhelm the homeostatic mechanisms available to the patient. Circulatory failure is multifactorial in origin, with vasodilation, the release of myocardial depressant factor (MDF), endothelial damage and microthrombi contributing to produce refractory hypotension. Cardiac failure results from the falling preload, hypoperfusion and direct myocardial dysfunction from MDF. Acute renal failure ensues from hypoxic acute tubular necrosis. Microthrombi destroy glomerular filtration secondary to the DIC, with immune complex deposition further compromising glomerular function. Adult respiratory distress syndrome (ARDS) results from pulmonary toxicity secondary to capillary leak and oxygen free radical injury. With progression, gastrointestinal tract integrity is lost with worsening of the endotoxin insult due to translocation of bacteria or endotoxins directly into the circulation, eventually producing hepatic dysfunction.

The patient will enter a gross catabolic state due to hypermetabolism and the overwhelming production of acute phase proteins, leukocytes and the process of wound healing. This hypercatabolic state is difficult to overcome despite aggressive nutritional support. Ongoing endothelial cell damage produces worsening DIC, and deterioration in the clinical status of the patient. Ultimately, blood pressure and urine output fall, tachycardia develops, and the serum lactate rises. These processes can proceed with the patient's clinical status becoming refractory to therapy, despite adequate control of the inciting focus of infection and intensive therapy with multisystem support.

The management of GNS is based on the triad

Circulatory failure	Congestive cardiac failure	Acute renal failure	Acute respiratory distress syndrome	Hepatic dysfunction	Loss of gut integrity	Hypercatabolic state

Figure 8.3

Organ dysfunction in Gram-negative sepsis.

of physiological support, appropriate antibiotic therapy and the removal of the source of sepsis. Physiological support involves fluid resuscitation, oxygen therapy and ventilatory support, dialysis, and vasoactive drugs, with further metabolic and nutritional therapy as required. Antibiotic therapy is initially broad spectrum with a β-lactam and aminoglycoside, or third-generation cephalosporin, as the mainstay until positive blood or urine cultures are available and antibiotic therapy can be tailored. The source of sepsis is identified and treated on an emergent basis as necessary. This may require drainage of an obstructed renal unit or debridement of an infective focus.

Mortality from GNS remains high in severe cases despite modern therapeutic and interventional techniques. Early diagnosis, aggressive therapy, and appropriate intensive care unit (ICU) referral will reduce this mortality rate significantly. Other measures that have been used to improve the outcome in this group of patients include antiendotoxin antibodies, anticytokine antibodies, monoclonal antibodies targeting leukocyte receptors, nitric oxide synthase inhibition and steroid therapy. To date, despite promising results in animal models of sepsis, no dramatic clinical benefit in human disease has been shown.

UPPER URINARY TRACT INFECTIONS

Upper UTIs are those infections related to the kidneys and perirenal structures, plus the collecting system including the calyces, renal pelvis and ureters, that is, those urological structures above the level of the bladder. The overlap between the various diagnoses related to these structures may be blurred at times. As with all UTIs it is of major importance to define whether the infection is uncomplicated or complicated, as this will have a major impact on subsequent investigation and treatment. The aim of management in upper UTI is to diagnose the pathology accurately and exclude obstruc-

tion, treat the infection with appropriate antimicrobials, and prevent ongoing renal damage with possible progression to chronic pyelonephritis and, potentially, renal failure. Infection in the presence of renal unit obstruction will invariably result in the onset of renal parenchymal destruction within 24 h if not relieved emergently.

ACUTE PYELONEPHRITIS

Acute pyelonephritis (APN) is an infection of the renal parenchyma and collecting system resulting in suppurative destruction of renal glomeruli and tubules. It is a relatively common condition in the community accounting for approximately a quarter of all UTI-related hospital admissions. This disease predominantly affects female patients, with an average age at presentation of approximately 30 years. APN is generally a unilateral rather than bilateral condition. The Gram-negative organism E. coli is the causative organism in approximately 85–90% of cases, with the P fimbria-producing strain the most commonly isolated. This selective advantage allows the bacterium to adhere more easily to the urothelium of the host with resultant ascending infection. Lewis antigen non-secretor status and expression of certain extended glycosphingolipids on vaginal epithelial cells increases bacterial adherence, and therefore susceptibility in uncomplicated APN. Vesicoureteric reflux can be responsible for ascending upper UTI, but infection with the P fimbriated E. coli may lead to APN without reflux because of the paralytic effect of lipid A on ureteral peristalsis.

Additional organisms commonly isolated include Klebsiella spp., P. mirabilis, Enterobacter, P. aeruginosa, Serratia and Citrobacter. P. mirabilis is a urea-splitting organism commonly associated with infection stone (struvite) production. UTI with a Proteus spp. must be treated thoroughly and the patient should have their urine cultured post treatment to ensure eradication of this organism. Furthermore, the presence of

Proteus necessitates imaging of the upper urinary tract to exclude concomitant urolithiasis with struvite calculi.

Prompt diagnosis and appropriate therapy decreases the risk of serious complications from APN. Patients with APN commonly present with fevers, rigors, dysuria and ipsilateral loin pain. Examination findings depend on the clinical status of the patient and the severity of infection. This can range from minor constitutional upset to signs of severe sepsis and cardiovascular compromise. On examination the patient may be febrile with loin tenderness and have reduced bowel sounds and occasionally generalized abdominal tenderness. Fluid status should also be assessed, as dehydration is a common finding due to fever and intolerance of oral fluids.

The investigation of APN depends upon the clinical picture. Midstream urine culture may grow less than 100 000 CFUs/ml in up to 20% of patients, however, a positive urine culture should be evident in all cases, with greater than 95% demonstrating the culture of a single organism. Appropriate urine culturing confirms the diagnosis and aids in prescribing suitable antibiotic therapy. The need for biochemical and hematological work-up can be assessed according to the case details.

The major aim of imaging the urinary tract in APN is to exclude complicating factors such as an infected hydronephrosis due to obstruction of the renal unit, or other anatomical and pathological variations. Imaging of the upper urinary tract with ultrasound as a first-line investigation is not mandatory if the clinical status of the patient is mild, and there is rapid improvement with initiation of appropriate antibiotic and supportive therapy. Most patients, however, who present for specialist urological care, should have imaging of their urinary tract. Failure to respond to adequate therapy after 24–48 h, deterioration in clinical status or past urological history suggestive of a complicated UTI (e.g. previous urolithiasis) should necessitate early radiological investigation. Alternative methods of imaging, such as IVU, CT and nucleotide renograms can be used if the ultrasound demonstrates an abnormality or insufficient information is yielded. CT is the increasingly preferred form of imaging in equivocal cases and in suspected complicated UTIs as it will define the extent of disease and exclude the presence of abscess formation and stone disease (Figure 8.4). Contrast media may be withheld if renal impairment contraindicates their use.

The aims of management in APN are to relieve symptoms, eradicate bacterial infection, treat complicating factors, prevent further renal damage, and prevent recurrence of infection. Patients with APN can usually be subdivided into three treatment groups: uncomplicated APN not requiring hospitalization, uncomplicated APN requiring hospitalization and complicated APN requiring admission to hospital and definitive management of the complicating factor(s). Initially, empiric broad-spectrum antibiotic cover should be administered with urine culture sensitivities determining subsequent prescribing. Oral antimicrobials that attain high renal tissue levels, such as trimethoprim alone or in combination with sulfamethoxazole, or fluoroquinolones are preferred in the treatment of patients with milder cases not requiring hospitalization. The optimal duration of antibiotic therapy for acute uncomplicated pyelonephritis has been relatively well established, with 14-day regimens commonly prescribed. Patients with severe infection will usually require hospitalization and intravenous antibiotic administration. Supportive therapy may be required according to the patient's clinical status. In these more severe cases the patient should be maintained on intravenous antibiotics until afebrile for approximately 48 h, and then switched to appropriate oral therapy according to culture sensitivities. Positive blood cultures will necessitate prolongation of intravenous antibiotic administration, the regimen for this should be planned in consultation with a clinical microbiologist. Generally *E. coli* bacteremia

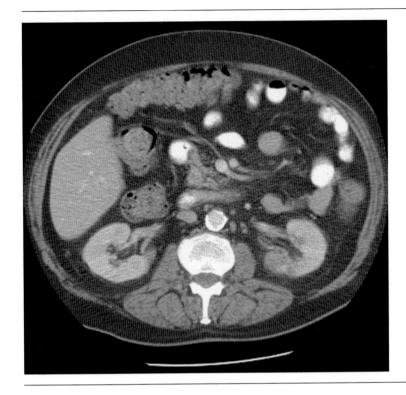

Figure 8.4

CT scan showing focal inflammatory lesion in a patient with acute pyelonephritis.

should be treated with intravenous antibiotics for 7 days or until the source is removed. The treatment of Gram-positive bacteremia will depend on whether the infecting organism is *S. aureus*. In cases of *S. aureus* infection and a known source 2 weeks of intravenous treatment is recommended. Furthermore, it is prudent to perform an echocardiogram (preferably trans-esophageal) to exclude subsequent endocarditis. If this is proved then at least 6 weeks of intra-venous therapy is required. In coagulase-negative staphylococcal infection 7–10 days treatment is usually appropriate and echocar-diography generally not indicated.

Complicated APN requires a longer period of antibiotic administration, usually 21 days, with management of the urinary tract abnormality a priority. This additional management may involve such measures as urinary bladder catheterization, nephrostomy drainage tube

insertion or more definitive endoscopic and open surgery.

Acute pyelonephritis in the elderly is caused less commonly by *E. coli* (60%). Symptoms also vary, with less genitourinary symptoms and more gastrointestinal upset. Furthermore, a leukocytosis is not alway evident. Because of this, the role of accurate urinalysis and culture takes on greater importance in the unwell elderly patient. The incidence of bacteremia and septic shock is higher in elderly patients with UTIs, however, these patients do respond well if an early diagnosis is made and appropriate therapy initiated. It is important to perform imaging of these patients to rule out complicat-ing factors such as stones and other causes of obstruction and urinary stasis.

Follow-up of patients after an episode of APN is aimed at confirming the complete resolution of infection. This requires repeat midstream urine culture, approximately 7 days after cessation of antibiotic therapy, to ensure urine sterility. Furthermore, definitive management of urinary tract abnormalities can be undertaken at this later stage once the infection is controlled. The importance of urine culture review is highlighted by a relapse rate in up to 25% of patients after treatment for APN.

LOBAR NEPHRONIA (ACUTE FOCAL BACTERIAL NEPHRITIS)

Lobar nephronia is a relatively uncommon, severe form of bacterial interstitial nephritis characterized by an acute **localized** infection without liquefaction. It is an inflammatory condition that has clinical, radiological and pathological similarities to both pyelonephritis and renal abscesses, and may be considered as part of a spectrum of disease. Patients with lobar nephronia are usually younger women who present systemically unwell with fever, rigors, abdominal pain, plus flank pain and tenderness. These patients are generally more unwell than those with simple APN. The source of infection is from an ascending rather than a hematogenous route in almost all cases.

The diagnosis of lobar nephronia relies on clinical suspicion, with appropriate microbiological and radiological investigations. All patients should demonstrate a positive urine culture and approximately 50% of patients have a positive blood culture for a single Gram-negative isolate. Generally, patients with lobar nephronia will undergo imaging, as indicated by their clinical condition. If the diagnosis is suspected then CT is the most accurate investigation, however, most patients will have had an ultrasound scan as first-line imaging. The ultrasound scan demonstrates an increased renal volume with a possible space-occupying, hypoechoic, mass or masses (Figures 8.5 and 8.6). The more widespread use of CT in the investigation of APN has resulted in an increase in the frequency of diagnosis of lobar nephronia. Prior to this trend patients were commonly

diagnosed as a severe form of APN and treated accordingly. CT typically demonstrates a hypodense or isodense mass with patchy focal enhancement in a wedge-shaped pattern. These appearances may be multifocal, and can be confused with cystic and solid renal lesions such as renal abscesses and renal cell carcinoma. A correlation between the spectrum of renal lesions and clinical severity of illness can be demonstrated and ranges from wedge-shaped lesions to focal mass-like lesions, and finally to multifocal lesions.

The management of lobar nephronia centers on an accurate diagnosis, with the exclusion of underlying obstruction. Subsequent treatment requires resuscitation, broad-spectrum parenteral antibiotics and adjuvant supportive therapy as clinically indicated. The use of intensive therapy is occasionally required for the more severe cases. Upon clinical improvement, oral antibiotic therapy should continue for a minimum 3-week duration. Confirmation of clearance of infection, with appropriate urine culture, is necessary upon completion of antibiotic therapy. Follow-up imaging in suspected renal tumor cases should demonstrate resolution of the lesion subsequent to improvement in the clinical condition of the patient. These lesions should resolve with appropriate antibiotic therapy over 1–3 months.

PYONEPHROSIS

An infected hydronephrosis is infection in a hydronephrotic kidney without suppurative destruction of the renal parenchyma. Pyonephrosis is suppurative destruction of an obstructed hydronephrotic kidney, which can result in near total or total loss of renal function. Pyonephrosis is the end-point in a clinical spectrum of infection in obstructed kidneys.

Pyonephrosis is a complicated UTI, most commonly associated with urolithiasis causing obstruction. Other benign and malignant causes of renal unit obstruction can also result in pyonephrosis. The obstructed infected renal

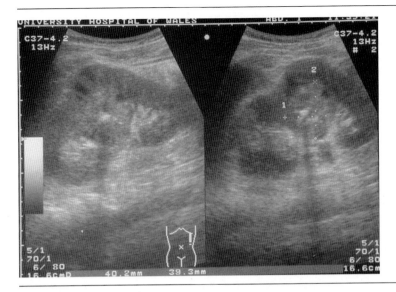

Figure 8.5

Ultrasound scan of a patient with renal sepsis showing a focal mass lesion with central calcification suggestive of lobar nephronia.

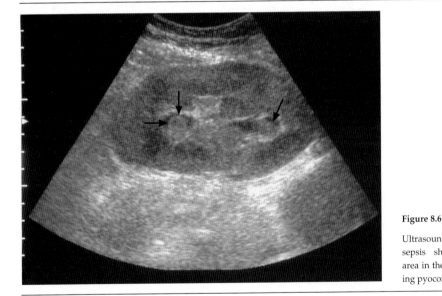

Figure 8.6

Ultrasound scan of a patient with renal sepsis showing increased echogenic area in the pelvicalyceal system indicating pyocongestion.

unit results in a significant source of bacteremia for the patient with septic sequelae.

The diagnosis of pyonephrosis is based on clinical, radiological and microbiological criteria. Patients typically present very ill with fever, rigors, flank pain and tenderness, and occasion-ally a palpable loin mass. Ultrasonography and CT are the most appropriate imaging modalities in the diagnosis of pyonephrosis and will show signs of obstruction with a fluid-filled collecting system. Contrast imaging such as IVU and CT will also demonstrate reduced or absent renal

135

function. Urine culture will identify the causative organism in almost all cases, with positive blood cultures found in a high proportion (~50%) of patients. The organisms identified in pyonephrosis include *E. coli*, and the other enterobacteria.

The aims of management in patients with pyonephrosis are to resuscitate the patient, initiate broad-spectrum Gram-negative antibiotic therapy, provide supportive therapy, confirm the source of sepsis, identify the cause of renal unit obstruction and treat this as appropriate. **Urgent** and **adequate drainage** of the obstructed kidney is the prime objective in pyonephrosis management. This can be performed through either retrograde ureteric stent insertion or percutaneous nephrostomy insertion, with system decompression and urinary diversion. Clinical status of the patient and center-specific expertise will usually determine which method of renal disobstruction is undertaken. In select circumstances nephrectomy is the most appropriate method to remove the source of sepsis and stabilize the patient.

Determination of residual renal function and definitive management of the source of obstruction will need to be deferred until all signs of sepsis have abated and an adequate period of time has been allowed for recovery of renal function. In poorly functioning renal remnants with adequate contralateral function, nephrectomy is generally advocated.

EMPHYSEMATOUS PYELONEPHRITIS

Emphysematous pyelonephritis (EPN) is a life-threatening, necrotizing, suppurative infection of the renal parenchyma and surrounding tissues caused by gas-forming organisms. EPN typically occurs in middle-aged (50 years) patients, usually women, with diabetes mellitus (80%) and/or ipsilateral urinary tract obstruction (<25%). The source of obstruction may be from varying sources such as stone disease, ureteric stricture disease (benign or malignant), and papillary necrosis. Approximately 10% of cases occur with

bilateral involvement, with a mortality rate approaching 45% in some series in those patients with both unilateral and bilateral disease. The higher mortality figures tend to occur in patients with underlying poorly controlled diabetes mellitus and more severe parenchymal destruction at diagnosis. Clinically, these are invariably adult patients presenting very unwell, with fever, flank pain, nausea and vomiting, and a palpable mass in approximately half the cases.

The gas in EPN is formed by the fermentation of glucose to CO_2 and H_2, with the most common organism being *E. coli*. Other organisms include *K. pneumoniae*, *Aerobacter* spp., *P. mirabilis*, and *P. aeruginosa*. Investigation of EPN will demonstrate positive urine cultures, with blood cultures being positive in up to 50% of patients. The most appropriate form of imaging is CT. The scan has a classic appearance of gas in the renal parenchyma, and frequently in the perinephric and pararenal tissues (Figures 8.7 and 8.8). This is quite distinct from gas solely in the collecting system, emphysematous pyelitis (EP), which usually indicates a less severe clinical course. Plain abdominal radiograph and ultrasound may demonstrate gas in the renal and perirenal tissues (Figure 8.9), with the sonographic features of bright echoes and a lack of post-acoustic shadowing (Figure 8.10).

Classification of CT findings into EPN1 and EPN2 (Figure 8.11) has recently been undertaken to better categorize the disease and define treatment protocols. Type 1 EPN is characterized by parenchymal destruction with either absence of fluid collection or the presence of streaky or mottled gas. Type 2 EPN is characterized by either renal or perirenal fluid collections with bubbly or loculated gas or gas in the collecting system. Generally, Type 1 EPN has a more fulminant course and requires more intensive medical and surgical management to prevent patient mortality.

Treatment initially involves aggressive supportive therapy and broad-spectrum parenteral antibiotics. As most patients are very ill at diag-

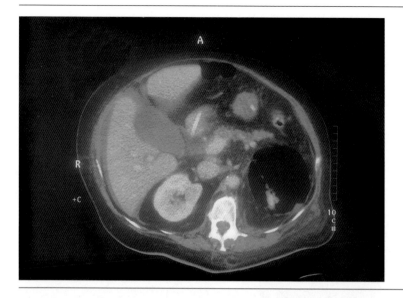

Figure 8.7

Emphysematous pyelonephritis (EPN). CT scan demonstrating gas within Gerota's fascia.

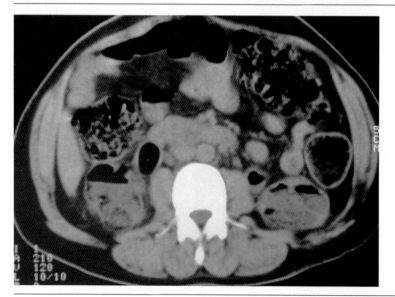

Figure 8.8

CT scan showing bilateral symmetrically shrunken kidneys with gas in the pelvicalyceal system in a patient with emphysematous pyelonephritis.

nosis, intensive care unit management is often needed for stabilization and optimization prior to any interventional procedures. In severe cases patient status may be refractory to intensive therapy and urgent nephrectomy may be required.

Thorough control of diabetes is an important aspect of treatment. Because the mortality rate is high in diabetic patients, emergency nephrectomy is often the treatment of choice. In non-diabetic patients, patients with a milder clinical presentation, patients with involvement of a solitary renal unit, and patients with gas in the collecting system and not in the parenchyma, adequate relief of obstruction and urinary diversion with percutaneous antegrade or endoscopic

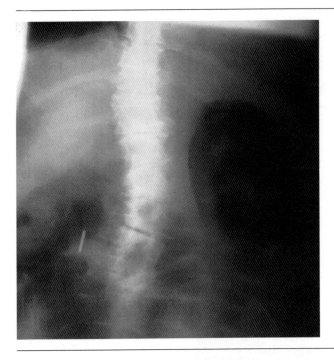

Figure 8.9

Emphysematous pyelonephritis (EPN). Plain abdominal x-ray demonstrating a gas renal pyelogram patient in the lateral position. (Courtesy of CRJ Woodhouse, UCL, London.)

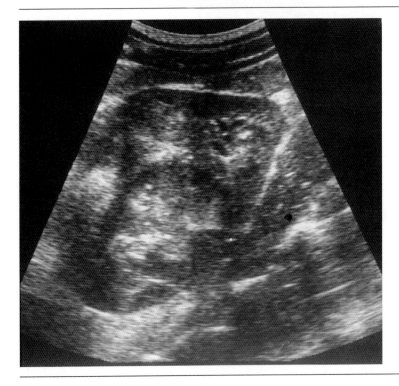

Figure 8.10

Emphysematous pyelonephritis: ultrasound scan showing a swollen kidney with patchy echogenic area in the renal parenchyma indicating collection of gas.

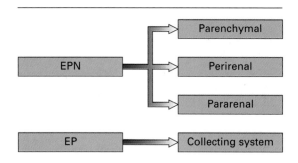

Figure 8.11

Classification of gas in emphysematous pyelonephritis (EPN) and emphysematous pyelitis (EP).

retrograde drainage may be attempted. This conservative treatment, with regular clinical assessment, may be trialed for 12–24 h, with a subsequent decision made as to the appropriateness of this form of conservative therapy based on the patient's clinical response. Many patients will however, ultimately require nephrectomy as definitive management, even if a satisfactory clinical response has occurred. Follow-up of this group of patients does involve determination of ipsilateral residual renal function, close medical management of renal and diabetic status, and prevention of further UTIs and obstructive uropathy from diseases such as urolithiasis.

RENAL ABSCESS

A renal abscess is a suppurative infection of the renal parenchyma that results in cavitation and abscess formation. Renal abscesses are uncommon severe UTIs, which are particularly dangerous because of their location and potential to spread to adjacent organs. A renal abscess is defined by its location within the renal parenchyma. Renal carbuncles are abscesses arising within the renal cortex, whereas a corticomedullary abscess involves both the cortex and medulla of the kidney. The latter comprise approximately 80% of all abscesses identified in the adult population. A renal abscess is gener-

ally the result of infection with Gram-negative organisms from an ascending UTI. Occasionally, abscesses can be secondary to hematogenous spread, usually of Gram-positive organisms; these classically occur in intravenous drug abusers. Differentiation of renal abscesses from acutely infected renal cysts is usually possible with adequate imaging. A rare cause of renal abscess formation is hydatid disease with *Echinococcus granulosus*.

Renal abscesses are more common in females than males with the average age at presentation being approximately 60 years. Clinically, these patients present unwell. Approximately 50% of patients will have a history of diabetes mellitus, with most of the remaining patients having a history of stone disease or have stones identified in their diagnostic work-up. Chronic pyelonephritis and recurrent UTIs are other common associations. Urinary stasis and obstruction are common underlying pathologies and usually secondary to calculi, with pregnancy and bladder neuropathy other uncommon problems. Initial diagnostic work-up aims at assessing the clinical status of the patient, defining the source of infection, and detailing underlying causes for a complicated UTI. Urine culture will isolate a causative organism in most patients. Imaging of the urinary tract with ultrasonography, usually the first-line method, demonstrates a fluid-filled renal parenchymal lesion (Figure 8.12a). Differentiation from a renal mass lesion is sometimes difficult with ultrasound alone. Once the diagnosis is suspected CT is the most appropriate imaging modality as it defines the extent of the abscess and aids in the diagnosis of underlying pathology (Figure 8.12b).

Treatment of patients with a renal abscess involves supportive therapy, broad-spectrum Gram-negative antibiotic cover, drainage of the renal abscess, plus treatment of any underlying urological pathology such as obstruction secondary to stone disease. Gram-positive antibiotic cover should be initiated in those patients at risk for hematogenous spread. Thorough

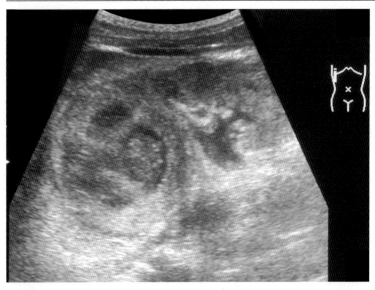

(a)

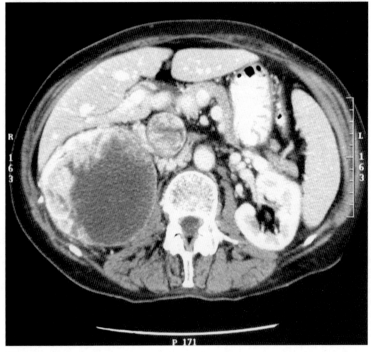

(b)

Figure 8.12

(a) Ultrasound scan showing a focal mass in the upper pole of the right kidney in a patient with sepsis suggestive of renal abscess.
(b) CT scan showing a large renal abscess.

assessment and management of poorly controlled diabetes, plus intensive care support will be necessary in the unwell patient with sepsis. Initial management of most renal abscesses involves adequate drainage, which can usually be satisfactorily achieved percutaneously under radiological guidance. Open surgical drainage may be required if the abscess cavity is multilocular, large (>5 cm) or percutaneous drainage has proved inadequate (Figure 8.13).

Conservative management of abscess cavities <3 cm, with appropriate antibiotics, has been shown in numerous series to be effective, but does require careful clinical and radiological monitoring. Larger renal abscesses have a higher rate of requiring multiple percutaneous procedures, and potentially, open surgical drainage. Occasionally, necrotic renal tumors can present as a renal abscess and should be considered in the differential diagnosis. Radiological follow-up is important to confirm complete resolution of the abscess cavity. Any concomitant ipsilateral renal tract obstruction will need to be treated with adequate stent or

nephrostomy drainage in the short term. Definitive management of all underlying pathology will be required to prevent recurrent problems. This may necessitate nephrectomy upon resolution of infection and ascertainment of a poorly functioning or non-functioning renal remnant. This should be deferred until the clinical status of the patient allows suitable intervention. A poorer prognosis is associated with elderly patients and those patients with chronic renal impairment.

PERINEPHRIC ABSCESS

A perinephric abscess is a suppurative infection with cavitation and abscess formation that is confined by Gerota's fascia to the perirenal tissues. It arises by direct extension from an infected kidney, commonly arising from rupture of an intrarenal abscess into the perinephric space. The source of infection is usually via the ascending route, however, hematogenous spread may occasionally be the source. Rarely, perinephric/paranephric abscesses can arise

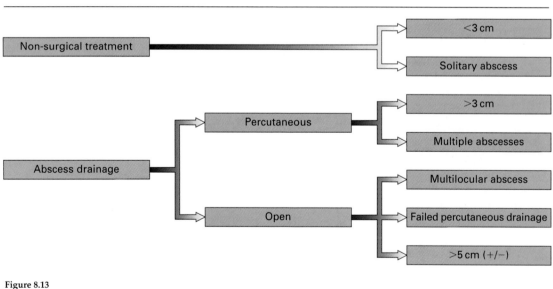

Figure 8.13

Treatment of renal abscess.

from gastrointestinal pathology such as a ruptured retrocecal appendix. Unlike most other severe UTIs, males are generally affected in equal proportion to females. Up to 5% of patients will be diagnosed with bilateral pathology. These abscess cavities can rupture through Gerota's fascia and result in a pararenal abscess. Perinephric abscesses are different from renal abscesses in that they are more difficult to diagnose and treat and generally have a poorer prognosis. Neurologically impaired patients, particularly those with high sensory levels, are at particular risk for the development and delayed diagnosis of this renal condition.

Clinically, patients with a perinephric abscess will often describe prolonged symptom duration of greater than 2 weeks, and delayed diagnosis is one of the major reasons for the high mortality rate associated with this condition. Common symptoms and signs include fever, rigors and chills, nausea, vomiting and anorexia, loin pain and tenderness, abdominal pain and tenderness and a loin mass in as many as 30–50%. Up to a third of patients will be afebrile at the time of presentation. As with many complicated UTIs, the common associations are diabetes mellitus and urolithiasis. Rare cases, subsequent to ESWL (extracorporeal shock wave lithotripsy) performed on patients with large infected stone burdens, have been reported.

Urinalysis may show no growth in up to 70% of patients and blood cultures are positive in approximately 50%. *S. aureus* was previously the most common bacterium isolated. Gram-negative enteric bacteria such as *E. coli*, *Proteus*, *Pseudomonas* and *Klebsiella* are the most common organisms cultured now, especially when obstruction or urolithiasis is present. Atypical organisms such as *Candida* spp. are generally isolated in immunosuppressed patients and have also been described in the perirenal tissues in autologous renal transplants. Imaging with renal ultrasonography is usually the first-line radiological investigation, and will demonstrate fluid-filled cavities in the perinephric space. Subsequently CT scan is the most useful modal-

ity as it helps diagnose the condition and gives accurate information as to the extent of the abscess, defines any loculations, identifies possible sources of obstruction and alerts to the possible involvement of adjacent retroperitoneal structures.

The management of a perinephric abscess is based on an accurate diagnosis with identification of any underlying causes such as diabetes mellitus. Broad-spectrum parenteral antibiotics are required in addition to supportive therapy as necessary. Antibiotic therapy may be tailored depending on urine culture results. The mainstay of treatment is adequate drainage of all abscess cavities. The options for drainage are percutaneous and open. The decision as to the most appropriate form of drainage will be based on the patient's clinical status and CT scan information. Traditionally, retroperitoneal open surgical drainage via a loin incision was definitive management. More recently, percutaneous placement of a drain under CT or USS guidance has proved successful. Multilocular abscess cavities and abscesses with thick purulent material are often best drained by an open technique with a drain left in situ upon completion. In cases with little remaining functioning parenchyma, nephrectomy may be the most appropriate method of management. Appropriate urgent management of any renal unit obstruction with internal or external drainage is an important adjunctive therapeutic aim. Definitive management of the obstructing lesion should be deferred until the patient's condition has improved satisfactorily. Despite adequate and relatively early intervention, the mortality from perinephric abscess formation has approached 50% in select series.

XANTHOGRANULOMATOUS PYELONEPHRITIS

Xanthogranulomatous pyelonephritis (XGP) is a severe, chronic variant of pyelonephritis characterized by destruction of the renal parenchyma and replacement with a chronic inflammatory infiltrate and lipid-laden macrophages, resulting in a poorly functioning or non-functioning enlarged kidney. XGP has been termed the great imitator due to the clinical and radiological features being difficult to characterize. Most cases of XGP are therefore diagnosed at the time of histopathological analysis after definitive management of the renal lesion by nephrectomy. The differential diagnosis of XGP includes renal cell carcinoma (RCC), renal abscess, infected renal cystic disease, tuberculosis, malakoplakia, and transitional cell carcinoma (TCC).

XGP is not common, with less than 1% of patients initially presenting with a clinical diagnosis of acute pyelonephritis being diagnosed with this condition. This disease generally involves the whole kidney, however, it may be segmental, multifocal and bilateral. Females are affected three times more commonly than males with most patients presenting subacutely. The average age at presentation is between 50 and 60 years, however, it can occur in any age group from pediatric to geriatric patients. The clinical presentation is remarkably non-specific and variable. Most patients present with fever, back or loin pain, palpable loin mass and constitutional symptoms of fatigue, malaise, weight loss and anorexia. On rare occasions these patients can present with a draining sinus.

The most common associated pathology is obstruction of the ipsilateral renal unit with concomitant urinary tract infection. This obstruction is most commonly secondary to underlying stone disease. Calculi in the renal pelvis or ureter are present in as many as 90% of cases. Staghorn calculi are present in up to 50% of these stone cases. Upper urinary tract obstruction resulting in XGP can be secondary to other pathologies, including benign and malignant causes such as congenital pelviureteric junction obstruction, malignancy such as TCC (far less commonly, RCC), and rarely ureteral schistosomiasis. Diabetes mellitus will be diagnosed in up to 15% of patients with XGP. Chronic liver disease with resultant liver insufficiency is a recognized association.

The events initiating XGP remain obscure, however, the features commonly associated with XGP are pelvicalyceal obstruction, ulceration of the urothelium, collection of necrotic material and bacterial infection. Multiple theories exist as to the pathogenesis of XGP including abnormal lipid metabolism, lymphatic obstruction, an altered immune response, arterial insufficiency and venous occlusion with hemorrhage. Macroscopically, these kidneys are enlarged, with a thick capsule and obvious parenchymal destruction. The renal pelvis and calyces are typically dilated and there is loss of corticomedullary differentiation. Microscopically, there is a polymorphonuclear infiltrate and edema around the calyces. These sections classically demonstrate lipid-laiden macrophages – xanthoma cells. In more longstanding cases, granulation tissue is present with necrotic debris, bacteria and plasma cells.

As stated, the diagnosis of XGP is usually based on pathological assessment, most commonly made after nephrectomy, although clinical suspicion may result in its inclusion in the differential diagnosis. The patients will have leukocytosis, hematuria, and commonly elevated creatinine, which may fall after management of the diseased kidney. Urinalysis will demonstrate pyuria in 90% of specimens with a positive culture in 60–80% of cases. Ten percent of urine specimens have mixed growth. The most common organisms grown are *Proteus* spp. and *E. coli*, however, anaerobic microorganisms can be occasionally isolated. Cultures from immunocompromised patients with XGP can grow atypical organisms such as *Candida* spp. Urine cytology may demonstrate xanthoma cells if this investigation is requested as part of the work-up for a renal mass. Renal tissue and stone culture should be performed upon nephrectomy.

Definitive imaging of XGP is essential for optimal management. XGP has no specific sonographic features upon which to base a diagnosis (Figure 8.14a). CT is the most appropriate radiological investigation because it allows imaging of the primary lesion and surrounding structures. Typically, the CT findings demonstrate an enlarged reniform lesion that is poorly functioning (Figure 8.14b). The 'bear-paw' sign is a CT feature of XGP and should raise suspicion for the lesion. The dilated calyces and renal pelvis, thinned parenchyma, and perinephric inflammatory reaction account for this radiological sign. A renal pelvis that tightly surrounds a calculus without dilatation can also be seen on imaging (Figure 8.14c). MRI does not appear to add any additional information compared to CT scan for the imaging of XGP. It is important to define whether the surrounding structures are involved prior to surgical intervention.

The treatment of XGP varies according to the timing of diagnosis. If this is made after nephrectomy then subsequent management will involve maintaining urine sterility, determining underlying risks for urolithiasis and preventing further stone formation. Furthermore, preservation of renal function in the remaining contralateral renal unit is necessary. If the diagnosis of XGP is suspected prior to any surgery then adequate imaging is necessary in an attempt to rule out involvement of adjacent organs by the inflammatory reaction. Renocolic fistula, as a complication of XGP, is an uncommon but potential intraoperative finding and may occur in the absence of colonic symptoms. If extensive retroperitoneal involvement is evident then disobstruction of the urinary tract and 4–6 weeks of appropriate antibiotics may reduce this inflammation and allow for less problematic surgical intervention to be undertaken. Due to the often-present perinephric inflammatory reaction, the benefits of laparoscopic nephrectomy should not be extended to XGP.

In most cases it is not possible to exclude malignancy by non-invasive means prior to surgery. These patients must undergo appropriate preoperative assessment and preparation. Nephrectomy in the setting of XGP can be a technically challenging procedure. Often appropriate bowel preparation and splenectomy prophylaxis for left-sided lesions are required prior

to intervention. Occasionally, assistance from allied surgical disciplines, such as general and vascular surgical colleagues, may be advantageous. Cases of segmental XGP and XGP in children being successfully treated by conservative means have been reported. Removal of the obstructing calculus and administration of long-term antibiotics, or partial nephrectomy in segmental disease can possibly control XGP.

LOWER URINARY TRACT INFECTIONS

Infections of the lower urinary tract are frequent cause for patients to present to medical practitioners. Lower UTIs are those infections that involve the urinary structures below the level of the ureters. This includes the bladder, the prostate in the male, and the urethra. Urethritis generally results from a separate pathophysiological process when compared to standard UTIs and is not included in this section but epididymo-orchitis is discussed.

ACUTE BACTERIAL CYSTITIS

Cystitis is a non-specific term indicating inflammation of the urinary bladder (Table 8.7). Cystitis can be diagnosed on clinical, microbiological, endoscopic and histological criteria. Acute bacterial cystitis is a superficial infection of the bladder mucosa, usually diagnosed clinically, with microbiological confirmation.

Acute bacterial cystitis is one of the most common problems for which young sexually active women seek medical attention and accounts for considerable morbidity and healthcare costs. These infections, however, also remain a significant cause of morbidity for all age groups. At-risk groups for acute bacterial cystitis, as well as the most effective management strategies have been well defined. Uncomplicated cystitis is caused, most commonly, by a predictable group of organisms, particularly *E. coli* (70–90%). Other organisms commonly isolated include *S. saphrophyticus, K.*

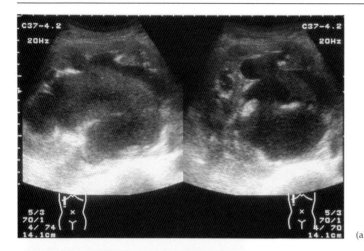

(a)

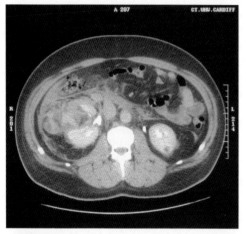

(b)

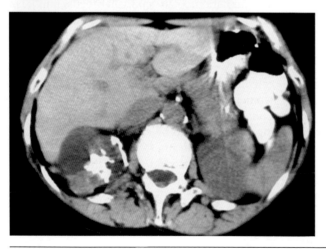

(c)

Figure 8.14

Xanthogranulomatous pyelonephritis (XPG). (a) Ultrasound scan showing distended calyceal system displaced by an underlying inflammatory mass. (b) Post contrast CT scan showing a focal heterogeneous inflammatory mass with extension into the perinephric space in a biopsy proven XPG with no renal calculi. (c) CT scan of a more typical XPG with a large renal calculus showing a small shrunken irregular kidney with focal calcification and an inflammatory mass.

Table 8.7 Atypical causes of cystitis and bladder pain

Iatrogenic	Infective	Inflammatory	Neoplastic	Other
Cyclophosphamide/ methotrexate	Tuberculous cystitis	Interstitial cystitis	Transitional cell caricinoma/ carcinoma in situ	Urethral diverticulum
Tioprofenic acid cystitis	Vaginitis	Eosinophilic cystitis	Gynecological malignancy	Detrusor instability
Radiation therapy	Malakoplakia	Endometriosis		
	Schistosomiasis	Stones – bladder/ distal ureteral		
	Viral – adenovirus			

pneumoniae, P. mirabilis, Group B streptococci, and *Enterococcus* spp. The type 1 mannose-sensitive pili are particularly important in adhesion of the *E. coli* to uroepithelial cells. These organisms remain susceptible to many oral antimicrobials, although resistance is increasing to some of the more commonly used agents.

Generally, patients with acute bacterial cystitis are diagnosed on the basis of classic presentation with symptoms of frequency, urgency, dysuria and suprapubic pain. Other symptoms including macroscopic hematuria, pyrexia, rigors and constitutional disturbance such as malaise may be present. In the elderly population less specific symptoms such as recent onset of confusion, newly diagnosed urge incontinence, offensive smelling urine, anorexia and nausea, and an acute failure to undertake the activities of daily living may be the only presenting signs and symptoms. Generally, cystitis in a male should be considered a complicated infection unless penetrative homosexual or heterosexual anal intercourse is practiced, or the female partner's vagina is known to be colonized with coliforms. Even in these circumstances it is prudent to exclude complicated infections in male patients presenting with lower UTIs.

Isolated acute bacterial cystitis, in most cases, is probably safe to treat without the need for specific urine cultures. Use of dipstick analysis, demonstrating pyuria (leukocyte esterase) and bacteriuria (nitrites), can suffice to confirm the clinical diagnosis of UTI. However, with a false-negative rate when used in combination of approximately 20%, a negative result does not exclude a UTI, and the opportunity to obtain a positive urine culture with appropriate antibiotic sensitivities may be lost. Recurrent infections, of any cause, do require quantitative and qualitative urine cultures to aid in the management strategy. A positive midstream urine culture for bacteria, with greater than 100 000 CFUs/ml of urine of a single isolate, pyuria (>10 white blood cells/mm^3), and no evidence of contamination (<10 epithelial cells/mm^3), is required for an unequivocal diagnosis of acute bacterial cystitis.

Radiological imaging of the urinary tract is generally not necessary in cases of uncomplicated bacterial cystitis in young, sexually active women. If the history is suggestive of functional or anatomical abnormalities then imaging may be undertaken as appropriate. Initial investigation, in these circumstances, should include an ultrasound scan of the urinary tract plus plain abdominal radiograph, once pregnancy is excluded (Figure 8.15). Determination of bladder emptying with a post-void residual volume is an important adjunctive investigational tool.

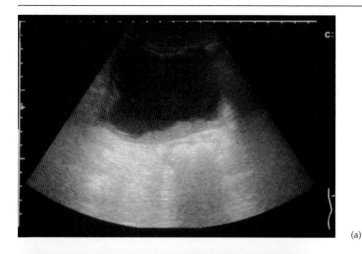

(a)

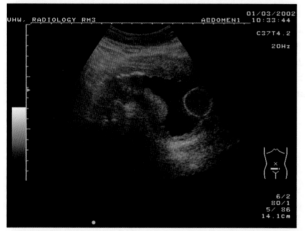

(b)

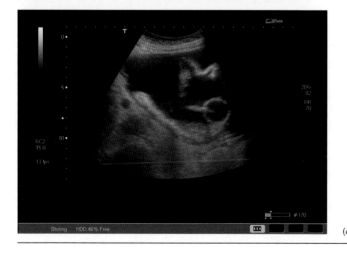

(c)

Figure 8.15

(a) Ultrasound scan of a bladder showing a thickened bladder trigone with debris in a patient presenting with acute cystitis. (b) Ultrasound scan of a bladder showing the whole bladder wall is thickened in a patient presenting with acute retention associated with acute cystitis. (c) Ultrasound scan of axial view of the bladder showing the whole bladder wall is thickened with irregular bladder mucosa in a patient presenting with hemorrhagic cystitis.

Published data suggest that a 3-day course of oral antibiotics, to which the isolated organism is sensitive, is more effective than a single-day regimen. The current standard of therapy for the empiric treatment of uncomplicated bacterial cystitis is trimethoprim-sulfamethoxazole, which appears more effective than β-lactams, regardless of the chosen duration of treatment. The better efficacy of trimethoprim-sulfamethoxazole is most likely related to its antimicrobial effect against *E. coli* in the rectum, urethra and vagina. Increasing resistance, in up to 20% of bacterial isolates, may be found towards this combination in certain regions. Although this regional resistance is quite variable, it does appear to be a generalized phenomenon increasing over time. Alternative antibiotic regimens, including nitrofurantoin (for 7 days), fluoroquinolones, or an oral third-generation cephalosporin may be a better choice in some regions with resistance in less than 10% of all isolates and less than 5% of *E. coli* in particular. Fluoroquinolones, with their low side-effect profile, convenient pharmacokinetics and high efficacy, are increasingly being prescribed as first-line therapy for uncomplicated cystitis. However, their increased use has resulted in an increasing incidence of fluoroquinolone-resistant uropathogens and judicious use is therefore recommended.

The problem with empiric antibiotic use arises in those patients who fail to respond to treatment, especially when the treatment has been based on urine dipstick analysis alone. For these patients no culture has been performed and accurate antibiotic sensitivities are not available. The added cost of treating these patients may be greater than the perceived savings with empiric treatment in the office setting. Of note the isolation of *K. pneumoniae*, and other uncommon bacteria, does increase the risk of antimicrobial treatment failure due to resistance.

Asymptomatic bacteriuria in elderly patients is not generally associated with increased morbidity and requires treatment only in select circumstances, such as high risk patients and those infected with *Proteus* spp. Those complicated infections diagnosed by quantitative urine cultures will require a longer course of antimicrobial therapy appropriate to the underlying pathology. Recurrent UTIs require exclusion of complicating factors prior to initiation of effective management strategies, such as topical estrogen therapy in post-menopausal women, antimicrobial uroprophylaxis, post-coital therapy, and self-start therapy. Antimicrobial uroprophylaxis appears is highly effective in preventing acute cystitis, and there does not appear to be tachyphylaxis with prolonged treatment periods in some studies with up to a 5-year follow-up.

PYOCYSTIS

Pyocystis is a suppurative bacterial infection, resulting in a contained collection of purulent material, in a poorly draining or defunctionalized bladder. It is a recognized complication of supravesical urinary diversion procedures, when the bladder is left in situ. Urinary diversion is performed to manage a variety of lower urinary tract pathologies, including intractable incontinence, interstitial cystitis, neuropathic bladder, chronic tuberculous cystitis, and radiation cystitis. The incidence of bladder infections and pyocystis in this group of patients ranges between 20 and 60% in selected series. This disease can also occur in anuric or oliguric haemodialysis patients although the incidence is much lower.

The diagnosis of pyocystis should be considered in any patient with a surgical history consistent with an intact but defunctionalized urinary bladder. The presentation can vary from a malodorous urethral discharge to being unwell with signs of sepsis, lower abdominal pain and tenderness, and possibly a palpable bladder. Investigation of these patients includes routine blood and bladder lavage cultures plus ultrasonography of the urinary tract, including the bladder (Figure 8.16). Exclusion of an

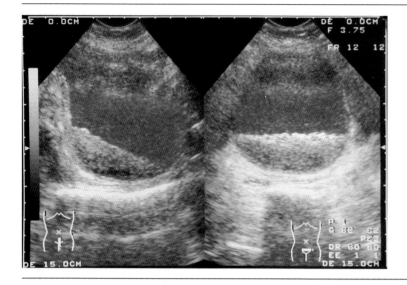

Figure 8.16

Ultrasound scan of a bladder showing the presence of increased echogenecity in a patient presenting with pyocystis.

infected bladder diverticulum, which is failing to drain, is important.

The acute treatment of pyocystis differs from acute bacterial cystitis in functioning bladders in that it requires catheterization with bladder irrigation, and enteral or parenteral, and often intravesical, antibiotic administration. Antibiotic therapy should initially be broad spectrum and than tailored to microbial culture and sensitivity. Bladder irrigation with diluted aqueous antiseptic solutions is also of value in the initial phase of treatment to rapidly reduce the intravesical bacterial burden. Most patients can usually be treated with conservative measures and do not require more definitive surgical treatment (Figure 8.17). Supportive therapy should be provided as the patient's clinical condition necessitates. Pyocystis, if undiagnosed can be life-threatening and result in severe sepsis and possibly death.

Long-term management of pyocystis if recurrent includes both conservative and surgical measures. A programme of self-administered bladder drainage and irrigation plus long-term antibiotics may prevent further recurrences of infection. With failure of conservative measures more definitive methods of treatment include transvaginal vesicostomy (iatrogenic vesicovaginostomy/vesicovaginal fistula), incorporating traditional and stapled techniques, and simple cystectomy. Transvaginal vesicostomy has been shown to fail in some patients requiring simple cystectomy as a salvage procedure.

EMPHYSEMATOUS CYSTITIS

Emphysematous cystitis (EC) is a rare, life-threatening, infective condition of the lower urinary tract in which pockets of gas are formed in and around the wall and lumen of the bladder by gas-forming organisms. It is a somewhat uncommon infective process in which early diagnosis and treatment play a key role in reducing the potentially high morbidity and mortality associated with this condition. It is most commonly caused by Gram-negative organisms such as *E. coli* and *Enterobacter aerogenes*, however, in rare circumstances other less common organisms can include *C. albicans, Clostridium perfringens* and other anaerobic bacteria. The gas found in EC is due to the conversion of glucose to carbon dioxide by bacteria. Commonly, underlying conditions such as diabetes mellitus

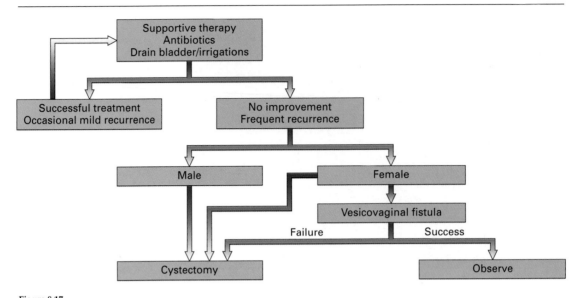

Figure 8.17

Treatment of pyocystis.

(50%) and glycosuria, chronic UTIs, prior treatment with broad-spectrum antibiotics, immunosuppression, bladder neuropathy, corticosteroid use, bladder outlet obstruction, chronic indwelling urinary catheters, and other debilitating medical conditions, predispose to this form of cystitis.

The spectrum of presenting features can range from a non-specific illness, cystitis-like signs and symptoms of irritative voiding and hematuria, to an acute abdomen with generalized life-threatening sepsis. Women are twice as likely to be diagnosed with EC compared with their male counterparts. A history of pneumaturia is highly suggestive, but is rarely offered by the patient without direct questioning. A degree of suspicion for this condition should be borne in mind in those patients known to be at risk, and in whom infective signs and symptoms do not settle promptly with conservative medical management.

Investigation of these patients involves routine microbiological culture of urine and blood.

Dipstick analysis of urine will generally show glycosuria, however, testing which is negative for glucose can be due to high bacterial consumption, even in poorly controlled diabetics. A plain abdominal radiograph may demonstrate gas in the bladder, bladder wall and possibly the perivesical tissues (Figures 8.18a). Ultrasonography will demonstrate the gas as hyperechogenicity, with potentially poor bladder emptying (Figure 8.18b). The most definitive radiological investigation is CT scan of the abdomen and pelvis. This will demonstrate the presence of gas within the wall and lumen of the bladder, plus identify the extravesicular extent of the disease. The identification of gas in the upper urinary tract and adrenal gland, in association with EC, heralds a poor prognosis. A plain abdominal radiograph is useful for follow-up imaging, as it will demonstrate the resolution of gas in the soft tissues of the pelvis. As the gas is carbon dioxide, prompt and effective treatment will result in quick clearance of the gas due to reabsorption. If cystoscopy is per-

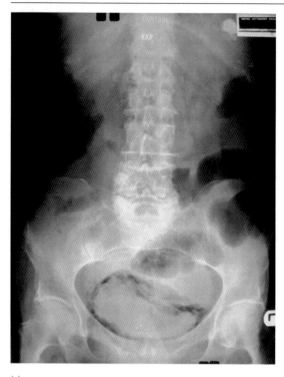

(a)

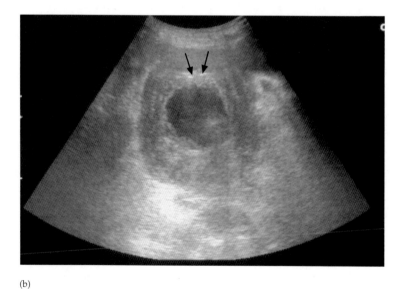

(b)

Figure 8.18

Emphysematous cystitis. (a) A plain film showing gas around the bladder. (b) Ultrasound scan showing a thick-walled bladder containing gas (arrowed).

formed the bladder will show a marked cystitis with hemorrhage and gas-filled vesicles arranged in clusters.

The foundation of treatment for patients with EC is prompt diagnosis and treatment of the underlying condition. Initial management of EC includes provision of appropriate physiological support and resuscitation as required, appropriate broad-spectrum antibiotic administration, establishment of urinary drainage, controlling underlying medical conditions such as diabetes, and exclusion of underlying pathology such as the presence of a bladder diverticulum or enterovesical and colovesical fistulas. Generally, most patients will respond to conservative medical therapy in the management of EC, however, non-responders may require surgical debridement, either as an endoscopic or open procedure. In rare cases of necrotizing cystitis, emergency cystectomy may be required.

ACUTE BACTERIAL PROSTATITIS

Acute bacterial prostatitis (ABP) is a well-described process characterized by infection of the entire prostate gland with typical uropathogens. It is considered as a separate pathological process to the chronic bacterial prostatitis and pelvic pain syndromes.

ABP arises from ascending infection or reflux of infected urine into the prostatic urethra and ducts. Uncommon causes are invasion of rectal bacteria directly into the prostate gland and hematogenous spread. Underlying bladder outlet obstruction with high voiding pressures is frequently associated. The common causative organisms are *E. coli*, *P. mirabilis*, *Klebsiella* spp., *Enterobacter* spp., *P. aeruginosa* and *Serratia* spp. *E. coli* strains that produce prostatitis tend to express the same virulence factors as those that cause uncomplicated acute pyelonephritis in females. Rarer organisms are *Gonococcus*, mycobacteria, *Chlamydia trachomatis*, *Candida* spp. and some parasitic infections can occur. Differentiation between simple bacterial cystitis in a male and APB should be based on clinical

findings as this alters the management strategies in these patients.

Patients with ABP generally present unwell with evidence of sepsis and possibly septic shock. The patient may describe dysuria, urgency and frequency with offensive urine. Pelvic, low back or perineal pain is a common association. Lower urinary tract symptoms suggestive of bladder outlet obstruction or complete urinary retention may be identified. On examination these patients will have signs of infection. Abdominal pain and suprapubic tenderness will often be present. It is also important to palpate for a distended bladder to exclude urinary retention. Digital rectal examination (DRE) should be performed with great care and will reveal an enlarged exquisitely tender prostate gland. Fluctuation on DRE is a clinical sign of prostatic abscess formation.

Patients with a diagnosis of ABP require standard urological investigations that should include midstream urine, blood cultures and urinary tract ultrasound (Figure 8.19). A positive urine culture should be identified in all antibiotic naive patients. With unresolved infections, further urine culture should be performed and antibiotic therapy tailored as appropriate. The serum prostate-specific antigen (PSA) may be acutely elevated and therefore acts as a surrogate acute phase marker. Serial monitoring of the PSA may be employed with a decreasing level indicative of resolution of inflammation with successful treatment. The aim of sonographic imaging is first, to ensure adequate bladder emptying, and second, to screen for upper urinary tract pathology in the setting of a lower UTI.

The treatment of acute bacterial prostatitis includes appropriate resuscitation in addition to the administration of broad-spectrum parenteral antibiotics to cover Gram-negative organisms. Atypical organisms should be suspected in those patients with chronic and immunosuppressive diseases such as diabetes mellitus and acquired immunodeficiency syndrome (AIDS). Antibiotic therapy requires prolonged high

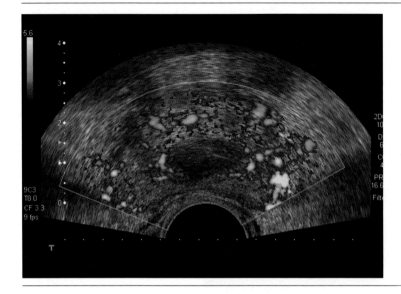

Figure 8.19

Acute prostatitis: ultrasound scan showing a periurethral low echogenic area with hyperemia on Doppler scan.

dosage to achieve adequate prostate parenchymal concentration, and careful monitoring to ensure bacterial eradication has been achieved. Intravenous antibiotics should be continued for at least 48 h after the patient becomes afebrile. In the presence of positive blood cultures prolongation of intravenous therapy is required. If there is a significant degree of urinary retention then a suprapubic urinary catheter should be placed to allow adequate bladder drainage. Insertion of a urethral indwelling catheter is not recommended for patients with urinary retention in the setting of ABP due to the increased risk of bacteremia at the time of catheter passage. Supportive therapy will include adequate hydration, analgesics and antipyretics, and stool softeners as required. If prompt improvement is not noted then further imaging should be performed to exclude prostatic abscess formation. Imaging modalities available are transrectal ultrasound (TRUS) and CT.

Oral antibiotics should be commenced once the patient is afebrile (>48 h) and voiding comfortably. The most appropriate oral antibiotics are the fluoroquinolones, and these should be continued for a total of 4 weeks. Ciprofloxacin is able to achieve high tissue levels in the acutely inflamed prostate and therapy for this prolonged period will significantly reduce the risk of progression to chronic prostatitis or the formation of a prostatic abscess. Alternative antibiotics include trimethoprim which is also able to achieve high tissue penetration, however, 6 weeks of therapy is recommended with this antibiotic. Accurate assessment of the male urinary tract, and diagnosis, with treatment as appropriate, of any underlying pathology is important to prevent recurrent disease.

PROSTATIC ABSCESS

A prostatic abscess is a suppurative infection with necrosis and cavitation of the prostatic parenchyma. Prostatic abscess formation is an uncommon condition with modern antibiotic prescribing. Generally, prostatic abscesses progress from untreated, inadequately treated, or severe acute bacterial prostatitis. Most patients diagnosed with ABP, however, are treated early in the course of their illness and progression to abscess formation is usually prevented. Other patients at increased risk of a prostatic abscess include diabetics, immuno-suppressed patients, those with chronic renal failure, and also those patients with a history of urethral instrumentation or chronic indwelling urethral catheters. These patients most commonly present between 50 and 70 years of age, however, any age group can be affected. Organisms commonly found in prostatic abscesses are *E. coli*, *S. aureus*, *P. aeruginosa*, *Klebsiella* spp. and occasionally obligate anaer-

obes. In the preantibiotic era *N. gonorrhoeae* was a common causative organism, although this would be considered rare today.

Prostatic abscesses can be difficult to diagnose with clinical assessment alone. The presenting signs and symptoms in patients with a prostatic abscess can vary from fulminant infection syndromes to a generally well patient with obstructive or irritative lower urinary tract symptoms. DRE will often demonstrate a tender enlarged

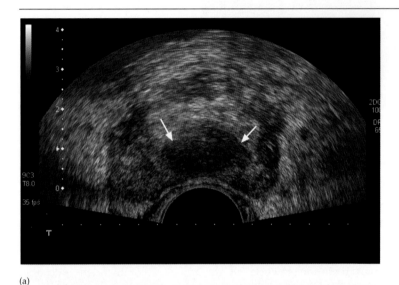

(a)

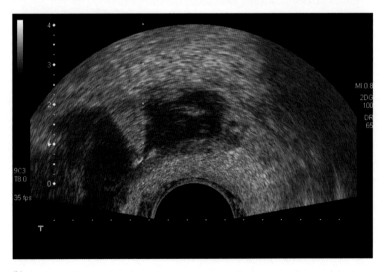

(b)

prostate gland with possibly a fluctuant region. Approximately 30% of patients will present in impending or acute urinary retention. Suspicion should be raised in any patient with a clinical diagnosis of acute bacterial prostatitis who fails to improve after adequate therapy thus necessitating further appropriate investigation.

Urine culture usually grows a single bacterial isolate infection, however, occasionally sterile pyuria is the sole finding. Collection of abscess fluid for Gram stain and culture and sensitivity including for *mycobacteria*, and fungal organisms such as *Candida* spp., *Histoplasma* and *Cryptococcus*, is warranted in atypical cases such as those patients with chronic disease and suppressed immunity. Imaging modalities include ultrasound imaging (Figure 8.20a,b), either transabdominally, or more appropriately transrectally (TRUS), and pelvic CT scan (Figure 8.20c,d). TRUS is the most sensitive investigation

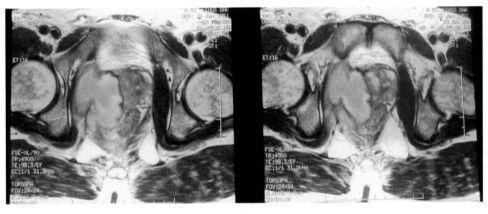

(c)

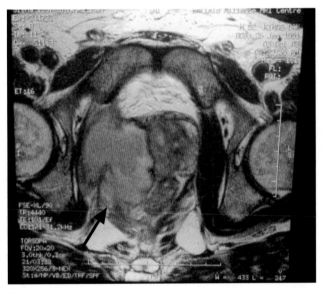

(d)

Figure 8.20

Ultrasound scan of the prostate in a patient with clinical evidence of prostatic abscess. (a) Axial view (abscess cavity arrowed). (b) Sagittal view showing a communication with extra prostatic collection arrowed. (c, d) MRI (anteroposterior and lateral views) showing a large prostatic abscess infiltrating the endopelvic fascia and obstructing the rectum. (Courtesy of Mr Faiz Mumtaz, Barnet and Chase Farm NHS Trust, Middlesex, UK.)

for diagnosing prostatic abscesses, however, patients will occasionally be unable to tolerate a transrectal probe without sedation or anesthetic, necessitating CT.

Treatment of a prostatic abscess is based upon adequate physiological support, broad-spectrum antimicrobial cover, and drainage of the abscess cavity as necessary. Conservative management of single small abscesses (<1 cm in diameter) has proved successful in select cases with close clinical and radiological follow-up. Various techniques of abscess drainage have been described including, transurethral unroofing, and transrectal or transperineal drainage under TRUS guidance (Figure 8.21). Generally, TRUS-guided aspiration of the abscess cavity, under antibiotic cover, has become the most commonly used first-line technique, and usually allows adequate drainage of most collections with very low morbidity. For larger abscess cavities and rare cases of emphysematous prostatic abscesses, transurethral unroofing with a resectoscope is advocated. Problems with the transurethral technique include the risk of anesthesia, increased bacteremia, incomplete

drainage of multiloculated collections or peripheral abscesses, and retrograde ejaculation.

Successful transrectal drainage of prostatic abscesses has been achieved under TRUS guidance, with infrequent recurrence, in many series. Follow-up TRUS imaging is recommended to follow resolution of disease and detect abscess recurrence. This allows repeat procedures to be performed if necessary, however, the recovery period may be prolonged in these cases. Fistula formation with transrectal drainage does not seem to be a recognized complication. For those patients in whom bladder outlet obstruction does not resolve after transrectal abscess resolution, transurethral resection of the prostate (TURP) may be performed.

In general both conservative and interventional management strategies are possible, with the technique used being based on individual case criteria. With chronic abscess formation sphincteric destruction with subsequent incontinence, after adequate treatment of the abscess, can occur. As with all severe UTIs, the identification and treatment of all underlying pathology is essential to reduce the risk of recurrence.

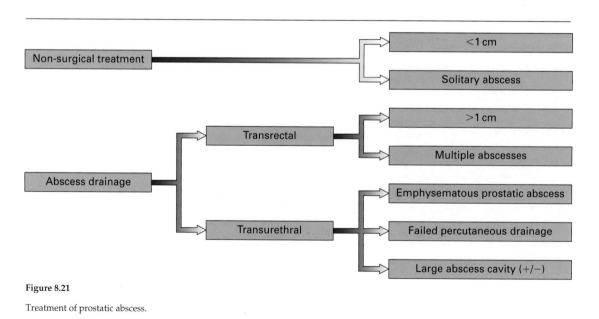

Figure 8.21

Treatment of prostatic abscess.

MALAKOPLAKIA

Malakoplakia is an uncommon benign granulo-matous inflammatory condition characterized, in the urogenital tract, by a chronic coliform bacteriuria. It can involve both urological and non-urological organs and means 'soft plaque'.

Malakoplakia is a disease process uncommonly diagnosed in the community. It affects female patients four times more commonly than men, with the typical diagnosis of genitourinary malakoplakia being in a woman >50 years of age. The etiology of malakoplakia is poorly understood. It is generally thought to arise as a result of defective macrophage liposome and micro-tubular assembly, resulting in dysfunctional intraphagosomal digestion of bacteria and therefore, an inability to overcome bacterial infection. Approximately a third of patients will have a systemic comorbidity such as immunosuppression, general debility or malignancy. The majority of patients with malakoplakia have involvement of the urinary tract (60–75%), with the bladder being involved in 40%, the kidneys in 15% and the ureters in approximately 10–11% of those diagnosed with genitourinary malakoplakia. Non-genitourinary sites include the gastrointestinal tract, the skin, lungs, bones, retroperitoneum and mesenteric lymph nodes. *E. coli* is the most common organism isolated in malakoplakia (80%), with *P. mirabilis* and *Klebsiella* spp. the other organisms likely to be cultured.

The diagnosis of malakoplakia is based on clinical, microbiological, radiological and histological features. Most patients present with a history of chronic UTI with malakoplakia diagnosed during investigations for associated signs and symptoms. Bladder malakoplakia usually presents with symptoms of cystitis such as dysuria and hematuria. Urine culture characterizes a coliform organism in most cases, irrespective of the extent of disease. Cystoscopy and subsequent bladder biopsy, when performed, will demonstrate the typical plaque lesions within the bladder. Macroscopically, these lesions are soft yellow-brown plaques with central umbilication and

ulceration. Peripheral hyperemia is also seen. Typical microscopic findings include von Hansemann's cells, which are lipid-laden macrophages with foamy eosinophilic cytoplasm. Michaelis-Gutmann bodies are intracellular and extracellular basophilic calculospheroles formed by the deposition of calcium phosphate crystals on a bacterial nidus, and are found upon histological sectioning of the lesions.

Ureteral involvement may be found incidentally during investigation of the patient with hematuria and infection or secondary to symptoms from ureteral obstruction. Ureteral and renal pelvic involvement is most commonly diagnosed in a patient with multiple filling defects or obstruction in the collecting system on IVU (Figure 8.22) or CT scan. As with bladder lesions, the urothelial lesions of the upper urinary tract may become enlarged and fungate or stricture causing obstruction and possibly loss of renal function. These patients can present with loin pain, and possibly a renal mass and sepsis. CT scan is the most appropriate form of imaging to confirm if the renal mass shows parenchymal involvement in these patients. Perinephric extension can be evident with imaging and also at the time of surgical exploration, but this is unusual. The differential diagnosis includes all causes of a reniform renal mass, including RCC, XGP and TCC.

The treatment and prognosis of malakoplakia is dependent on the extent of the disease and the response to conservative therapy. The extent can be defined by whether it involves the bladder in isolation or also the upper tracts and furthermore if the renal parenchyma is involved in a unilateral or bilateral distribution. The choice of antibiotic therapy in malakoplakia is based on the use of intracellular active agents such as trimethoprim, rifampicin and ciprofloxacin. Reports of the use of vitamin C and bethanechol as adjunct therapy have shown possible benefit. Vitamin C is felt to increase intracellular cAMP and bethanechol, a cholinergic agent, increases cGMP. Both these cyclic compounds are thought to be important in bacterial killing.

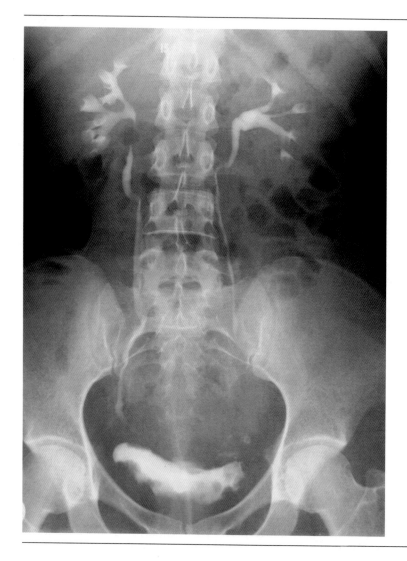

Figure 8.22

Intravenous urethrogram showing signs of Malakoplakia. (Courtesy of David Lloyd, University Hospital of Wales.)

In the treatment of bladder disease, control of the UTIs with long-term appropriate antibiotic therapy generally results in a resolution of symptoms and stabilization of the disease. Progression within the bladder may necessitate endoscopic surgical resection and more aggressive antibiotic therapy. Upper tract collecting system involvement, when unilateral and not involving the renal parenchyma, can usually be successfully treated with removal of any obstructing focus and control of infection with antibiotics.

With disease progression surgical intervention may be required. Cases of successful treatment with open partial ureterectomy and reimplantation have been reported for unilateral disease.

Renal parenchymal disease signifies a poorer outcome with medical management. Unilateral renal malakoplakia is generally best treated with an ipsilateral nephrectomy, however, up to 50% of patients with parenchymal disease will show bilateral involvement. The risk of subsequent contralateral renal involvement is rare but difficult to predict. Bilateral renal malakoplakia is a difficult condition to treat, with long-term antibiotics being advocated, and good disease control possible. However, a very high mortality rate is frequently reported in early series with bilateral renal parenchymal involvement, due to disease progression. Appropriate exclusion and definitive management of any urinary tract obstruction is essential. Overall, with widespread and multifocal disease the mortality from malakoplakia approaches 50% despite thorough medical and surgical therapy.

ACUTE EPIDIDYMO-ORCHITIS

Acute epididymitis is an inflammatory condition of the male epididymis, of less than 6 weeks duration, which can progress to involve the testicle – epididymo-orchitis (EO).

Acute EO is a clinical syndrome of inflammation, pain and epididymal swelling. The causes of EO can generally be classified into infective and non-infective. Infective causes of EO can be sexually transmitted or non-sexually transmitted. Non-bacterial infection can arise secondary to infection with mumps virus. Non-infective causes of EO include trauma, chemical causes and drugs such as amiodarone. Free reflux of sterile urine in young males is presumed to be a precipitant of chemical epididymitis, with patients usually being afebrile or having a low-grade temperature at presentation. Common risk factors of acute infective EO include urethritis, indwelling urethral catheters, prostatitis, urethral stricture disease and urinary tract instrumentation.

Two major groups of adult patients are at risk of acute bacterial epididymitis. First, younger men (<35 years) develop this condition, most commonly as a result of unprotected intercourse, resulting in a sexually transmitted disease (STD). In this group of patients symptoms of urethritis should be sought. STDs resulting in EO include *chlamydial* infection (*C. trachomatis*), gonorrhoea (*N. gonorrhoeae*), and occasionally infection with *U. urealyticum*. *C. trachomatis* is

estimated to be present in approximately 1% of males aged 18–35 years.

The second major group at risk includes older men with dysfunctional voiding, commonly due to bladder outlet obstruction. In this setting organisms ascend via the vas deferens or perideferential lymphatics, into the tail of the epididymis. A less significant cause of epididymitis (with the modern use of prophylactic antibiotics), is instrumentation of the lower urinary tract. The coliform organisms, including *E. coli*, are most commonly isolated in these last two settings. In homosexual males EO can be associated with both coliform infections and STDs (chlamydial and gonorrhoea). Other less common causes of acute EO include tuberculosis, BCG after intravesical therapy and systemic diseases such as cryptococcosis and brucellosis.

The clinical presentation of acute epididymitis is that of a gradual onset of unilateral epididymal pain and swelling. This may become more generalized and involve the ipsilateral testicle or hemiscrotum. Fevers, rigors and constitutional symptoms may be present in the more severely affected patients. Clinical examination reveals a swollen, tender epididymis and on occasion the spermatic cord, with possible involvement of the ipsilateral testicle. Elevation of the ipsilateral testicle and epididymis often provides symptomatic pain relief (Prehn's sign). Patients may complain of pyuria and urethral discharge, and furthermore, symptoms of acute prostatitis and cystitis may be evident. Historical information such as recent sexual contacts, lower urinary tract instrumentation, and premorbid lower urinary tract symptoms should be obtained. The differential diagnosis of unilateral hemiscrotal pain includes testicular torsion, testicular appendage torsion, orchitis (viral), trauma, malignancy, referred pain (T10), acute inguinal hernia, scrotal cellulitis and Fournier's gangrene. The exclusion of acute testicular torsion as a diagnosis in those patients presenting with unilateral orchalgia is essential.

Investigation of patients with acute EO is based on the history and clinical assessment, and targets the most likely cause of the infective episode. Urine culture for coliforms and *C. trachomatis* as required, should be obtained. Endourethral swabs for *N. gonorrhoeae* and *C. trachomatis*, and urine polymerase chain reaction (PCR) for chlamydial DNA amplification should be obtained in those patients at risk of genital infection from STDs. Ultrasonographic imaging of the scrotal contents is a routine investigation in the management of patients with EO (Figure 8.23a). Increased blood flow with enlargement of the epididymis is typically found. Duplex imaging, which includes echo color Doppler examination, is more sensitive than ultrasonography alone for revealing testicular inflammation (Figure 8.23b). Acute phase reactants such as erythrocyte sedimentation rate (ESR) and C-reactive protein are useful in monitoring resolu-

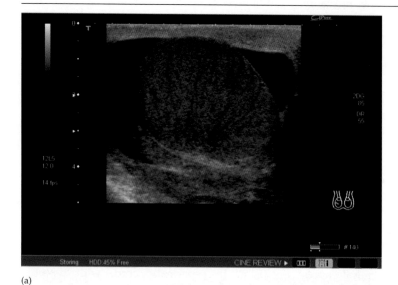

(a)

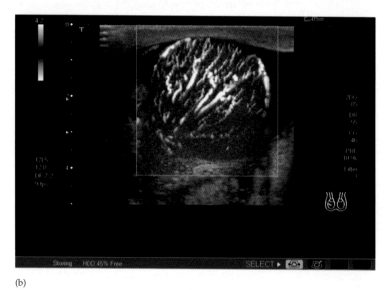

(b)

Figure 8.23

Acute epididymoorchitis. (a) Ultrasound scan showing enlarged oedematous testis with thickened reactive hydrocele. (b) Color Doppler showing hyperemic testis.

tion of inflammation. In those patients diagnosed with a coliform UTI, further investigation to exclude lower urinary tract pathology and voiding dysfunction is warranted. In those patients suspected of mumps orchitis appropriate serology should be obtained.

The aims of treatment for patients diagnosed with EO include symptomatic relief, eradication of infection, prevention of long-term complications, identification and treatment of predisposing factors, plus treatment of infected partners where appropriate. First-line therapy for EO includes scrotal support, analgesics, antipyretics, bed rest, and appropriate antibiotics. Broad-spectrum antibiotic therapy should be continued for approximately 2 weeks in total. Doxycycline to treat chlamydial infection, and Gram-negative cover with an oral agent such as ciprofloxacin or trimethoprim-sulfamethoxazole is appropriate. Parenteral antibiotic therapy may be required in those patients unable to tolerate oral therapy. Recently, azithromycin, a macrolide antibiotic, has been introduced as an alternative to doxycycline in the treatment of *C. trachomatis* infection due to its improved tolerability and ease of use. Proven or suspected gonorrhoeal infection should be treated with intramuscular ceftriaxone. Adjustments in antibiotic prescribing should be made according to the culture results and regional microbiological resistance profiles. When counseling patients with EO, it is important to outline the protracted time course for resolution of the swelling.

Complications secondary to acute EO include abscess formation, testicular infarction, chronic pain, infertility and chronic infection. Finally, thorough counseling and investigation of the partners of those patients with a proven or suspected STD is important to prevent reinfections and associated complications. Complications possible in female partners of patients with chlamydial infection include pelvic inflammatory disease, infertility, ectopic pregnancy, pelvic pain syndromes and perinatal infections in their children.

FUNGAL URINARY TRACT INFECTIONS

Fungal infections of the urinary tract are relatively uncommon in the acute outpatient and emergency department setting. However, up to 8% of nosocomial infections are caused by fungal organisms, 75% of which are, *Candida* spp. including *C. albicans*, *C. tropicalis* and *C. parapsilosis*. Other organisms causing fungal UTIs include *Aspergillus* and *Cryptococcus*, are essentially opportunistic.

Many factors increase the risk of developing a fungal UTI including diabetes mellitus, chronic illness, steroid use and other forms of immunosuppression including human immunodeficiency virus (HIV) infection, antibiotic use, multidrug therapies, urine flow turbulence, and other anatomical and functional abnormalities of the urinary tract including ileal conduits and neuropathy. In immunosuppressed patients sites predisposed to fungal infection including the prostate, epididymis and testicles, adrenal gland, kidney, distal urethra and bladder (Figure 8.24).

The clinical presentation of patients with fungal infections can be quite variable and ranges from an absence of symptoms to irritative voiding, dysuria, pyuria and hematuria, classic APN, oliguria and genital infection with balanitis. Appropriate urine microscopy with urine and blood cultures and consultation with a clinical microbiologist will identify the causative organisms. Imaging should be undertaken as indicated. IVU (Figure 8.25) and CT may identify filling defects in the bladder or upper urinary tract.

The management of fungal infections is first aimed at treating any underlying pathology, and second, at targeting the fungal organism with an appropriate antimicrobial agent. The most commonly used agents in the management of fungal infection include amphotericin B and fluconazole. Advice from a clinical microbiologist should be taken when considering administration of antifungal agents due to the lack of familiarity of most clinicians with their use and side effect profiles. Both these agents can be administered

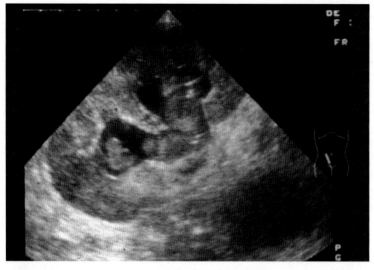

(a)

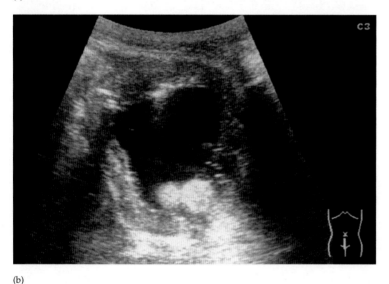

(b)

Figure 8.24

Fungal balls in a transplanted kidney in (a) calyces and (b) bladder.

intravenously. Fluconazole, a triazole, has the added advantage over amphotericin B in that it is available in an oral formulation. Oral fluconazole appears to be as efficacious as intravesical amphotericin B (which is highly nephrotoxic), for the treatment of mild candidal cystitis. Amphotericin B can also be delivered via urethral catheter and nephrostomy catheter irriga-tions (Table 8.8) for high urine concentrations and prolonged dwell times in those patients with significant funguria often with fungal ball disease. More invasive management of fungal ball disease of the upper urinary tract with percutaneous surgical procedures is occasionally necessary. The prognosis of critically ill patients with persistent funguria is generally poor.

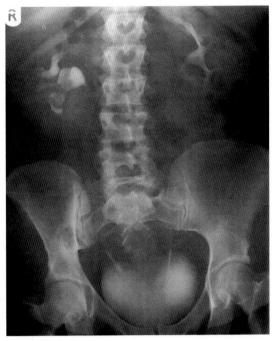

Figure 8.25

Intravenous urogram of a diabetic patient showing large fungal balls in the kidney.

Table 8.8 Amphotericin B irrigations in the management of funguria.

Bladder irrigation	Nephrostomy irrigation
50 mg/l of sterile water	50 mg/l of sterile water
Instill at 100 ml of solution	Instill at 40 ml of solution
per h over 10 h	per h over 24 h

FURTHER READING

Walsh PC, Retik AB, Darracott-Vaughan Jr E, Weing J (eds). *Campell's Urology* 8th edn. Philadelphia: Saunders, 2002.

GENERAL

De Man P, Jodal U, van Kooten C, Svanborg C. Bacterial adherence as a virulence factor in urinary tract infection. *APMIS* 1990; **98**: 1053–60.

Mulholland SG. Urinary tract infection. *Clin Geriatr Med* 1990; **6**: 43–53.

Walsh P et al. (eds) Campbell's Urology. 8th edition. Philadelphia: WB Saunders. Volume 1, Section 4, Chapters 14 and 15.

IMAGING

Berklund I, Truls E. Diagnosis and imaging in urinary tract infections. *Curr Opin Urol* 2002; **12**: 39–43.

Dalla-Palma L, Pozzi-Mucelli F, Ene V. Medical management of renal and perirenal abscesses: CT evaluation. *Clin Radiol* 1999; **54**: 792–7.

Herbener TE. Ultrasound in the assessment of the acute scrotum. *Clin Ultrasound* 1996; **24**: 405–21.

Kawashima A, Sander CM, Goldman SM, Raval BK, Fishman EK. CT of renal inflammatory disease. *Radiographics* 1997; **17**: 851–66.

Kawashima A, Sandler CM, Goldman SM. Current roles and controversies in the imaging evaluation of acute renal infection. *World J Urol* 1998; **16**: 9–17.

Kim JC. US and CT findings in xanthogranulomatous pyelonephritis. *J Clin Imaging* 2001; **25**: 118–21.

Thornbury JR. Acute renal infections. *Urol Radio* 1991; 12: 209–13.

Rabushka LS, Fishman EK, Goldman SM. Pictorial review: computed tomography of renal inflammatory disease. *Urology* 1994; **44**: 473–80.

Tiu CM, Chou YH, Chiou YH, et al. Sonographic features of xanthogranulomatous pyelonephritis. *J Clin Ultrasound* 2001; **29**: 279–85.

ACUTE PYELONEPHRITIS

Garrison J, Hooton TM. Fluoroquinolones in the treatment of acute uncomplicated urinary tract infections in adult women. *Expert Opin Pharmacother* 2001; **2**: 1227–37.

Nickel JC. The management of acute pyelonephritis in adults. *Canadian J Urol* 2001; **8** (Suppl 1): 29–38.

Roberts JA. Aetiology and pathophysiology of pyelonephritis. *Am J Kidney Dis* 1991; **17**: 1–9.

Roberts JA. Management of pyelonephritis and upper urinary tract infections. *Urol Clin N Am* 1999; **26**: 753–63.

Tenner SM, Yadven SM, Kimmel PL. Acute pyelonephritis. Preventing complications through prompt diagnosis and proper therapy. *Postgrad Med* 1992; **91**: 261–8.

Valiquette L. Urinary tract infections in women. *Canadian J Urol* 2001; **8** (Suppl 1): 6-12.

ACUTE LOBAR NEPHRONIA

Boam WD, Miser WF. Acute focal bacterial pyelonephritis. *Am Fam Physician* 1995; 52: 919–24.

RENAL AND PERINEPHRIC ABSCESS

Dembry LM, Andriole VT. Renal and perirenal abscesses. *Infect Dis Clin North Am* 1997; **11**: 663–80.

Yen DH, Hu SC, Tsai J, et al. Renal abscess: early diagnosis and treatment. *Am J Emerg Med* 1999; **17**: 192–7.

XANTHOGRANULOMATOUS PVELONEPHRITIS

Brown Jr PS, Dodson M, Weintrub PS. Xanthogranulomatous pyelonephritis: report of nonsurgical management of a case and review of the literature. *Clin Infect Dis* 1996; **22**: 308–14.

Mittal BV, Badhe BP. Xanthogranulomatous pyelonephritis – (a clinicopathological study of 15 cases). *J Postgrad Med* 1989; **35**: 209–14.

Osca JM, Piero MJ, Rodrigo M, Martinez-Jabaloyas JM, Jimenez-Cruz JF. Focal xanthogranulomatous pyelonephritis: partial nephrectomy as definitive treatment. *Eur Urol* 1997; **32**: 375–9.

BACTERIAL CYSTITIS

Echols RM, Tosiello RL, Haverstock TC, Tice AD. Demographic, clinical, and treatment parameters influencing the outcome of acute cystitis. *Clin Infect Dis* 1999; **29**: 113–19.

Gossius G, Vorland L. A randomized comparison of single-dose vs. three-day and ten-day therapy with trimethoprim-sulfamethoxazole for cystitis in women. *Scand J Infect Dis* 1984; **16**: 373–9.

Gupta K, Scholes D, Stamm WE. Increasing prevalence of antimicrobial resistance among uropathogens causing acute uncomplicated cystitis in women. *JAMA* 1999; **281**: 736–8.

Hooton TM, Running K, Stamm WE. Single-dose therapy for cystitis in women. A comparison of trimethoprim-sulfamethoxazole, amoxicillin, and cyclacillin. *JAMA* 1985; **253**: 387–90.

Hooton TM, Stamm WE. Management of acute uncomplicated urinary tract infection adults. *Med Clin N Am* 1991; **75**: 339–57.

Hooton TM, Stamm WE. Diagnosis and treatment of uncomplicated urinary tract infection. *Infect Dis Clin N Am* 1997; **11**: 551–81.

Hooton TM, Winter C, Tiu F, Stamm WE. Randomized comparative trial and cost analysis of 3-day antimicrobial regimens for treatment of acute cystitis in women. *JAMA* 1995; **273**: 41–5.

Orenstein R, Wong ES. Urinary tract infections in adults. *Am Fam Physician* 1999; **59**: 1225–34, 1237 review.

Ronald AR. Standards of therapy for urinary tract infections in adults. *Infection* 1992; **20** (Suppl 3) S164–70; discussion S175–80.

Stamm WE, McKevitt M, Roberts PL, White NJ. Natural history of recurrent urinary tract infections in women. *Reviews of Infectious Diseases* 1991; **13**: 77–84.

PROSTATITIS

Andreu A, Stapleton AE, Fennell C, et al. Urovirulence determinants in Escherichia coli strains causing prostatis. *J Infect Dis* 1997; **176**: 464–9.

Leigh DA. Prostatitis – an increasing clinical problem for diagnosis and management. *J Antimicrob Chemother* 1993; **32** (Suppl A): 1–9.

PROSTATIC ABSCESS

Bachor R, Gottfried HW, Hautmann R. Minimal invasive therapy of prostatic abscess by transrectal ultrasound-guided perineal drainage. *Eur Urol* 1995; **28**: 320-4.

Barozzi L, Pavlica P, Menchi I, De Matteis M, Canepari M. Prostatic abscess: diagnosis and treatment. *AJR AM J Roentgenol* 1998; **170**: 753–7.

Collado A, Palou J, Garcia-Penit J, et al. Ultrasound-guided needle aspiration in prostatic abscess. *Urology* 1999; **53**: 548–52.

Gan E. Transrectal ultrasound-guided needle aspirations for prostatic abscesses: an alternative to transurethral drainage? *Tech Urol* 2000; **6**: 178–84.

Granados EA, Riley SG, Salvador J, Vincente J. Prostatic abscess: diagnosis and treatment. *J Urol* 1992; **148**: 80–2.

Lim JW, Ko YT, Lee DH, et al. Treatment of prostatic abscess: value of transrectal ultrasonographically guided needle aspiration. *J Ultrasound Med* 2000; **19**: 609–17.

Ludwig M, Schroeder-Printzen I, Schiefer HG, Weidner W. Diagnosis and therapeutic management of 18 patients with prostatic abscessess. *Urology* 1999; **53**: 340–5.

Weinberger M, Cytron S, Servadio C, et al. Prostatic abscess in the antibiotic era. *Rev Infect Dis* 1988; **10**: 239–49.

PYOCYSTIS

Adeyoju AB, Thornhill J, Lynch T, et al. The fate of the defunctioned bladder following supravesical urinary diversion. *BJU* 1996; **78**: 80–3.

Adeyoju AB, Lynch TH, Thornhill JA. The defunctionalized bladder. *Int Urogynecol J Pelvic Floor Dysfunct* 1998; **9**: 48–51.

Doherty AP, Bellringer J. Stapled vaginal vesicostomy for pyocystis in the defunctioned female bladder. *BJU Int* 1999; **83**: 339–40.

Granados EA, Salvador J, Vicente J, Villavicencio H. Follow-up of the remaining bladder after supravesical diversion. *Eur Urol* 1996; **29**: 308–11.

Singh G, Wilkinson JM, Thomas DG. Supravesical diversion for incontinence: a long-term follow-up. *BJU* 1997; **79**: 348–53.

EMPHYSEMATOUS CYSTITIS

Katz DS, Askoy E, Cunha BA. Clostridium perfringens emphysematous cystitis. *Urology* 1993; **41**: 458–60.

O'Connor LA, De Guzman J. Emphysematous cystitis: a radiographic diagnosis. *J Am J Emerg Med* 2001; **19**: 211–13.

Quint HJ, Drach GW, Rappaport WD, Hoffmann CJ. Emphysematous cystitis; a review of the spectrum of disease. *J Urol* 1992; **147**: 134–7.

EPIDIDYMO-ORCHITIS

Dale AW, et al. management of epididymo-orchitis in Genitourinary Medicine clinics in the United Kingdom's North Thames region 2000. *Int J STD AIDS* 2001; **12**: 342–5.

Horner PJ. European guideline for the management of epididymo-orchitis and syndromic management of acute scrotal swelling. *Int J STD AIDS* 2001; **12** (Suppl 3): 88–93.

Templeton K, Roberts J, Jeffries D, Forster G, Aitken C. The detection of Chlamydia trachomatis by DNA amplification methods in urine samples from men with urethritis. *Int J STD AIDS* 2001; **12**: 793–6.

9. Penile trauma

Faiz Mumtaz, Giles Hellawell and David Ralph

Penile injuries can be classified as blunt, penetrating or ischemic. The most common presentation is a blunt injury of the erect penis leading to a fracture of the cavernous bodies. Penetrating trauma which can be the result of self penile amputation, animal or human bites, missile and zipper injuries are seen less frequently. Rarely, ischemic injuries can result from a penile prosthesis, priapism, corporeal injections of pharmacotherapeutic agents, diabetes and chronic dialysis. Severe penile injuries are uncommon, with approximately one to two cases reported per annum in large centers.

The management of penile injuries attracts considerable controversy due to the lack of clear guidelines in the literature. However, as the reluctance of patients to report such injuries appears to be decreasing and with the increased publication of such cases a more informed description of management has been developed. The aim of this chapter is to discuss the presentation and provide guidelines for management of various forms of penile trauma.

BLUNT TRAUMA

PENILE FRACTURE

ETIOLOGY AND PRESENTATION

In the West, the most common blunt injury to the penis is a fracture of the tumescent shaft during vaginal penetration. It is often caused by the erect penis striking against the symphysis or perineum after the penis has slipped out of the vagina usually in the woman-on-top position. In the Middle East and Mediterranean regions fractures of the penis are predominantly due to masturbation. The fracture is commonly seen as a tear in the ventral or lateral aspect of the tunica albuginea of the penis. During erection, the intracavernous pressure may exceed 150 mmHg when the normally resilient tunica albuginea decreases in thickness from 2 mm to 0.25 mm. This thinning of the tunica albuginea puts the cavernous bodies at risk of blunt trauma. In addition, structural abnormalities of the tunica albuginea may alter the elasticity of the cavernous bodies which may further increase the risk of penile rupture.

Patients typically present acutely with a history of a snapping or popping sound accompanied by sharp pain and rapid detumescence following blunt trauma to an erect penis. Clinical findings include penile swelling, deformity and ecchymosis which produces the 'aubergine sign' that is highly diagnostic for this injury (Figure 9.1). Additional features are the 'rolling sign' in which a clot at the fracture site can be palpated as a firm, immobile lump over which the penile skin can be rolled. Coexistence of urethral injuries may cause hematuria and tearing of Buck's fascia permits extravasation of blood into the scrotum and pubic areas. This may present with the characteristic 'butterfly sign' in the perineum.

The diagnosis of penile fracture relies almost entirely upon clinical findings. The site of fracture can often be identified on physical examination by a palpable defect in the tunica albuginea. Cavernosography can also accurately diagnose and localize the fracture site, but it is rarely used as it is time consuming, invasive, difficult to interpret and there is potential to induce infection. Ultrasonography has a limited role as negative results do not exclude a rupture. However, a good ultrasound can usually identify the site of the fracture and allows the site of repair to be decided. Although magnetic resonance imaging has been used, its benefit is limited to the rare cases with an atypical presentation. Urethral and corporal damage is best

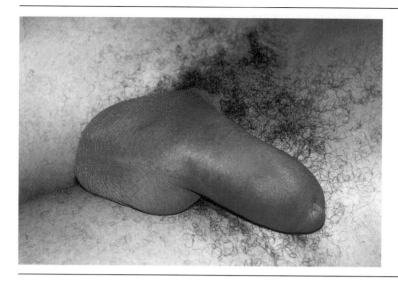

Figure 9.1

A swollen and a bruised penile shaft following fracture of the penis.

identified by intraoperative urethral and corporeal saline injections, which can accurately delineate the damage.[2] Reliance upon preoperative urethrography may result in false-negative urethrograms and, hence, does not preclude the need to assess the urethra peroperatively. The frequency of urethral injuries associated with blunt penile trauma varies from 1–3% in the Middle East to 20–30% in the West. This difference is attributed to the preponderance of coitus-related penile injuries in the West that are associated with a higher force of penile manipulation.

MANAGEMENT

Previously, treatment of penile fracture consisted of conservative measures such as penile splints and compression bandages. Such simple measures were associated with significant complications that included Peyronie's-like plaques, penile bend, impotence and arteriovenous fistulas. In contrast, contemporary management involving prompt exploration with surgical repair has shown better results. Surgical repair uses a variety of penile incisions that provide access to the cavernous bodies. These include a degloving incision, a direct longitudinal incision, and a midline high scrotal raphe incision.

The degloving incision provides the best access to the three corpora and permits easy repair of urethral injuries. The incision site is also dependent on the site of fracture. Catheterization may also aid localization of the fracture site in the presence of hematuria. Intraoperative saline cavernous injection can also be used to confirm the location of a laceration and to ensure no leaks occur post repair. Injuries are repaired with either nylon suture with a buried knot or an absorbable suture of high tensile strength; both have equal efficacy. A circumcision may be required to decrease the amount of postoperative edema and it ensures exposure of the suture sites thus allowing hematoma drainage and decreasing risk of infection. Following repair, consider the use of antiandrogens to suppress erections postoperatively especially if a urethral injury has been repaired. However, their routine use is controversial, as there may be a psychological benefit of subsequent erections in patients concerned about impotence due to the injury.

COMPLICATIONS

There are few reports of infection following uncomplicated penile fracture but with urethral rupture the risk of infection increases considerably and hence antibiotic prophylaxis is indicated. Fibrosis at the site of trauma may lead to painful erections, pain during intercourse and erectile dysfunction similar to Peyronie's disease. The complication rate with conservative management tends to be higher (ranging from 10 to 53%). Thus, surgical degloving and prompt repair represents standard care.

PENETRATING TRAUMA

AMPUTATION

Today, genital self-mutilation remains the most common cause of penile amputation. Other causes include accidental and iatrogenically induced amputations. An epidemic of penile amputations was reported in Thailand in the 1970s when women amputated the genitalia of their unfaithful husbands. This experience provided the key principles involved in the replantation of the penis.

SELF-INFLICTED PENILE AMPUTATION (FIGURE 9.2)

The majority of patients with self-inflicted penile amputation are acutely psychotic at the time of injury and nearly all have a history of psychiatric illness. Thus, the psychological condition or degree of intoxication of the patient may substantially delay the initial presentation of such cases. However, regardless of late presentation or active psychosis, all patients with amputated genitals should be considered for repair. Therefore, immediate resuscitation of the patient is warranted as significant blood loss may have occurred prior to presentation. Coexisting injuries may exist, especially in the psychotic patient and drug overdose must always be suspected. The acutely psychotic patient may require sedation and early psychiatric assessment should always be sought. The two most commonly recognized psychiatric conditions are schizophrenia (51%) and depression (19%). However, a significant group who mainly have personality disorders or transsexual concerns have also been described. This latter group represent the more difficult group to treat as ambivalence towards their injury makes management following surgery problematic. Importantly, further attempts at amputation following repair have been observed even after appropriate psychiatric treatment, thus emphasizing the need for continued psychiatric support.

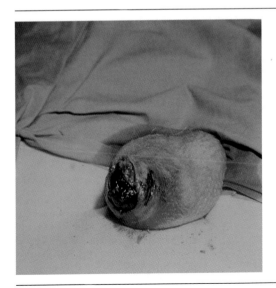

Figure 9.2

Complete avulsion of the penis.

PENILE REPLANTATION

The severed penis is thoroughly cleansed in a sterile saline solution following retrieval. It is then wrapped in saline-soaked gauze and placed in a sterile bag which is immersed in iced water to maintain hypothermic conditions. This important procedure minimizes warm ischemic time which allows replantation to be performed within 24 h. A pressure dressing or tourniquet should be applied to the proximal stump and the patient transferred to a unit that can provide microsurgical expertise.

An understanding of the penile blood supply is essential for successful revascularization of the amputated penis. Briefly, the arterial blood supply to the penis is derived from the common penile artery, a branch of the internal pudendal artery just distal to Alcock's canal. This artery divides within the corpus cavernosum to become the deep cavernosal arteries and the superficial dorsal penile arteries (Figure 9.3). The repair commences with the dorsal arteries followed by the dorsal vein, tunica albuginea and urethra, the nerves being the last to be repaired. Since the cavernosal arteries are small, revascularization is best performed using the larger dorsal arteries. This reconstruction uses microsurgical techniques to achieve higher rates of penile viability and erectile function. Vascular anastomoses is performed using 9/0–11/0 non-absorbable suture. In contrast, microsurgical repair of the dorsal nerve (with 11/0 non-absorbable suture) has not consistently improved erectile function. Urethral continuity is restored with a 5/0 or 6/0 absorbable suture prior to reanastamosis of the corporal spongiosum with similar sutures. The fascia and skin are closed and a urethral and suprapubic

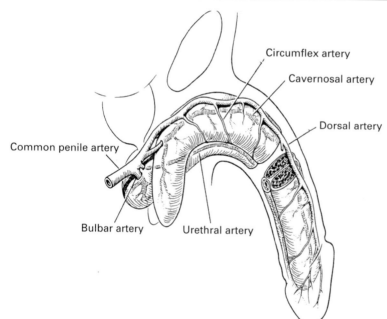

Circumflex artery

Cavernosal artery

Dorsal artery

Common penile artery

Bulbar artery   Urethral artery

Figure 9.3

Distribution of the common penile artery – the arterial supply to the deep structures of the penis. (Reproduced with permission from *Men's Health*, second edition. Kirby et al. (eds). London: Martin Dunitz, 2004.)

catheter placed until recovery is complete. A penile implant may need to be inserted for the treatment of erectile dysfunction at a later date.

PENILE RECONSTRUCTION

Loss of the amputated penis or excessive time delay to replantation may require reconstruction using microsurgical free flap techniques. Tubularized pedicle grafts have been described for penile reconstruction since the 1930s, but the advent of microsurgical techniques has permitted the creation of a useable penile using forearm flaps. The radial forearm flap described by Chang is now the standard for penile reconstruction. This method can be a one or two stage procedure and arterial anastamosis may be achieved using either the inferior epigastric artery or by saphenous interposition grafts to the femoral artery. Venous drainage to saphenous grafts is made and sensory innervation achieved by anastamosis of the ilioinguinal nerve with the cutaneous nerves of the forearm (Figure 9.4).

The majority of reports on the outcome of penile reconstruction come from transsexual surgical operations. These have identified sig-nificant long-term urethral complications such as urethrocutaneous fistulas and stricture formation. Complication rates tend to be higher in cases associated with urethral damage. Once the normal sensation is restored insertion of penile prostheses can be considered. However, long-term outcome of sexual satisfaction is variable.

ACCIDENTAL AMPUTATION

Accidental amputation injuries of the penis are very rare. Reports describe farm accidents, animal or human bites, vehicle accidents or war injuries as the main causes. The principles of surgical management are similar to those following self-penile amputation. In addition, however, meticulous debridement and the use of broad-spectrum antibiotics are necessary following accidental amputation injuries. Extensive penile skin loss may necessitate the use of skin grafts, which should be of full thickness to permit expansion of the penis during erection.

IATROGENIC AMPUTATION

The main cause of iatrogenic penile amputation is circumcision, particularly in children because

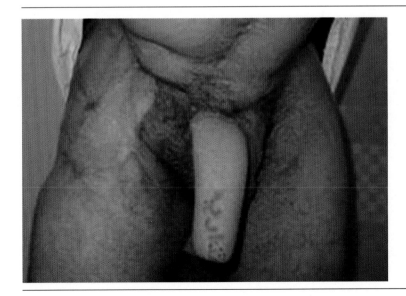

Figure 9.4

Phalloplasty following a total loss in a farm accident.

of the inappropriate use of electrocautery. The extensive sloughing of the penis complicates such injuries, which makes replantation a non-realistic option. Reconstruction usually involves the difficult and controversial decision of sex reassignment, which is associated with poor psychological outcome especially after the age of 2 years. Penile reconstruction has, however, been undertaken in older children using the techniques already described with encouraging results.

BITE INJURIES

These injuries are primarily caused by dog bites and most wounds are minor with few victims seeking medical assistance (Figure 9.5). In all cases the wound is thoroughly cleaned and debrided when indicated. Subsequently, the wound is best closed primarily under antibiotic cover. A partial penectomy may be an option when complete avulsion of the genitalia has occurred (Figure 9.6). A sex reassignment surgery is not usually required. The patients with urethral injury may have poor outcome as a result of urethral stricture and fistula formation. The additional trauma sustained to tissues,

as well as the increased risk of tissue contamination from bite injuries combine to increase the risk of both short- and long-term complications.

The most common pathogens associated with dog and cat bites are the *Pasteurella* spp., followed by anaerobic organisms. The most appropriate antibiotics for these injuries are amoxicillin and a β-lactamase inhibitor. The tetanus immunization status of the patient should be ascertained and where indicated tetanus immunoglobin and toxoid should be given. The risk of rabies can be determined from observing the behaviour of the animal – in certain countries rabies infection is endemic in the domestic animal population and prophylaxis is required. The incubation period may be 9–90 days and hence prophylactic measures can be taken even months after a bite. The vaccine involves a series of six inoculations and is given with intramuscular and local infiltration of rabies immunoglobulin.

PENOSCROTAL INJURIES

The traumatic laceration injuries described so far may include partial or complete loss of scrotal skin with testicular injury. The same general

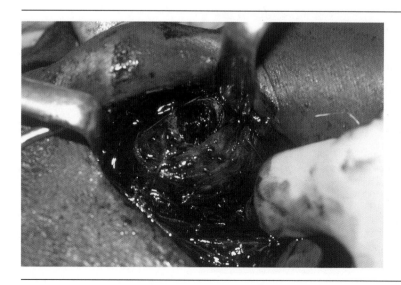

Figure 9.5

Partial penectomy following an animal bite.

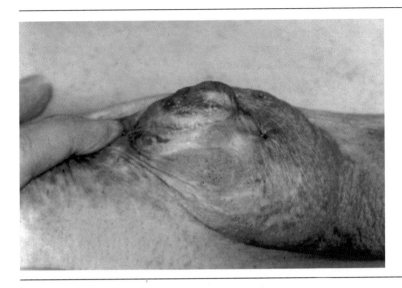

Figure 9.6

Final appearance of the penis following partial penectomy and reconstruction.

principles of treatment apply: appropriate resuscitation of the patient, thorough irrigation of the wound and removal of devitalized tissue. Complete loss of the scrotal skin may initially be managed with daily applications of saline dressings until skin grafts are possible onto the granulating scrotum. Local skin flap mobilization is possible and if repositioning of the testis is undertaken prior to scrotal reconstruction, the testes can be anchored in place and placed in a bile bag until granulation tissue appears. Thorough debridement with removal of contaminating materials and appropriate broad-spectrum antibiotic prophylaxis is necessary to minimize infection.

PENILE SKIN EMERGENCIES

The loss of penile skin due to degloving injuries can initially be addressed by burying the denuded penis into the scrotum. Subsequent skin grafting will be necessary and, as previously described, these should be of full thickness to prevent pain and discomfort during erections.

Fournier's gangrene is a form of necrotizing fasciitis that usually begins in the scrotum or penis and rapidly spreads along fascial planes to encompass the entire perineum and abdominal wall. The onset of symptoms may occur over 3–5 days and the patient presents with fever and malaise. On examination there is pathognomonic blistering of the genital skin with a cellulitic area with yellow-brown fluid. Progression of infection occurs rapidly and gangrenous sloughing rapidly ensues. The spectrum of microbes involved is wide with Gram-positive cocci, Gram-negative rods and anaerobes often implicated. Patients may often be immunosuppressed with a history of diabetes or alcoholism.

Prompt treatment is required with extensive debridement, broad-spectrum antibiotics and meticulous wound care prior to delayed skin grafting. Despite adequate treatment, this infection still has significant mortality approaching 50% and hence early diagnosis and treatment are essential.

Sensitivity to applied medications, lubricants or contraceptives may lead to severe allergic contact dermatitis. Severe cases may require systemic corticosteroids and identification of the allergen to avoid subsequent responses. Immediate IgE-mediated hypersensitivity to natural rubber latex has been reported and may result in life-threatening anaphylaxis.

PENILE AND SCROTAL BURNS

Thermal burns to the penis and perineum are usually the result of fire and to a lesser extent from boiling liquids. They rarely occur in isolation and usually in association with extensive burns that generally exceed 40% of the total body surface area. Isolated burns to the penis are rare and are usually the result of assault or child abuse. Scrotal burns are mostly first- and second-degree burns whereas penile burns tend to be full thickness burns as the penile shaft skin is thin.

Initial evaluation includes complete physical examination, laboratory evaluation, tetanus prophylaxis, intravenous antibiotics and estimation of the overall extent and depth of the burn.

Immediate management consists of aggressive fluid and electrolyte resuscitation. Diversion of urine by either urethral or suprapubic catheterization is performed to prevent urinary retention and monitor urine output. Urethral catheterization, although usually appropriate may not be desirable in patients with full thickness of the glans penis. To avoid pressure necrosis of the anterior urethra, suprapubic catheterization is recommended.

All non-viable penile tissue should be removed by prompt skin debridement and immediately replaced by primary skin grafts. This immediate intervention reduces the risk of infection, shortens recovery time and hospital stay and also prevents delayed scar contracture. However, burns to the glans penis should not be debrided and grafted unless obviously necrotic. The burnt glans penis usually heals satisfactorily with time.

SUSPENSORY LIGAMENT INJURY

Injury to the suspensory ligament of the penis is more common than fracture of the penis. It results during a forced ventral manipulation of the penis in a position with the woman on top and leaning back. Although, there is usually no crack heard and no sign of bruising is noted, the penis is extremely painful. Interestingly, following injury to the suspensory ligaments the penis remains erect. However, it can lead to chronic painful erections, penile instability and penile torsion, and as a result, complete lack of sexual activity. The diagnosis is made on the basis of a palpable defect in the base of the penis. The treatment includes an urgent surgical repair with 3/0 Ethilon suture.

PEDIATRIC PENILE TRAUMA

Please see chapter 11 (Pediatric Urological Trauma).

PRIAPISM

Priapism is a rare urological emergency that is defined as the presence of a prolonged penile erection lasting for >6 h and not accompanied by sexual desire or stimulation. Priapism can be primary or idiopathic (40% of cases) or secondary to various causative factors (Table 9.1). Although, priapism can occur at any age it mainly occurs in two age groups: in children 5–10 years old where the etiology is sickle cell disease or hematological malignancies and in those between 20 and 50 years of age where the cause is unknown. Priapism tends to occur at night or after prolonged sexual activity when the cavernosal smooth muscle is maximally relaxed. Most cases involve the full length of the corpora cavernosa, while the corpora spongiosum and glans remain flaccid. Two types of priapism are recognized: a low-flow and a high-flow priapism. The episodes may be minor lasting less than 3 h or major lasting 12–24 h. The latter is associated with significant morbidity. Most cases are of the low-flow type; high flow priapism is exceptionally rare.

Table 9.1 Etiology of priapism

Primary	Idiopathic	
Secondary	Hematological	Sickle cell disease, leukemia, lymphoma, thalassemia, myeloma
	Neurogenic	Spinal cord injury or lesions, cauda equina compression syndrome
	Neoplastic	renal, bladder, prostate, lung, melanoma
	Traumatic	Genital/perineal
	Iatrogenic	Intracavernosal injections of papaverine
	Infections	Malaria, rabies, scorpion bites
Medications	Antipsychotics	Chlorpromazine, thioridazine, trifluperazine, haloperidol
	Antidepressants	Fluoxetine, sertraline, trazodone
	Anticoagulants	Heparin
	Recreational drugs	Cocaine, alcohol abuse
	Total parenteral nutrition	Intralipid

The management of priapism depends upon the type and the underlying contributing pathology.

LOW-FLOW PRIAPISM

PATHOPHYSIOLOGY

Low-flow priapism can be further classified as acute, intermittent (stuttering) and chronic. In acute low-flow priapism the corpora are usually fully rigid as a result of the sludging of blood. A history of cavernosal self-injection, hematological disorders or specific medications associated with a painful erection permit the rapid identification of low-flow priapism. Prolonged veno-occlusion due to the causes listed in Table 9.1 results in anoxia and edema of the cavernosal trabeculae as illustrated in Figure 9.7. The resultant increase in intracavernosal pressure leads to further anoxia, smooth muscle necrosis with eventual scarring and fibrosis of the corpora. Even with prompt diagnosis and management the long-term potency rates may only be 50%.

Sickle cell disease is the main hematological disease associated with low-flow priapism and is the most common cause of priapism in children. Priapism results from sickling of red cells within the sinusoidal spaces during normal erection. A large study of boys with sickle cell disease reported the incidence of priapism as 18–27% and a distinct lack of parental knowledge of this complication.

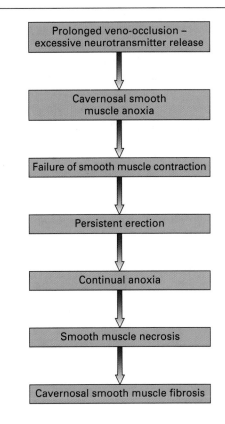

Figure 9.7

Pathophysiology of low-flow priapism.

Intracavernosal injections of vasoactive drugs for the treatment of impotence are a major cause of low-flow priapism. The risk of priapism with the initial diagnostic use of papaverine is higher (5%) compared to when used therapeutically (0.4%). The use of prostaglandin E_1 is associated with a much lower risk of priapism (<1%) and the transurethral form of the drug appears to have an even lower risk (<0.1%). Sildenafil, now widely used in the treatment of impotence, has been rarely reported to be associated with priapism. Priapism occurs in a small percentage of patients taking oral antihypertensive agents (e.g. hydralazine, guanethidine and prazosin) and antipsychotic drugs such as chlorpromazine. Cessation of heparin therapy (e.g. patients on hemodialysis) may result in a hypercoagulable state that may also lead to priapism.

Direct or metastatic malignant infiltration by bladder or prostate cancer may result in priapism, possibly through obstruction to venous drainage. Treatment is directed at controlling the relevant primary disease. Neurological disorders (Table 9.1) are a rare cause of priapism. Surgical spinal decompression has been recommended to alleviate priapism associated with lumbar spinal stenosis.

Although perineal trauma commonly results in high-flow priapism, low-flow priapism due to venous compression secondary to penile hematoma or edema is also recognized. Intermittent or stuttering priapism, an uncommon condition, is described as recurring periods of nocturnal prolonged erections usually associated with hemoglobinopathies. These were first reported in a group of Jamaican patients homozygous for the sickle cell trait. The recurrent nature of stuttering priapism has been suggested to be a result of disequilibrium between arterial inflow and venous outflow, but the underlying pathophysiology is still unclear.

MANAGEMENT

The aim of treatment is to initiate rapid detumescence, relief of pain and preservation of potency. Early diagnosis and treatment reduces the risk of fibrosis and erectile dysfunction, which are directly related to the duration of priapism. A detailed history should be taken particularly when addressing the risk factors described above to distinguish between low- and high-flow priapism. Table 9.2 highlights the distinguishing features of the two types of priapism.

A cavernosal blood gas measurement is helpful to distinguish between high-flow (arterial blood) and low-flow (venous blood) priapism. Color flow Doppler ultrasonography is currently the imaging investigation of choice (Figure 9.8).

Initial management within the first 24 h consists of increased exercise and corporeal aspiration of 20–50 ml of blood using a 19–21 gauge butterfly needle and irrigation with heparinized saline. If this simple measure fails to cause satisfactory detumescence intracorporeal injection

---

Table 9.2 Distinguishing features of low- and high-flow priapism

	Low-flow priapism	High-flow priapism
Frequency	High	Low
Etiology	Multiple	Trauma
Pathophysiology	Obstruction of corporeal blood flow	Arteriolacunar fistula
Symptoms	Painful	Mild discomfort
Aspiration	Thick and dark	Bright red
	Low P_{O_2}	P_{O_2} 12 kPa
	Acidic pH	pH 7.4
Doppler scan	Low/no arterial flow	High arterial flow
Treatment	Urgent	Deferred

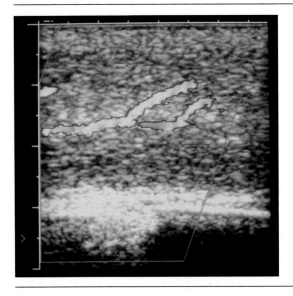

Figure 9.8

Color Doppler demonstrating high-flow in penis in a patient with priapism.

of an α-adrenergic agonist is indicated. A tourniquet is placed at the base of the penis and one of the following α-adrenergic agonists is used:

- Phenylephrine: 10 mg (1 ml) vial diluted to 10 ml with saline. 0.5 mg (0.5 ml) doses injected to a maximum of 2.5 mg (2.5 ml)
- Epinephrine and lignocaine (lidocaine) mixtures: 0.5% or 1% lignocaine with 1:20 000 (5 mg/ml) epinephrine. 1 ml given and repeated once if necessary.
- Ephedrine: 30 mg in 1 ml vial. 15 mg (0.5 ml) given and repeated once if necessary.

It is essential that blood pressure and pulse are monitored continuously. Furthermore, exercise extreme caution in patients with coronary heart disease, uncontrolled hypertension or cerebral ischemia and those taking monoamine oxidase inhibitors. Supportive measures can be used at the same time and include narcotic analgesics, hypotensive agents and intravenous ketamine. Ketamine has been reported to achieve up to 50% successful detumescence in early cases and avoids the need for more invasive procedures. By its non-specific inhibition of cyclic GMP, intracavernosal injection of methylene blue (50 mg) has been used as an alternative to α-adrenergic receptor agonists for the treatment of low-flow priapism. Transient penile burning and blue discoloration are the reported side effects.

Specific treatments for sickle cell disease include rehydration, oxygenation, alkalinization and exchange transfusion to reduce intra-corporeal acidosis and hence sludging. Etilefrine is an oral α-adrenoceptor agonist that in the form of maintenance therapy may help prevent further attacks, with little effect on the systemic blood pressure.

These measures are successful in up to 70% of cases but corporeal surgery may be required if these techniques fail. A variety of shunt techniques (Table 9.3) have been described once pharmacotherapy fails, although their benefit remains controversial due to the smooth muscle damage that has already occurred and the high postoperative erectile dysfunction rate.

The creation of a fistula between the corpora and glans can be achieved by the insertion of a Trucut needle (Winter; Figure 9.9) or scalpel

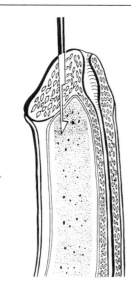

Figure 9.9

Winter shunt for priapism.

blade (Hashmat's) through the glans into the corpora.[12] A more extensive shunt is achieved by the El-Ghourab procedure (Figure 9.10) that removes small strips of tunica albuginea from each corpus. More complicated shunts have

Table 9.3 Techniques for shunt surgery in priapism	
Shunt surgery	**Reference**
Cavernosal–glandular	Winter
	El-Ghourab
Cavernosal–spongiosal	Quackels
Cavernosal–saphenous	Grayhack
	Barry

been described such as dorsal vein to corpora or saphenous vein to corpora (Grayhack), but these appear to be associated with higher incidence of erectile dysfunction. A Quackels is a proximal corporal shunt best carried out via the perineal approach to reduce the risk of urethral injury (Figure 9.11). A 7.5 cm perineal incision is made to expose the bulbar urethra and adjoining corpora cavernosa. A 2 cm incision is made on the bulbospongiosus and corpus cavernous. The two bodies are then anostomosed with a running 5/0 prolene suture.

PROGNOSIS

Corporal fibrosis with erectile dysfunction resulting from priapism is inevitable in low-

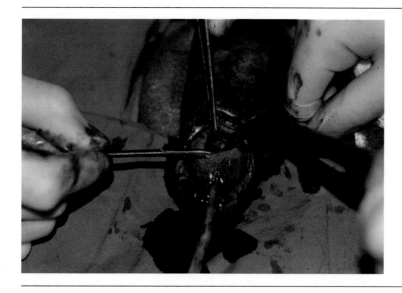

Figure 9.10

El-Ghourab shunt for priapism.

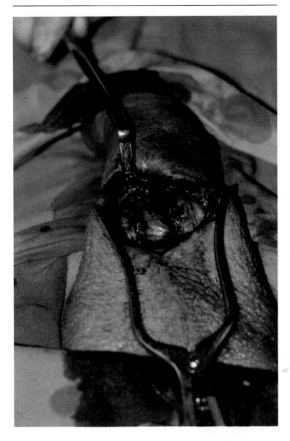

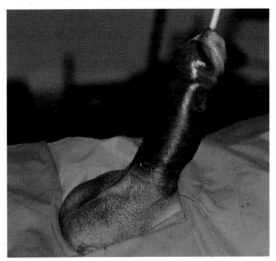

Figure 9.12

Appearance of the penis in a case of delayed treated low-flow priapism.

Figure 9.11

Spongiosal (Quackels) shunt for priapism.

flow, untreated priapism (Figure 9.12). However, even with swift intervention postpriapism potency rate has been reported to be less than 50%. A poor prognosis is associated with older patients (>50 years), duration of priapism (>24 h), post-heparin treatment, alcohol or antipsychotic-associated priapism and those that fail conventional treatment.

The treatment of postpriapism erectile dysfunction is made difficult by the inevitable associated fibrosis. The placement of malleable prostheses is the mainstay of treatment but extensive fibrosis may restrict placement and subsequent function of such devices. Recent literature suggests that penile prosthesis should be placed early (i.e. within few days to weeks) following failure to treat priapism satisfactorily. The clear advantage is that it maintains penile length and allows easy insertion. A late placement, i.e. 6 months later, results in significant penile shortening and placement of the prosthesis is more difficult.

HIGH-FLOW PRIAPISM

CAUSES
The high uncontrolled arterial inflow into penile sinusoidal spaces usually results from perineal trauma during which the cavernosal artery is damaged. The subsequent development of priapism may be of gradual onset as the flow of arterial blood into the cavernosal space produces priapism.[10] The penile tissue does not become ischemic as venous outflow continues and the patient is usually free of pain.

MANAGEMENT

The clinical presentation of high-flow priapism is less acute and patients may present after many months with a history of chronic semi-rigidity. Normal arterial blood gas analysis and a high maximum systolic velocity on Doppler ultrasound (see Figure 9.8) will confirm the diagnosis of high-flow priapism. Therefore, treatment can initially be conservative with the administration of ice packs and observation being all that is required in some cases. If erection persists, selective internal pudendal arteriography is carried out to identify the site of the arteriovenous fistula (Figure 9.13). Embolization of communicating vessels can be undertaken simultaneously using autologous blood clot, polyvinyl alcohol or N-butylcyanocyalate. Open arterial ligation using intraoperative ultrasonography for guidance may be required if less invasive procedures fail.

Figure 9.14 presents an algorithm for the management of priapism.

MANAGEMENT OF RECURRENT (OR STUTTERING) PRIAPISM

In this rare condition, spontaneous resolution commonly occurs, but on occasions medical management is necessary. Resolution by one of the medications listed below is usually successful although potency is usually impaired.

- Cyproterone acetate: 100 mg nocte
- Flutamide
- Leutinizing hormone-releasing hormone analogs (e.g. Zoladex)
- Procyclidine
- Phenylepherine (self-injected)
- Terbutaline
- Etilefrine (α-adrenoceptor agonist)

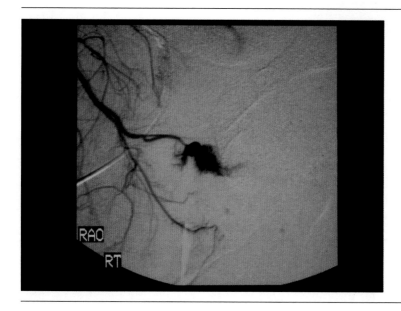

Figure 9.13

Arteriovenous fistula in high-flow priapism.

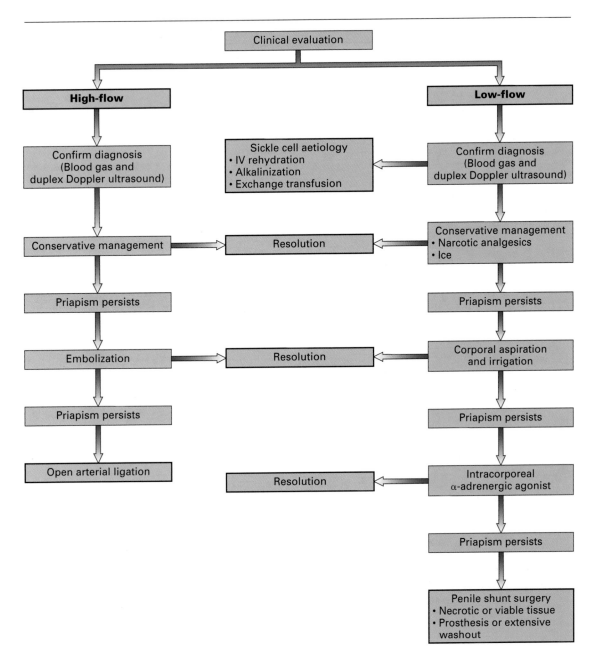

Figure 9.14

An algorithm for the management of priapism.

REFERENCES

1. Zargooshi J. Penile fracture in Kermansha, Iran: report of 172 cases. *J Urol* 2000; **164**: 364–6.
2. Mydlo JH, Harris CF, Brown JG. Blunt, penetrating and ischemic injuries to the penis. *J Urol* 2002; **168**: 1433–5.
3. Cortellini P, Ferretti S, Larosa M, Peracchia G, Arena F. Traumatic injury of the penis: surgical management. *Scand J Urol Nephrol* 1996; **30**: 517–19.
4. Kalash SS, Young JDJ. Fracture of the penis: controversy of surgical versus conservative treatment. *Urology* 1984; **24**: 21–4.
5. Mydlo JH, Gershbein AB, Macchia RJ. Nonoperative treatment of patients with presumed penile fracture. *J Urol* 2001; **165**: 424–5.
6. Bhanganada K, Chayavatana T, Pongnumkul C et al. Surgical management of an epidemic of penile amputations in Siam. *Am J Surg* 1983; **146**: 376–82.
7. Jezior JR, Brady JD, Schlossberg SM. Management of penile amputation injuries. *World J Surg* 2001; **25**: 1602–9.
8. Kalsi JS, Arya M, Rees R, Minhas S, Ralph DJ. Radial artery phalloplasty in penile reconstruction in female to male transsexuals. *BJU Int* 2002; **90**: 50.
9. El-Bahnasawy MS, El-Sherbiny MT. Paediatric penile trauma. *BJU Int* 2002; **90**: 92–6.
10. Ricardi R, Bhatt GM, Cynamon J, Bakal CW, Melman A. Delayed high flow priapism. Pathophysiology and management. *J Urol* 1993; **149**: 119–21.
11. Fowler JE, Koshy M, Strub M, Chinn SK. Priapism associated with the sickle cell haemoglobinopathies. Prevalence, natural history and sequelae. *J Urol* 1991; **145**: 65–8.
12. Ercole CJ, Pontes JE, Pierce JMJ. Changing surgical concepts in the treatment of priapism. *J Urol* 1981; **125**: 210–11.

10. Scrotal emergencies

Mark E Sullivan and Robert J Morgan

Acute scrotal problems represent potential urological emergencies. They require urgent and accurate evaluation which may lead to emergency surgical management. They present a diagnostic challenge as difficulties often exist in identifying normal physical landmarks and pain may limit the physical examination. The most important entity that needs to be excluded or treated as an emergency is testicular torsion. The history and physical examination are often helpful in determining the underlying diagnosis (Table 10.1). In some boys, laboratory and/or radiographic studies are useful in confirming or ruling out various conditions.

TESTICULAR TORSION

Torsion of the testicle is a urological emergency because of the risk of testicular loss. It can occur at any age, but is most common during adolescence (12–18 years; peak incidence 14–16 years) with an estimated incidence of 1:4000 in men <25 years. In adolescents and adults the torsion is intravaginal while in neonates it is usually extravaginal. The

---

Table 10.1 Etiology of the acute scrotum

Testicular torsion
Torsion of appendix testis
Torsion of appendix epididymis
Acute epididymitis
Acute orchitis
Acute hydrocele
Strangulated inguinoscrotal hernia
Testicular hematoma
Acute scrotal hematocele
Acute idiopathic scrotal edema
Testicular infarction
Idiopathic fat necrosis
Hemorrhage or infarction of testicular neoplasm
Fournier's gangrene
Scrotal trauma

---

left testis is more frequently involved than the right (6:4), possibly due to the greater length of spermatic cord on the left. Bilateral synchronous occurrence is ≤1%. Testicular torsion is also more common in cold weather possibly due to cremasteric contraction allowing elevation and rotation. When torsion occurs, the venous blood supply to the testicle is obstructed, secondary edema and hemorrhage develop with subsequent arterial obstruction. This eventually leads to testicular necrosis. Animal studies suggest that the duration and degree of torsion affect the severity of ischemic damage to the testis.

EXTRAVAGINAL TORSION

First described by Taylor in 1897, this condition can occur both pre- and postnatally; 75% occur prenatally and the other 25% within 30 days of birth. The attachments between the tunica vaginalis and the scrotum in the neonatal period are loose and flimsy and allow the testis and tunica to twist. The insertion of the tunica vaginalis is normal, thus explaining why an intravaginal torsion is rarely seen at this stage.

Patients can present in a number of ways depending at which fetal age the torsion occurs and whether the testis was intra-abdominal or scrotal. If the torsion of a single testicle occurs early in the prenatal period, whether intra-abdominal or inguinal, patients are born with monorchia. Patients with the vanishing testis syndrome are thought to have suffered bilateral torsion of intra-abdominal testes sometime after the twelfth week of intrauterine life. If the torsion of an intra-abdominal testis occurs just before or soon after birth the patient may present with an abdominal crisis.

The most common group is those who present with a hard scrotal mass at the time of delivery. The time of the torsion is variable.

Some infants have an oedematous, erythematous scrotum with a black testis and little surrounding inflammatory reaction. Others have minimal scrotal reaction and marked fibrosis around the testis seen at surgery, suggesting the torsion is of some days duration. The diagnosis is usually straightforward, although scrotal and testicular trauma suffered during a difficult delivery can be difficult to differentiate. Rarely, neonates who have had a normal postnatal examination are then found to have a swollen tender testes within 1 month of life.

The management of these patients is controversial. The torted testicle is invariably non-viable and because of the extravaginal nature of the torsion, some surgeons recommend no exploration. However, some surgeons recommend exploration to fix the contralateral testicle in view of the risk, albeit very small, of torsion on that side. It also allows assessment of the torted testicle and orchidectomy is usual. The method of fixation of the contralateral testis is debatable. Three-point fixation using a monofilamentous non-absorbable suture has been recommended but more recent evidence supports the eversion of the tunica vaginalis and placement of the testis in a dartos pouch without suture. This approach may reduce potential testicular injury caused by suturing.

INTRAVAGINAL TORSION

This was first reported by Delasiauve in 1840. The incidence appears to be increasing with 1 in 158 men experiencing a torsion by the age of 25 years in the Bristol series.[1] The mean age of torsion in this series was 16.7 years and torsion was as common in men in their twenties as peripubertally. Scudder drew attention to the horizontally lying testis within a cavernous tunica vaginalis and a high investment of the tunica producing the 'bell clapper' deformity (Figure 10.1).[2] It has been reported to be present in 54–100% of cases and this anomaly is seen on both sides and probably explains the significant later risk of testicular torsion on the contralateral side. Scorer and Farrington have suggested that torsion occurs because of a narrow mesenteric attachment from the cord onto the testis and epididymis.[3] The narrow mesentery allows the testicle to fall forward and freely rotate like a clapper within a bell. This would also explain why torsion is more likely to occur during puberty as the testis increases in volume by

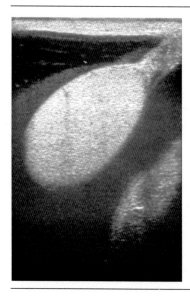

Figure 10.1

Scrotal ultrasound scan showing the 'bell clapper deformity'. The narrow testicular pedicle is visible because of the associated hydrocele.

five to six-fold. This anomaly is also usually bilateral.

The classic presentation is of sudden pain and swelling on the affected side. However, in infants, symptoms may be absent such that the patient presents only with irritability, restlessness and loss of appetite. Previous episodes of acute scrotal pain with spontaneous resolution imply prior testicular torsion (often referred to as 'intermittent torsion'). Irritative urinary symptoms and pyuria are universally absent in testicular torsion. Physical examination should start with the scrotal skin. The scrotal wall may be erythematous and swollen in testicular torsion and epididymitis but not with tumor. Examination of the scrotal contents aims to define the testis and epididymis as separate structures and their relation to each other. If the physician finds a non-tender epididymis displaced anteriorly and a swollen tender testis, testicular torsion is most likely. If the epididymis can be defined in its normal posterior position, tenderness is localized to the epididymis and the testis is normal, epididymitis is the likely diagnosis. Many cases, however, tend to present somewhere between these two classic presentations. Two twists of the spermatic cord will produce a posterior position for the epididymis, although it may be somewhat transverse in its orientation. Several hours of testicular torsion produce pronounced swelling of both the testis and epididymis so that they cannot be defined as separate structures. Severe epididymo-orchitis, testicular abscess or testicular tumor can present similarly, but acute epididymitis will not.

The effect of testicular elevation may be helpful early in the course of testicular torsion. In the supine position, the affected testis is gently elevated by the examiner. This will relieve the pain of epididymitis by removing tension from the spermatic cord. It will not alleviate the pain of testicular torsion (which is ischemic in nature) and may worsen it. There is usually no fever and urinalysis is normal.

The most common misdiagnoses are torsion of the testicular/epididymal appendages or acute epididymitis. If testicular torsion cannot be ruled out by the examining physician surgical exploration should be undertaken immediately. Interest has developed in the use of radionuclide imaging and Doppler ultrasonography (Figure 10.2) in an effort to reduce the number of unnecessary explorations. Neither

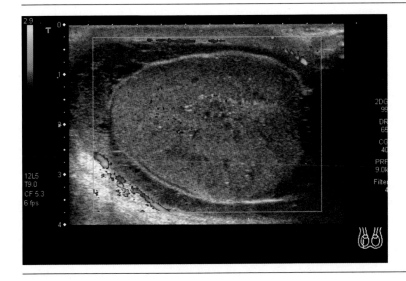

Figure 10.2

Torsion of approximately 8 h duration. A color Doppler ultrasound scan showing flow in the scrotal wall but none in the inhomogeneous swollen testis. Epididymis also appears swollen.

method is 100% accurate and this, taken together with the time taken to perform the test, precludes their use in the acute setting. They may have a role in patients with longer-standing symptoms where the chance of salvaging a torted testicle is very small or the likelihood of testicular torsion is felt to be very small.

The diagnosis of testicular torsion warrants immediate exploration, detorsion and a dartos pouch or three-point non-absorbable suture fixation of a viable testis together with orchidopexy of the contralateral testis. Consent must be taken for possible orchidectomy and bilateral orchidopexy as well. Prognosis is good if the patient is operated on within 4–6 h and contralateral orchidopexy performed. If viability is uncertain following detorsion, the tunica albuginea can be incised and if fresh bleeding is seen, it is worth leaving the testicle in situ and fixing it. Reperfusion of the detorted testicle can also be assessed with intravenous fluorescein or Doppler ultrasound where doubt exists. Nonviable testis are removed and a testicular prosthesis can be inserted at the same time or later. Salvage rates for torsion have increased from 45% in the 1960s to 67% in the 1980s.

An alternative approach to immediate surgical intervention involves manual external detorsion, followed by elective orchidopexy. The manual detorsion is usually performed in an anticlockwise direction. This approach has been criticized as it is often very painful for the patient and testis and can be incomplete allowing for retorsion in the intervening period.

The outcome of testicular torsion and surgical intervention is usually assessed by examination of the testicle to detect atrophy. Testicular volume mostly reflects the response of the germ cell population of the testis to ischemic injury. Despite apparent viability at the time of surgery, progressive atrophy can occur postoperatively and, therefore, follow-up at 3–4 months is recommended.

After torsion many patients have oligospermia. Initial studies suggested this was due to autoimmunization secondary to antisperm antibodies. More recent work, however, suggests the oligospermia is related to a pre-existing testicular defect.

TORSION OF THE TESTICULAR APPENDAGES

The most common testicular appendage susceptible to torsion is the appendix testes, a remnant of the müllerian duct. The presentation is usually the same as that for testicular torsion. Patients are usually adolescents and present with sudden onset of testicular pain. It is sometimes possible, when edema has not developed, to palpate the twisted appendage as a 3–5-mm tender mass near the upper pole of the testis (Figure 10.3) and the characteristic 'blue dot' sign may be seen on the skin of the scrotum. However, once edema develops palpation of the appendage becomes impossible. If certainty about the diagnosis exists, these patients can be managed conservatively with bed rest and analgesics.

ACUTE EPIDIDYMITIS

This is a clinical syndrome resulting from inflammation, pain and swelling of the epididymus of less than 6 weeks. Studies have suggested that it is a major cause of loss of work in the military and other complications include abscess formation, testicular infarction, development of chronic pain and infertility. It accounts for 1:350 of all medical consultations in men ≥18 years and is the fifth commonest genitourinary diagnosis in men between 18–50 years. Peak incidence is at 20–29 years although all ages can be affected. Right and left sides are affected with equal frequency and it is rarely bilateral. There is no racial predilection but it is more common in homosexual men who engage in unprotected anal intercourse. Exposure to sexually transmitted diseases is usually evident in the history, but this can be months before the onset of symptoms.

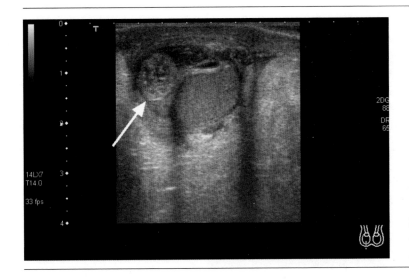

Figure 10.3

Torted testicular appendix (appendix arrowed).

Clinically, fever (>37.5 °C) is present in 75% of patients, chills in a quarter of those with fever and dysuria is reported by a third of the patients. Typically in acute epididymitis the inflammation and swelling begin in the tail of the epididymis (Figure 10.4a) and may spread to the rest of the epididymis and the testicular substance (epididymo-orchitis) (Figure 10.4b). The spermatic cord is usually swollen and tender. Involvement of the adjacent testis and development of an inflammatory hydrocele is common. Orchitis occurs in 58%, erythema of the scrotal skin in 62% and this erythema correlates with epididymal swelling. The external urethral meatus needs to be examined for redness or discharge. Co-existant prostatitis is rare (8%).

Peripheral leukocytosis is found in 64%. The microbial cause can usually be determined by examination of a Gram-stained urethral smear and Gram staining of a mid-stream urine specimen for Gram-negative bacteriuria. These tests should be performed for all men with suspected acute epididymitis. Ideally, a smear from the urethra should not be taken within 2 h of bladder emptying as it reduces the sensitivity of the test. The presence of intracellular Gram-

negative diplococci on the smear is diagnostic of neisseria gonorrhoea. White blood cells on urethral smear only indicate a non-specific urethritis, and *Chlamydia trachomatis* is isolated in two-thirds of these. It is imperative to make the differential diagnosis between testicular torsion and acute epididymitis. Difficulties tend to occur in men under 35 years in whom both diagnosis are common. The presence of urethritis probably indicates the patient has epididymitis and not torsion.

The causes usually fall into two categories. In men under 35 years, acute epididymitis is caused by sexually transmitted organisms, while most cases in children and older men are due to common urinary pathogens. Previously, the majority of cases of acute epididymitis in young men were considered to be idiopathic. It was thought the inflammation resulted from sterile urine being forced down the vas deferens whilst the patient strained against a closed external urethral sphincter. Further studies in both military and civilian populations have shown that this is not the case.

Acute epididymitis is usually caused by spread of infection from the urethra or bladder. The most common cause of acute epididymitis

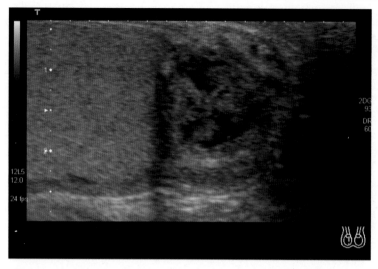

(a)

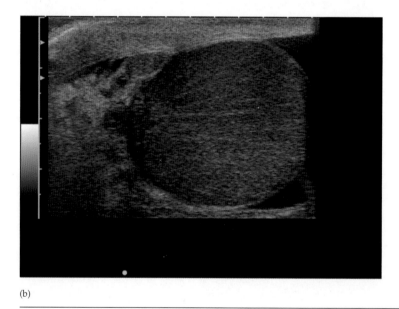

(b)

Figure 10.4

(a) Epididymitis: with a very swollen epididymal tail. (b) Swollen oedematous epididymis and testis consistent with a clinical diagnosis of epididymo-orchitis.

in any group is usually the most common cause of genitourinary infection in that group. In children, where acute epididymitis is uncommon, coliforms are the usual cause and lead to bacteriuria. In heterosexual men under 35 years, bacteriuria is uncommon, while urethritis due to *Neisseria gonorrhoeae* (21%) and *Chlamydia tra-* *chomatis* (47%) is common. In approximately two-thirds of heterosexual men under 35 years with non-coliform, non-gonococcal epididymitis, *Chlamydia trachomatis* is the cause. In homosexual men practicing anal sex, coliforms appear to be the most common cause of acute epididymitis. In men over 35 years, sexually transmitted infection is uncommon, whilst bacteriuria secondary to acquired bladder outflow obstruction, e.g. benign prostatic hyperplasia, prostate cancer and urethral stricture, is relatively common. The most common cause of acute epididymitis in older men is the organism that causes bacteriuria. *Escherichia coli* is most common (32%), followed by *Pseudomonas* (14%) and *Proteus* (4%).

Rarely, in all age groups, the acute epididymitis is due to systemic disease such as tuberculosis, cryptococcosis and brucellosis. A non-infectious cause of acute epididymitis is the drug amiodarone. With this drug only the epididymal head is involved and the condition responds to a lowered dose of amiodarone but not antibiotic therapy. Orchitis is most commonly viral in origin, e.g. mumps. A history of recent viral-like illness should be sought. Epididymo-orchitis, however, is rarely due to a viral cause. The onset is more like epididymitis than the sudden nature of torsion. Examination reveals a tender and swollen testis, but the epididymis and spermatic cord are normal on palpation.

Radionuclide scanning is probably the most accurate imaging method for diagnosing acute epididymitis, although color Doppler ultrasound is the imaging modality of choice for the acute scrotum. Doppler ultrasound in experienced hands has a sensitivity of 82% and specificity of 100% in torsion, whilst for acute epididymitis, sensitivity is 70% and specificity 88% (Figure 10.5).

Few randomized trials exist to inform decision making in acute epididymitis. Antibiotic selection should be based on age, sexual history, recent instrumentation or catheterization and local guidelines for antibiotic sensitivities of sexual and urinary pathogens. Treatment is directed at the specific etiologic organism. Bed rest, analgesia and scrotal elevation can all improve symptoms. If urethritis is present, a single dose of penicillin V to cover *N. gonorrhoeae* and a 10-day course of tetracycline/doxycycline is required. Recent sexual partners need to be examined and treated. Patients with urethritis caused by infective microorganisms rarely have urological structural abnormalities.

Men with bacteriuria require a 10-day course of broad-spectrum antibiotics such as ciprofloxacin. Intravenous antibiotics should be considered if systemic illness is present and culture and sensitivities followed. Failure to

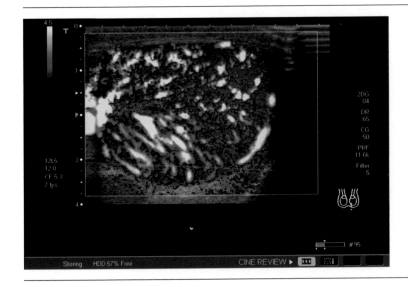

Figure 10.5

Orchitis: color Doppler ultrasound demonstrating intratesticular hyperemia.

respond after 3 days of treatment necessitates reassessment. Diagnostic doubt or worsening testicular pain are indications for surgical intervention. Younger men and boys with epididymitis and bacteriuria often have structural urological abnormalities and should undergo KUB (kidney, ureter, bladder) ultrasound, radiographic examination and cystoscopic evaluation.

OTHER CAUSES OF ACUTE SCROTAL SWELLING

Hydroceles can occasionally present as acute swellings, often associated with acute rise in intra-abdominal pressure due to constipation or upper respiratory tract infections. The swellings are usually non-tender and scrotal contents can be seen with transillumination (Figure 10.6) and on scrotal ultrasound (Figure 10.7). Incarcerated hernias can be diagnosed by examination of the inguinal canal and scrotum. The intestine and testis may both be at risk for infarction and manual reduction under sedation is usually successful and allows for subsequent elective surgical correction. Testicular hematoma and acute

scrotal hematocele usually occur following trauma, although they can occasionally arise spontaneously.

Idiopathic scrotal edema was first described by Qvist in 1956. It is an uncommon cause of acute scrotal swelling, though its incidence may be as high as 20–30% of all scrotal swellings in prepubertal boys. It has been reported in adult men. Patients are either asymptomatic or have minimal scrotal discomfort. The scrotum may be itchy initially followed by the swelling and erythema. It occurs as often unilaterally as bilaterally. The affected scrotum is edematous and erythematous (from a pink discoloration to violaceous). The erythema commonly extends beyond the scrotum to involve the groin, perineum, penis and suprapubic abdomen. The underlying testis, epididymis, prostate and spermatic cord are non-tender and normal in size. Sometimes the edema can be so severe to preclude palpation of the testis and epididymis. All laboratory tests are normal except scrotal ultrasonography that shows the characteristic marked thickening of the scrotal wall and dartos (Figure 10.8). The edema and erythema are self-limiting and resolve completely within 6–72 h. Reassurance, activity restriction, scrotal elevation

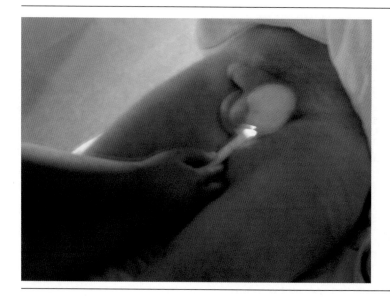

Figure 10.6

Transillumination of the scrotum showing a large hydrocele.

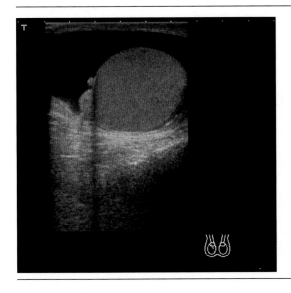

Figure 10.7

Hydrocele clearly seen on ultrasound.

and observation for 24–48 h are required. Recurrences occur in up to 21% of cases.

Testicular infarction is a rare event. It has been reported in association with a number of conditions such as sickle cell disease, sickle cell trait, chronic lymphocytic leukemia, protein S deficiency, angiitis, polycythemia, malakoplakia of the epididymis, thrombotic endocarditis of Wegener's disease and acute epididymitis. The condition can present acutely and be indistinguishable from testicular torsion or develop slowly over a few weeks where Doppler ultrasonography (Figure 10.9) may aid in diagnosis. In the acute scenario, scrotal exploration may reveal a viable testis and bivalving may allow excision of necrotic tissue with salvage of the remaining testicular tissue.

Idiopathic fat necrosis was described by Hinman in 1939. It is a very rare cause of acute scrotal swelling. It occurs in prepubertal children in association with minor trauma, cold temperatures and salt water. It can be unilateral or bilateral. Presentation is usually with pain with or without tenderness and erythema of the scrotum. A mass is usually palpable but may not be obviously separate from the testis. Again if doubt arises scrotal exploration is mandatory.

The necrosis occurs in the lipomatous tissue present in the prepubertal scrotum.

Testicular tumors present with scrotal enlargement, but are rarely tender. Their presentation is rarely acute but they have been reported in association with testicular torsion, infarction and hemorrhage following apparent minor trauma. A history of undescended testicle or orchidopexy should alert the physician to the possibility of a malignancy.

FOURNIER'S GANGRENE

This is a true urological emergency that needs to be recognized and treated immediately. It is a form of synergistic polymicrobial necrotizing fasciitis involving the perineum and external genitalia. It may be genitourinary, colorectal or idiopathic in origin. It is also known as idiopathic gangrene of the scrotum, streptococcal scrotal gangrene, perineal phlegmon, and spontaneous fulminant gangrene of the scrotum. It was originally reported by Baurienne in 1764 and then by Fournier in 1883. Classically, it is characterized by an abrupt onset of a rapidly fulminating genital gangrene of idiopathic

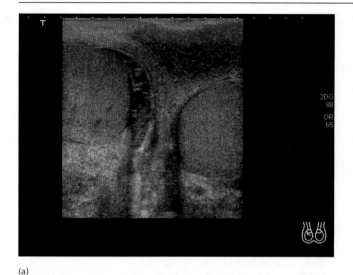

(a)

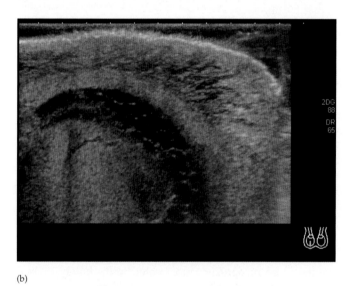

(b)

Figure 10.8

Idiopathic scrotal oedema. (a) A general view of a thick scrotal wall on ultrasound scan with a normal underlying testis and epididymis. (b) Localized view of the swollen scrotal wall.

origin in previously healthy young patients. It can, however, occur at any age including older people, follow a more indolent course and the source is identifiable in 95% of cases. The infection usually arises from the skin, urethra or rectal regions. An association between urethral obstruction associated with strictures and extravasation and instrumentation is well documented. Other predisposing factors include local trauma, paraphimosis, perirectal or perianal infections particularly abscesses, colonic perforation secondary to cancer, trauma and diverticulitis, periurethral extravasation of urine and surgery such as circumcision or herniorraphy. A history of some sort of immunosuppression, such as diabetes mellitus (32–66%),

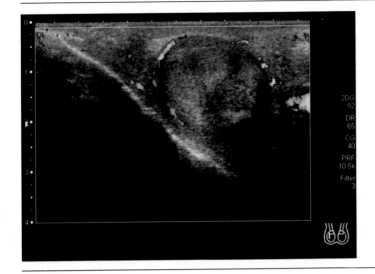

Figure 10.9

Testicular infarction: a color Doppler ultrasound scan demonstrating no blood flow into the testis.

alcoholism (25–68%), systemic disease or human immunodeficiency virus (HIV) infection is common. Other associations include prolonged hospitalization, malignancy, intravenous drug abuse or malnutrition. Patients frequently have a history of recent perineal trauma, instrumentation, urethral stricture associated with sexually transmitted disease or urethral cutaneous fistula. Specific genitourinary symptoms associated with the condition are dysuria, urethral discharge and obstructive voiding symptoms. Pain, rectal bleeding and a history of anal fissures suggest a rectal source of infection. Dermal sources are suggested by a history of acute and chronic infections of the scrotum and spreading recurrent hidroadenitis suppurativa or balanitis.

The clinical presentation of Fournier's gangrene is highly variable. A high index of suspicion and awareness of the clinical appearance aid recognition. The infection often begins with cellulitis close to the portal of entry, though cyanosis, blistering, bronzing or skin induration may be the earliest cutaneous manifestations (Figure 10.10). The involved area is swollen, erythematous and tender as the infection starts to involve the deep fascia. Pain is a prominent symptom and fever and systemic toxicity are

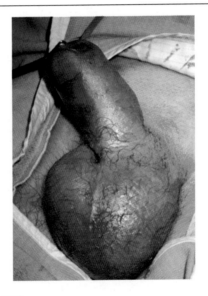

Figure 10.10

Fournier's gangrene: early presentation with a hyperemic penile swelling.

marked. The swelling increases, crepitus becomes more obvious and dark purple areas appear and progress to extensive gangrene. Pain often decreases with the onset of gangrene

(Figure 10.11). Spread up the abdominal wall can be very rapid, particularly in the immunocompromised. Gram-negative sepsis is suggested by alterations in mental status, temperatures above 38 °C or below 35 °C, tachycardia and tachypnea.

Careful evaluation of the urethra and rectum is required, either preoperatively or in the operating theatre, if there is any suspicion of involvement. The urethra should be assessed by urethroscopy and those with significant penile involvement, urethral trauma or urinary extravasation require suprapubic cystotomy. The rectum is assessed by proctoscopy and patients with rectal or colonic perforation require a diverting colostomy. Anemia may be present secondary to sepsis and thrombosis and ecchymosis. Hyponatremia, elevated creatinine and hypocalcemia are common.

A plain abdominal film will often demonstrate the crepitus and may point to an intraperitoneal or retroperitoneal source of infection. Scrotal ultrasonography can similarly show the scrotal crepitus, often with a normal testes and thickened scrotal wall (Figures 10.12 and 10.14). CT or MRI scanning can also detect subcutaneous gas and define the source of infection.

The cause is a synergistic infection comprising enteric Gram-negative organisms, Gram-positive staphylococci or streptococci and anaerobes. Through a process of spreading inflammatory reaction the local infection extends to the deep fascial planes and rapidly progresses to the characteristic obliterative endarteritis resulting in cutaneous and subcutaneous vascular necrosis. The creation of a

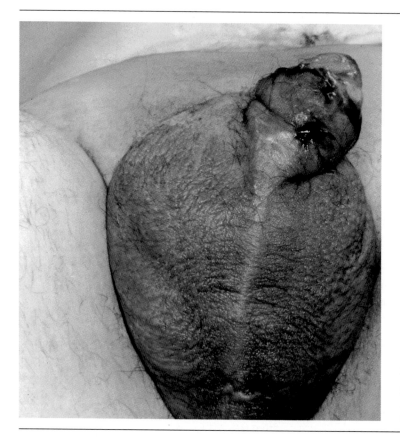

Figure 10.11

Fournier's gangrene: a late presentation. A late consequence is painless necrosis of the skin and non-viable tissues.

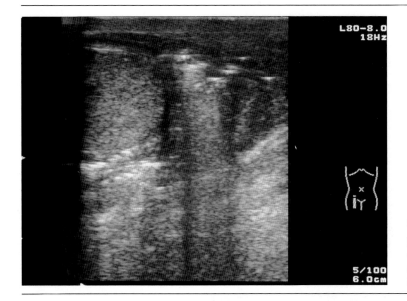

Figure 10.12

Fournier's gangrene; patient presented with epididymitis. Gas bubble seen in the epididymis which later spread to the perineum.

hypoxic milieu is crucial to the pathogenesis of Fournier's gangrene.

Early diagnosis and treatment is vital because of the speed with which the process can spread. The difficulty often lies in differentiating clinically between Fournier's and cellulitis as both often present with pain, erythema and edema. The presence of systemic signs out of proportion with the local findings or a lack of response of the cellulitis to appropriate antibiotics should alert the clinician.

The patient needs to be aggressively rehydrated or resuscitated with intravenous fluids and should be given intravenous antibiotic therapy. Penicillins or third-generation cephalosporins, clindamycin or metronidazole and an aminoglycoside are all needed to cover the spectrum of pathogens that may be present until specific culture sensitivities are available. Immediate surgical debridement is required. Consent needs to cover extensive debridement and the possibilities of urinary diversion, fecal diversion and laparotomy. In theater, the patient is placed in a dorsal lithotomy position and an extensive area of skin and subcutaneous tissue needs to be excised going beyond the involved areas until normal fascia is identified. Necrotic fat and fascia is excised and the wound is left open. Orchidectomy is not usually required as the testes have their own blood supply independent of the affected fascial and cutaneous circulation. If the testis is involved it is important to consider an abdominal process that has led to thrombosis of the testicular artery. The testes can either be placed subcutaneously in groin pouches or wrapped in saline gauze. The patient should be taken back into theater 24–48 h later to reassess wounds and carry out further debridement if required. Hyperbaric oxygen may be helpful in improving outcomes by reducing gangrenous spread, wound healing and shorter hospital stay. When wound healing is complete the patient should be referred to a plastic surgeon for consideration of reconstruction of the skin and subcutaneous defect.

The mortality rate is in the order of 20% but ranges from 0 to 75%. The mortality rate is higher in the elderly, alcoholics, extensive disease, shock or sepsis at presentation, positive blood cultures and those without a colostomy following debridement.

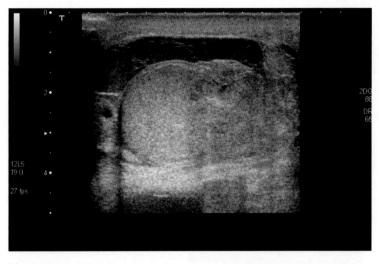

(a)

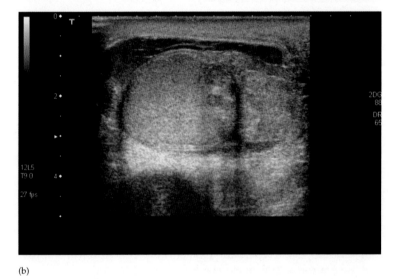

(b)

Figure 10.13

(a, b) Ultrasound scan showing a testicular rupture at the lower pole of the testis.

SCROTAL TRAUMA IN THE ADULT

Trauma to the scrotum may be divided into blunt, penetrating and scrotal skin loss. Management of these injuries are dictated by the goals of salvage of the function of the testes and cosmesis. An attempt is made to salvage maximal numbers of seminiferous tubules and maintain continuity from the seminiferous tubules to the seminal vesicle. The physiologic requirements of the testicle in terms of its blood supply and temperature dependency are also deciding factors.

BLUNT SCROTAL TRAUMA

The causes of blunt scrotal trauma vary widely from road traffic accidents, sports injury, violence or work-related causes. The presentation is, however, usually the same. There is severe testicular pain often associated with nausea and vomiting. The symptoms are due to compression of the seminiferous tubules and tearing of the tunica albuginea. If the tunica albuginea is ruptured but the tunica vaginalis remains intact, the patient may have only minimal swelling or ecchymosis. Marked tenderness can easily be elicited on physical examination. If there has been minimal trauma causing severe symptoms the possibility of pre-existing pathology must be entertained.

The differential diagnosis of testicular pain after trauma includes testicular torsion, torsion of the appendix testis or appendix epididymis, reactive hydrocele, epididymitis, injury to the testicular artery, nerve or vein and testicular tumor. Blunt trauma may also cause a hematoma of the epididymis, cord or a hematocele with or without tunica albuginea rupture. If the examination reveals an enlarged, tender testis it is difficult to differentiate between these conditions.

Initial studies reported that ultrasound is effective at showing the extent and type of injury. The tunica albuginea could be easily identified with a 90% diagnostic accuracy for rupture. The tunica albuginea is usually able to withstand 50 kg of blunt trauma. Sonographically, the finding most likely to indicate tunica albuginea rupture is hypoechogenicity of the parenchyma subtending the region of injury and this is supported by focal disruption of the echogenic tunica (Figure 10.13). More recent studies, however, put the sensitivity at 75% and specificity at 64%. Although ultrasound may be helpful, it should not deny or delay surgical exploration. Straddle injuries to the scrotum also put the bulbar urethra at risk of injury. Missed urethral injuries can be disastrous and it is wise to perform retrograde urethrograms for these types of injury. Testicular torsion needs to be ruled out and if this has been done a management decision for the testicular injury is required. Studies have suggested that conservative non-operative management of testicular rupture results in a subsequent orchidectomy

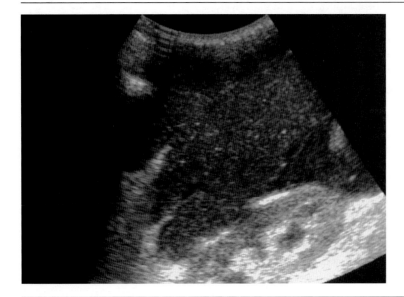

Figure 10.14
Fournier's gangrene: an ultrasound scan of perineum with gas pockets causing shadowing and comet tails).

rate of 45% compared with 5% of patients operated early. The operated patients also had a shorter convalescence period. Early surgical exploration and repair is, therefore, recommended primarily to maximize testicular salvage. The consent form needs to include possible orchidectomy. The surgical approach should be via the midline raphe. The hematoma is evacuated and the edges of the ruptured tunica albuginea debrided. Devascularized and extruded seminiferous tubules are excised and the tunica albuginea is closed with an absorbable suture (interrupted or continuous). A drain is placed under the tunica vaginalis and brought out via a separate stab incision in the scrotum. Marsupialization of the tunica vaginalis is recommended to prevent further hydrocele formation. Closure of the dartos and skin is done in standard fashion. Broad-spectrum antibiotics are required for 7 days.

PENETRATING SCROTAL TRAUMA

Penetrating injuries to the scrotum are classified as simple or complicated. Simple injuries penetrate the skin but do not injure deeper structures. Complicated injuries imply urethral involvement, testicular injury, amputation or near amputation. Ideally, simple lacerations of the testicle are primarily closed, with meticulous closure of all layers and control of any spermatic cord bleeding. If doubt exists about testicular vascularity, Doppler ultrasound evaluation is required. If the wound is contaminated, open dressing and delayed closure is advisable.

Deep penetrating scrotal trauma requires exploration. Gunshot wounds are the most common cause of this type of injury. Through and through wounds may cause injuries to the cord structures, epididymis and testes. Ultrasound can be helpful regarding injury to the tunica albuginea but the patient's associated injuries usually preclude these studies.

The surgical approach is via a median raphe which allows good access to the cord structures

and orchidectomy if necessary. Closure of a ruptured tunica albuginea can be performed after judicious debridement of extruded tubules. Injuries to the spermatic cord usually require little more than meticulous hemostasis. If testicular viability is questioned the tunica albuginea can be incised and bleeding from the testicular parenchyma is reassuring. Testicular amputation injuries can be managed with a micro-replantation procedure. Vasovasostomy using a two-layer or single-layer 'tricorner technique', microarterial coaptation and venous anastomosis, and reapproximation of the external spermatic fascia should be performed. It appears that for testicular replantation to be successful it needs to be achieved within 6–8 h of the injury. Vasal injuries should not be primarily repaired for fertility as the extent of tissue ischemia especially with gunshot injuries may not be clearly demarcated at the time of exploration. Silk sutures can be used at the cut ends to aid identification if infertility mandates repair at a later stage.

When repair of structures following a gunshot wound is being undertaken a number of principles need to be followed. The blast effect causes more tissue necrosis than may be evident at exploration. The bullet may also carry with it fibers of clothing, hair or debris and the wound must be considered contaminated. Thorough wound irrigation, intravenous antibiotic cover and wound drainage must be employed. Repair of the tunica albuginea can be performed after a gunshot wound, but requires generous tissue apposition of the fascial layer as later necrosis from the blast effect may occur. High-velocity missile injuries have been associated with testicular salvage in only half of the cases.

SCROTAL SKIN LOSS

The scrotal wall contains multiple layers of connective tissue and a thin-layered muscle separating the skin from the testis and underlying structures. The scrotal skin can thus be 'violently' removed without subsequent damage to underlying structures including the testis. It most often occurs when the scrotum is caught in clothing entangled in farm equipment or machinery.

Partial skin loss can be treated with debridement and primary closure. The wound must be irrigated and all necrotic and foreign tissue fully debrided. Grossly contaminated wounds are packed with sterile gauze dressings. Cleaner wounds are drained and closed in several layers with absorbable sutures. The scrotal skin is very compliant and well vascularized allowing coverage of large defects.

More severe avulsion injuries can take skin from the abdomen, genitalia and thighs as well as deeper structures. A complete evaluation of the urethra, rectal examination and possible sigmoidoscopy to assess the anal sphincter and the integrity of the anus and rectum are required. Management of total scrotal skin loss is directed to protecting the underlying testis. The testis can be initially managed by placing saline soaked dressings over them with frequent change of dressings. This can continue until there is adequate scrotal granulation tissue to permit application of a mesh or split skin graft. Alternatively, when the patient has stabilized from associated injuries, the testes can be definitively protected by placing them in superficial thigh pouches. The thigh pouch is a temporary measure until definitive scrotal reconstruction is undertaken (if possible). Each testis is placed subcutaneously in the medial aspect of the thigh on its respective side. The pouches need to be asymmetrical in position so that during walking they do not contact and cause pain. It seems to be important to place the testes superficial to the subcutaneous tissue as the reduced temperature allows spermatogenesis to be maintained.

Split-thickness skin grafting may be used as a secondary procedure for scrotal skin replacement with excellent results. Thigh-based cutaneous flaps are an alternative option, though the extensive mobilization needed for these flaps have led some groups to advise that they should be reserved for failed split-thickness skin grafts.

REFERENCE

1. Anderson JB, Williamson RCN. Testicular torsion in Bristol: a 25-year review. *Br J Surg* 1988; **75:** 988–92.
2. Scudder CL. Strangulation of the testis by torsion of the cord. *Ann Surg* 1901; **34:** 234–8.
3. Scorer CG, Farrington GH. *Congential deformities of the testis and epididymis.* London: Butterworth & Co, 1971.

FURTHER READING

Baskin LS, Carroll PR, Cattolica EV, McAninch JW. Necrotizing soft tissue infections of the perineum and genitalia. *Br J Urol* 1990; **65:** 524–9.

Berger RE, Alexander ER, Harnisch Paulsen CA, Monda GD, Ansell J et al. Aetiology, manifestations and therapy of acute epididymitis: prospective study of 50 cases. *J Urol* 1979; **121:** 750–4.

Clinical Effectiveness Group (Association of Genitourinary Medicine and the Medical Society for the Study of Venereal Diseases). National guidelines for the management of epididymo-orchitis. *Sex Trans Inf* 1999; **75:** S51–S53.

Collins MM, Stafford RS, O'Leary MP, Barry MJ. How common is prostatitis? A national survey of physician visits. *J Urol* 1998; **159:** 1224–8.

Delvillar RG, Ireland GW, Cass AS. Early exploration following trauma to the testicle. *J Trauma* 1973; **13:** 600–1.

Fournier JA. Gangrene foudroyante de la verge. *Med Practique* 1883; **4:** 589–97.

Hadzisilemovic F, Snyder H, Duckett J, Howards S. Testicular histology in children with unilateral testicular torsion. *J Urol* 1986; **136:** 208–10.

Herbener TE. Ultrasound in the assessment of the acute scrotum. *J Clin Ultrasound* 1996; **24:** 405–21.

Kratzik C, Hainz A, Kuber W, Donner G, Lunglmayr G et al. Has ultrasound influenced the therapy concept of blunt scrotal trauma? *J Urol* 1989; **142:** 1243–5.

Paty R, Smith AD. Gangrene and Fournier's gangrene. *Urol Clin North Am* 1992; **19:** 149–62.

11. Pediatric urological trauma

Gerald C Mingin and Hiep T Nguyen

Trauma remains the most common cause of death in the pediatric population.[1] In particular, the genitourinary tract is susceptible to blunt injury from motor vehicle accidents, falls and sports injuries, and other causes include sexual abuse or rarely penetrating trauma. Upper tract trauma predominately involves the kidney while isolated ureteral injuries are a rare event. Blunt lower tract trauma occurs in children with concomitant pelvic fractures and is usually associated with non-urological injuries. Scrotal trauma and circumcision injuries account for the smallest portion of pediatric urological trauma.

Although we are not the first physicians to initially treat these children, as urologists our expertise may be called upon to help in the management of these genitourinary injuries. Understanding the pathology, combined with effective evaluation and treatment ensures the best care for these children.

RENAL TRAUMA

Blunt trauma is responsible for more than 90% of all renal injuries.[2] The kidney is injured in 10% of all abdominal trauma and is the most frequent genitourinary organ to be effected as a result of blunt trauma. Motor vehicle accidents and deceleration injuries account for most of these injuries. Roughly equal numbers of children are struck by or are passengers in a motor vehicle (31–35%), while falls account for approximately 28% of renal injuries.[3]

The child's kidney is more susceptible to trauma compared with the adult kidney due to its proportionally larger size, limited thoracic cage and decreased perinephric fat.[4] The child's kidney while being larger also projects further below the twelfth rib when compared with adults. The ribs in small children are flexible and fail to provide the same rigid protection seen in adults and their abdominal and trunk muscles are less developed and provide decreased protection. Children with hydronephrosis due to ureteropelvic junction obstruction or an ectopic kidney are also at increased risk for injury,[5] as are children who have had prior renal surgery. Children are more likely to suffer a ureteropelvic disruption during deceleration injuries because of increased flexibility and mobility of the kidney.

The majority of blunt renal injuries are not isolated events. Eighty percent of all children with renal injuries have an associated organ injury. These include splenic injuries, followed by head and orthopedic injuries.[3] More than 80% of renal injuries are classified as contusions or minor lacerations[6] (grade I, see Figure 6.1) and can be treated conservatively. More severe injuries (grades II-V, see Figure 6.1) are associated with urinary extravasation or rupture of the vessels. These injuries require staging and may require intervention. There are no standardized criteria for the radiographic and laboratory evaluation of children. Since hypotension has traditionally been a poor indicator of major renal injury, most children with hematuria have been imaged.[7] However, the degree of hematuria does not correlate with the extent of the injury and minor contusions are as likely to present with hematuria as is a major injury. Interestingly, only 2.6% of children with renal injuries do not have hematuria. Unfortunately there is no set number of red blood cells (RBCs) in the urine that correlates with injury. A cut-off of <20–50 RBCs high-power field with no associated injuries appears to exclude almost all renal injury[8] and further radiographic evaluation will yield little information. A recent study evaluating children with microscopic hematuria (>3 RBCs high-power field) after blunt trauma, identified only three of 65 patients with significant renal injury. All three of these patients had a mechanism of injury as well as clinical signs consistent with associated injuries requiring radiographic evaluation.[9] Currently, only those children with microscopic hematuria and associated injuries and or suspicious findings on clinical examination require immediate imaging. Other children presenting with microhematuria, who do not fall into the above category may be safely observed, reserving imaging for those with persistent or worsening hematuria.

The imaging modality of choice for the detection of renal injury is the computed tomography (CT) scan with intravenous contrast, which has been shown to rapidly stage most cases[8] (Figure 11.1).[8] CT scan has the advantage of differentiating the degree of injury by allowing for a functional assessment of the renal parenchyma. CT scan is also sensitive in detecting associated abdominal/pelvic injuries. Although renal bladder ultrasound is widely used in pediatric urology, it is not ideal for evaluating traumatic injury due to its inability to adequately image the renal parenchyma. A still older modality, the intravenous pyelogram (IVP) is not used for

routine imaging. A disadvantage of the IVP is that it may be misinterpreted as normal in up to 20% of patients with a major renal injury.[10] The IVP still has a role in evaluating the functional status of the contralateral kidney. This is especially true during emergent exploration for associated injuries in a patient who has not undergone a CT scan. In this case the IVP study can be performed on the operating room table.

The treatment of blunt renal trauma is dependent on the grade of the injury (Figure 11.2). Patients with contusions (grade I, see Figure 6.1) can be managed conservatively with bed rest and do not require follow-up imaging. Children with grades 2 and 3 lacerations present with a perinephric hematoma. The hematoma is contained by Gerota's fascia which tamponades the bleeding. These patients are managed with bed rest and repeat imaging to ensure that the hematoma is not expanding. In the rare instance of continued bleeding, angiography and selective embolization of the vessel is often successful.[11]

More severe lacerations lead to the disruption of the collecting system and formation of a urinoma (grade IV, see Figure 6.1). There is no

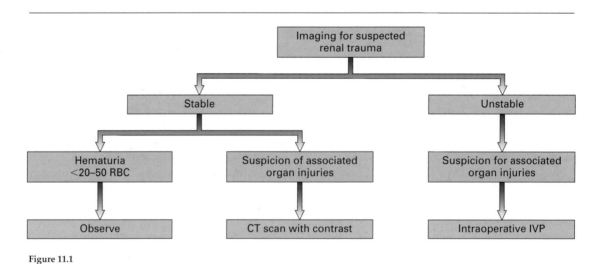

Figure 11.1

Algorithm for imaging for a suspected renal injury in children. RBC, red blood cells; CT, computed tomography; IVP, intravenous pyelogram.

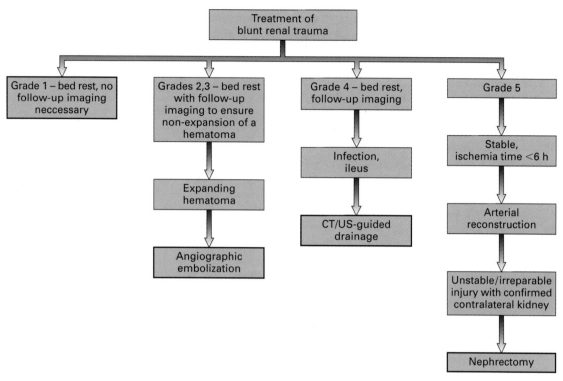

Figure 11.2

Algorithm depicting the steps in the treatment of renal injury.

clear consensus on the management of collecting system injuries with an associated urinoma. In the past urinary extravasation was an indication for laparotomy. Recently these injuries have been managed with initial observation. In adults, spontaneous resolution of urinary extravasation has been reported in 87% of patients followed after major renal trauma.[12] Russell et al reported their results in children;[13] overall 60% of cases with grade 4 renal injuries required no intervention. When intervention was required, it consisted of either percutaneous drainage of the urinoma or endoscopic placement of a ureteral stent.[13] Observation of these injuries can lead to infection and/or a prolonged ileus. In these cases CT scan or ultrasound-guided placement of a nephrostomy tube

to drain the urine collection is appropriate. We do not advocate ureteral stent placement, especially in small children where stents are not well tolerated. In addition, the small caliber may not be sufficient for adequate drainage.

Renal vascular injuries account for the remainder of blunt renal trauma. Injuries involving the renal artery are rare occurring in 1–3% of all blunt renal trauma. The mechanism of these arterial lesions is a rapid deceleration of the kidney with subsequent stretching of the renal artery. The adventia and the muscularis layers of the artery will stretch, however the intimal layer is prone to rupture. This rupture leads to clot formation and eventual renal ischemia. The diagnosis of these grade 5 injuries is not straightforward. Renal pedicle injuries are usually associated with injuries of other organs and hematuria is often not present. A non-perfused kidney on CT scan is an indication for obtaining angiographic confirmation of an arterial injury.

Management of these injuries is controversial and depends on the time elapsed since the injury, the other organs involved and, ultimately, the skill and experience of the surgeon. In cases where the warm ischemia time is greater than 6 h or the patient has a normal contralateral kidney but is too unstable to risk an operation, no attempt should be made to salvage the injured kidney. If the decision is made to proceed with surgery, exposure is obtained through a midline abdominal incision (see Figures 6.6–6.8). The first step requires obtaining control of the renal vascular pedicle. Vascular control is achieved by incising the posterior parietal peritoneum just medial to the inferior mesenteric vein. The left renal vein is identified and elevated to expose the underlying arteries. Vessel loops are placed around the appropriate artery and vein to facilitate control of bleeding should it become necessary. The colon can then be reflected and the kidney exposed. Arterial reconstruction is performed via an end-to-end anastamosis, by graft repair or autotransplantation.[14] In cases where the pedicle injury is irreparable or the patient becomes unstable nephrectomy is performed. However, even in the best hands the success rate for repairing renal arterial lesions is poor and should only be performed by surgeons with experience in this type of surgery.

URETERAL TRAUMA

Ureteral avulsion resulting from blunt trauma is extremely rare, and the clinician must have a high index of suspicion, since there is a delay in diagnosis in up to 60% of patients with these injuries.[15] The majority of cases occur in younger children, usually as a result of an automobile accident. The most common site of disruption is the ureteropelvic junction followed by the proximal and mid-ureter, respectively.[16] The mechanism of injury is similar to that seen in renal trauma with hyperextension followed by deceleration and avulsion of the ureter. Symptoms are non-specific and hematuria is often absent. The diagnosis of ureteral injury is made using either IVP or CT scan. The latter has the added benefit of detecting associated organ injuries. Whichever modality is used, it is important to obtain delayed studies because urinary extravasation may not be detected on the initial films.

Treatment of ureteral injuries depends on time the injury is discovered, the extent of the injury and the location of the injury. If the injury is discovered several days after the initial trauma, the radiographic findings will often reveal a urinoma. If the injury is a partial laceration, a ureteral stent can be placed with percutaneous tube drainage of the urinoma.

A complete laceration which has been diagnosed late is treated by placing a nephrostomy tube into the kidney and percutaneously draining the urine collection. At a later date, after hematoma resorption and resolution of the inflammation the injury can be repaired. The type of surgical repair depends on the position of the injury and the amount of ureter lost. Proximal injuries are best repaired by performing a pyeloplasty or transureteroureterostomy. Distal injuries with sufficient healthy ureter are treated by primary anastamosis. A psoas hitch or boari flap can be used if more length is needed. A ureteral stent should be left in place until complete healing has occurred, this usually takes 3–4 weeks. In rare cases the extent of the injury may warrant autotransplantation of the kidney or interposition of a bowel segment. When surgery is performed at the time of the injury the same techniques are used depending on the position and amount of the ureter involved. If reconstruction is difficult or the patient becomes unstable, the ureter is ligated and a nephrostomy tube placed until such time as formal reconstruction is performed.

BLADDER TRAUMA

Bladder injury is relatively uncommon in adults because it is positioned in and protected by the pelvis. In children the bladder is an abdominal organ, without the benefit of protection and is more susceptible to blunt trauma. Bladder rupture is most often associated with a pelvic fracture sustained during a motor vehicle accident. However, the incidence of bladder rupture in children in the absence of a pelvic fracture is higher than in adults;[17] this is explained by the bladder's relatively exposed position. Bladder rupture can be classified as either intraperitoneal or extraperitoneal. Intraperitoneal rupture is more common in children. This occurs when the bladder sustains a blow and the sudden increase in pressure leads to rupture of the bladder dome. With rupture of the overlying peritoneum urine will extravasate into the peritoneal cavity. Extraperitoneal rupture is almost exclusively associated with a pelvic fracture. In this type of injury the bladder may suffer a laceration with the inclusion of bone fragments within the bladder.

Clinically, bladder rupture is almost always associated with gross hematuria,[18] other associated findings include suprapubic tenderness and inability to void. A Foley catheter should not be passed blindly into the bladder until a urethral injury has been ruled out. Children who present with gross hematuria and a concomitant pelvic fracture or associated injuries require imaging, either a retrograde cystogram or a combination of retrograde and CT cystography is appropriate. It is important to make sure that the bladder is fully distended or the injury may be missed. This requires estimating the patient's bladder capacity and instilling this amount of contrast into the bladder under drainage by gravity. CT cystography alone without retrograde instillation of contrast may not adequately distend the bladder. The diagnosis of an intraperitoneal rupture is made when contrast is seen outlining the peritoneal cavity.

Serum chemistries may also reveal an increase in blood urea nitrogen, creatinine and potassium. Extraperitoneal rupture will not lead to changes in serum chemistry; however, the cystogram will show a flame type pattern of contrast extravasation in the pelvis.

The treatment of the ruptured bladder is based on whether the injury is intraperitoneal or extraperitoneal. Intraperitoneal rupture requires surgical closure of the bladder, with or without placement of a suprapubic catheter. In most cases extraperitoneal rupture can be managed with urethral catheter drainage for 2–3 weeks. However, evidence of bone fragments within the bladder mandates surgical debridement and closure, as the bladder will not heal adequately with retained bone fragments. In either case the patient should remain on a prophylactic antibiotic while the suprapubic tube/urethral catheter remains. Before removing the suprapubic tube a cystogram is performed to ensure that the bladder has healed.

URETHRAL TRAUMA

The majority of urethral injuries are associated with pelvic fractures. The incidence of urethral injury in children with pelvic fractures ranges from 7.4 to 13.5% with one recent study reporting a 0.9% incidence.[19] The majority of children who sustain pelvic fractures are pedestrians hit by a motor vehicle, or passengers in a motor vehicle.[19]

The anatomy of the male child contributes to the uniqueness of the urethral injuries. The prostate in children is immature and not well formed. Unlike in adults this leads to shearing of the urethra between the bladder and the prostate and the prostatic urethra itself. Shearing of the urethra will lead to bleeding resulting in a pelvic hematoma, as well as extravasation of urine. The combination of the two leads to a gap between the proximal and distal urethra. Clinically the patient may present with blood at the urethral meatus, gross hematuria or inability to void.

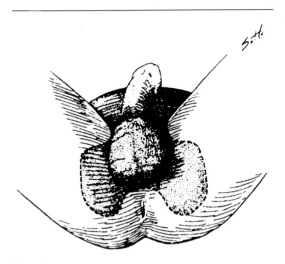

Figure 11.3

Illustration of the extent of the hematoma seen in a bulbar ure-thral straddle injury. (Reproduced from Walsh et al (eds). *Campbell's Urology* 5th edn. Philadelphia: WB Saunders, 1986 with permission from Elsevier.)

In addition to posterior urethral injuries, the bulbous urethra is often injured during straddle trauma while bike riding, or by direct injury to the perineum. These injuries cause the urethra to be crushed instead of transected and bleeding is contained within Colles' fascia, giving rise to the classic butterfly hematoma pattern seen on the perineum (Figure 11.3).[9]

Blunt injury to the urethra in girls is less common, this may be due to its mobility as well as its shorter course behind the pubic bone. Because of the relative infrequent occurrence of this injury, it is often missed. Unlike in boys, urethral injuries associated with a pelvic fracture result in a complete rupture which can occur anywhere along the entire length of the urethra.[20] Vaginal injuries are associated with urethral injuries in up to 87% of girls. These injuries vary from partial disruption of the anterior vaginal wall to a circumferential vaginal rupture.[20]

Evaluation of the urethral injury begins with inspection of the urethral meatus for blood. If no blood is noted, gentle passage of a urethral catheter can be attempted. If there is blood at the meatus, a retrograde urethrogram is performed to delineate the site and extent of the injury. The patient should be positioned obliquely in order to image the entire urethra as well as the bladder neck. A rectal exam and a pelvic exam are included as part of the work-up to ensure there are no associated vaginal or rectal injuries.

The management of urethral injury is controversial. Traditionally these injuries have been managed with suprapubic bladder decompression and delayed primary end-to-end urethral anastamosis. Placement of a suprapubic tube leads to urethral stricture formation in 97% of adult cases.[21] After delayed primary repair in adults, the urethral restricture rate is between 11 and 30%, with continence rates between 90 and 95%.[21] Strictures have been seen in 67% of children after delayed repair,[22] however, almost all are continent with a final success rate of over 90%.[23]

Alternatives to delayed repair include immediate surgical repair of the urethra and bladder neck. This type of repair unfortunately is associated with a high incidence of bleeding and incontinence.[21] Yet another option would be initial primary realignment over a catheter. This is performed with concomitant suprapubic access. A sound is passed into the proximal urethra from above in order to pass beyond the injured segment, then a catheter can be passed over a guide wire and left in place until healing is complete in 4–6 weeks. The rate of incontinence is very low with this type of repair but the stricture rate remains high.[24] It appears that delayed repair and immediate realignment are equally efficacious and treatment depends primarily on the condition of the patient. If the patient is unstable, primary realignment should not be attempted. This type of patient is best treated with a suprapubic diversion and delayed repair.

The management of female urethral injuries is no less controversial. This is due to the small number of cases reported in the literature.

Immediate surgical repair is advocated by some because delayed repair in patients with vaginal injuries may lead to urethral vaginal fistula formation or vaginal stenosis. However when primary realignment was performed in one series the stricture rate was 100%.[25] In a recent study by Podesta and Jordan. girls treated with initial suprapubic drainage and subsequent delayed primary repair had a 100% stricture free rate as well as a low rate of incontinence.[20] In girls, it appears that delayed repair may be the preferred treatment.

PENILE TRAUMA

Trauma to the penis is a rare event; due to its mobility and position it is rarely affected during a blunt traumatic injury. Most injuries are due to circumcision, dog bites or child abuse. Iatrogenic circumcision injury is by far the most common type of penile injury.[26] These injuries range in severity from degloving of the shaft to partial glanular amputation to total penile amputation. Three-quarters of circumcision-related trauma is in the form of a urethral cutaneous fistula, which occurs when excess ventral skin and urethra are trapped in the circumcision clamp.[26]

If the fistula is proximal to the glans, it may be repaired by primary closure. When the fistula is subcoronal, primary closure should be avoided due to the overlapping suture lines which can lead to a recurrence.[27] Subcoronal fistulas are repaired by splitting the glans with formation of a neourethra using a ventral Mathieu flap. Alternatively, the fistula is repaired using a vascularized pedicle onlay flap 9 (Figure 11.4). This flap can be either a ventral or dorsal vascularized penile skin pedicle flap.[27] Partial amputation or complete amputation of the glans presents a more serious challenge. In most cases the initial treatment of a partial glans amputation involves debridement with healing by secondary intention. Long-term issues are those of

cosmesis and a deviation of the urinary stream. Correction can be done at a later date by advancing the urethra and mobilizing it to a more normal position. Complete transection of the glans requires early reattachment. Reanastamosis is recommended even with a delay of up to 8 h.[28] The amputated glans must be recovered and placed in moist, chilled saline-soaked gauze. The wound should be debrided and excessive hemorrhage controlled with a topical solution of 1:100 000 epinephrine. The repair can be performed under a microscope, however, loupe magnification is sufficient. The goal of the reattachment is to provide a source of arterial blood to the amputated end. This is done by advancing the dorsal penile artery and anastamosing it to the corpus spongiosum. The urethra is reapproximated with chromic gut, and a shunt is created between the glans and the corporeal bodies to ensure adequate venous return (Figure 11.5).[29] Alternatively, the glans and distal penile amputation may be treated as a composite graft by anastomosing the urethra and the corpora and then suturing the skin. There have been reports of success with this technique, which depends on corporeal sinusoidal blood flow.[30] In the unfortunate case of a complete penile amputation, no thought should be given to gender conversion. Although controversial, it is our belief that those converted children who are genotypically male adjust poorly to being raised female. Reattachment of the completely amputated penis is similar to that already described. In the event that there is a non-recoverable loss of the penis, the existing urethra and corporeal bodies can be mobilized to fashion a functional penis. The operation is performed in two stages. A circumferential incision is made around the urethral meatus, and the corporeal bodies, the spongiosum and urethra are mobilized. The suspensory ligaments are cut and the corpora are passed under a midline scrotal tunnel. Two to six months later the penis can be detached from the scrotum and either the scrotal skin or skin grafts can be used for coverage of the penile shaft.

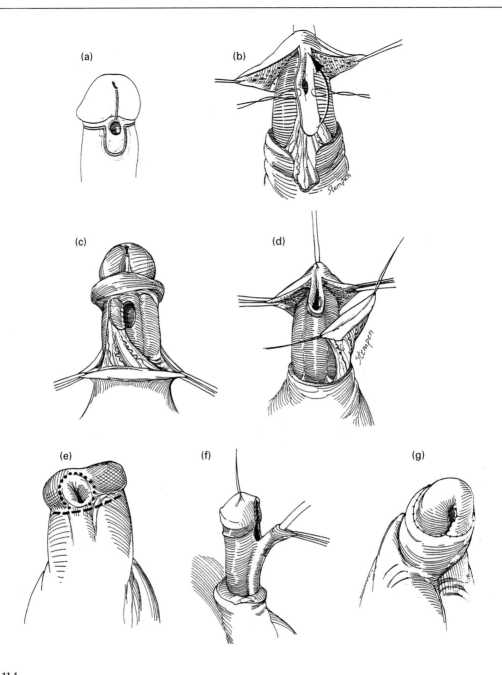

Figure 11.4

Technique for repair of an iatrogenic urethral cutaneous fistula and partial penile glans amputation. (a, b) Repair of urethral fistula using a Mathieu flap. (c, d) Repair of urethral fistula using an onlay island flap. (e–g) Repair of a partial amputation of the glans by urethral mobilization and advancement. (Reproduced from Baskin et al. *J Urol* 1997; **158**: 2269–71.[27])

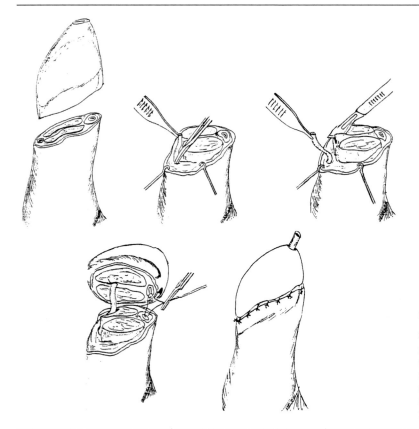

Figure 11.5

Steps in repairing a complete penile amputation, beginning with approximation of the urethra and dorsal penile artery to the distal corpora spongiosum. (Reproduced from Okan and Gurpinar. *J Urol* 1997; **158**: 1946–7.[45])

SCROTAL TRAUMA

Trauma to the scrotum and intrascrotal contents can be divided into blunt injury and penetrating injury. Blunt trauma to the scrotum leading to testicular rupture is seen in the setting of a straddle or sports injury. Although the testicles are mobile they may be compressed up against the pubic bone during the injury. These children usually present with acute pain and scrotal swelling. It is important to evaluate the patient for urethral injury, as well as considering the alternative diagnosis of testicular torsion and torsion of the appendix epididymis. Scrotal ultrasound can help to differentiate a testicular rupture. However, ultrasound has been found to be only 56% accurate in diagnosing a rupture of the tunica albuginea.[31] We recommend surgical exploration and closure of the tunica when the possibility of rupture cannot be ruled out. Penetrating injuries or skin avulsion occur much less frequently. The most common injury of this type is a dog bite. Bites account for approximately 1% of all emergency room visits, of which 60–70% involve children.[32] The microbiology of dog bites has been well studied and the most common isolates are *Pasteurella*, *Streptococcus* and *Staphylococcus* in addition to anaerobic organisms. Therefore all wounds should be covered prophylactically with an appropriate cephalosporin. These wounds should never be closed primarily due to contamination.

When evaluating non-bite lacerations, the area and surrounding structures should be surveyed. It is important to rule out testicular and urethral injuries. Testicular injury can be confirmed with a scrotal ultrasound. Blood at the urethral meatus, hematuria or retention suggests a urethral injury and necessitates retrograde urethrography. Penetrating trauma with exposure of the testicle and chord is best managed by exploration and repair of the injured structures.[33] In the case of complete avulsion of the scrotum the testicles may be placed in a thigh pouch. In the absence of gross contamination the wound can be debrided and closed primarily. If the injury results in significant loss of scrotal skin, reconstruction with skin grafts or flaps may be necessary. The best cosmetic and functional outcome results from the use of a split-thickness skin graft obtained from the thigh or the abdomen.[34]

DIAGNOSIS AND ACUTE MANAGEMENT OF URINARY TRACT INFECTION

Acute febrile urinary tract infections (UTIs) are common and are associated with significant morbidity. Approximately 3–8% of girls and 1% of boys will be affected.[35,36] Of these children 20–60% will be diagnosed with vesicoureteral reflux[37,38] and 3–25% will have an anatomic abnormality such as ureteropelvic junction obstruction.[39]

The diagnosis of UTI depends upon obtaining an uncontaminated urine culture. Suprapubic aspiration is the least likely to be contaminated, however, in most cases a catheterized specimen is sufficient. A urine culture with a colony count of >100 000 of a single organism is considered positive for infection. Treatment depends on the presentation of the child. If the child appears acutely ill (dehydrated with inability to tolerate liquids), hospitalization and treatment with parental antibiotics is indicated. In those children who appear less ill, oral antibiotics are acceptable. In either case the patient should receive 7–10 days of treatment. If the patient requires intravenous therapy, a third-generation cephalosporin or a combination of ampicillin and an aminoglycoside, such as gentamicin is appropriate. If oral therapy is selected the patient can be placed on a sulfa-based antibiotic and the medication changed to reflect the culture results. If the patient fails to improve within 48 h of treatment the urine should be recultured. All young children who present with a febrile UTI require ultrasound imaging of the kidneys and bladder as well as a voiding cystourethrogram to rule out an anatomical abnormality or vesicoureteral reflux.

BALANOPOSTHITIS AND PARAPHIMOSIS

Paraphimosis is defined as an inability to retract the foreskin over the glans penis. If this state persists, the glans will become edematous due to prolonged venous engorgement. These children will present with pain and in rare instances with urinary obstruction.[40] Physical examination reveals a swollen collar of foreskin just proximal to the corona. Treatment depends on the duration and extent of the swelling. In the older child or infant with a moderate amount of edema, the foreskin can be manually replaced over the glans. Before starting, a topical anesthetic such as Emla cream is applied. Alternatively, the penis can be wrapped in an elastic dressing for several minutes before attempting manual reduction. Surgical therapy should be considered in those patients presenting with a large amount of edema or ischemic changes of the glans. Circumcision is the treatment of choice, performed under general anesthesia or with a penile block.

Balinoposthitis, although not a surgical emergency may present with pain or difficulty with urination. The cause is often a bacterial infection secondary to poor hygiene in uncircumcised boys. Treatment consists of retraction of the foreskin and cleansing with soap and water. A topical antibiotic ointment may also be applied to the affected area. If there is penile discharge or the patient is febrile a course of oral antibiotics is appropriate. If it is not possible to retract the foreskin, topical low-dose steroids can be applied to the affected area with gentle retraction of the skin after 1 week of treatment. Continued phimosis not responding to steroid treatment necessitates circumcision.

AMBIGUOUS GENITALIA

The evaluation of an infant with ambiguous genitalia is a true emergency. The diagnosis and treatment is approached in a stepwise fashion by a team consisting of a pediatric urologist and others with expertise in this area.

Physical examination is the first step in the evaluation. If the child has bilateral palpable gonads in the scrotum (even in the presence of hypospadias) the child should be considered a male and no karyotype is needed. If the child has hypospadias and only a single palpable gonad, this rules out female pseudohermaphroditism (congenital adrenal hyperplasia) but not other intersex states. These children will need to be karyotyped. If there is no palpable gonad, serum electrolytes should be obtained emergently to rule out salt-wasting in a patient with congenital adrenal hyperplasia. Once the most severe form of congenital adrenal hyperplasia is ruled out, a karyotype and serum studies (17-hydroxyprogesterone and deoxycorticosterone) are obtained to determine if a 21-hydroxylase or 11-hydroxylase deficiency is present. Other helpful but less emergent studies include an ultrasound of the abdomen and pelvis to identify the presence or absence of a uterus. A genitogram is also useful to delineate the anatomy in those children suspected of having a concomitant urogenital sinus.

Treatment and the timing of treatment remain controversial. Gender conversion should not be considered in a child with an XY karyotype. In children who are mosaics the sex of rearing is best determined by the external genitalia as well as the presence of at least one normal testicle. To

this end diagnostic laparoscopy is essential in determining the presence of a normal testicle. At the time of surgery a biopsy of the gonad is taken. If a normal testicle is seen, the gonad is left in place or brought down into the scrotum. Streak or dysgenic gonads necessitate gonadectomy due to the risk of gonadoblastoma. Clitoral reduction in the case of congenital adrenal hyperplasia or the creation of a vagina is better approached surgically at a young age, however this remains a point of controversy.

POSTERIOR URETHRAL VALVES

The diagnosis of posterior urethral valves is most often made in utero. Prenatal ultrasound will reveal a dilated bladder and kidneys. The newborn patient may present with an inability to void and a palpable abdominal mass or rarely, with sepsis and failure to thrive. The initial goals in the management of valve patients are to relieve obstruction and preserve glomerular filtration. At presentation a small 5 Fr feeding tube should be placed through the urethra in order to relieve obstruction. The position of the catheter is then confirmed with a bladder ultrasound. A serum creatinine is obtained after several days of hydration. A serum creatinine of 0.8 mg/dl or less suggests a good prognosis and is followed by endoscopic valve ablation. When the urethra is too small to accommodate a pediatric cystoscope a vesicostomy is performed. In children, whose serum creatinine nadir is greater than 1 mg/dl the management is not straightforward. Options include a vesicostomy or supravesicle diversion in the form of a nephrostomy tube or cutaneous loop ureterostomy. However, no clear objective data support the use of these operations in the recoverability of renal function.

BLADDER EXSTROPHY

Bladder exstrophy presents as a spectrum of disease affecting the urinary bladder, genitalia and intestinal tract. Although rare, with an incidence of 3.3 per 100 000 births[41] the diagnosis of bladder exstrophy requires transfer to a center with expertise in the management of this condition. In preparation for surgery these children should receive adequate fluid resuscitation, and the exposed bladder needs to be covered with a clear plastic wrap. This covering will protect the bladder mucosa. A new wrap should be applied and the bladder irrigated with saline at each diaper change. Surgery is performed within the first 24–48 h. Osteotomies are often performed prior to closure. If closure is delayed beyond 48 h, osteotomies are necessary for proper positioning of the bladder in the pelvis. The bladder and external genitalia can be repaired in one surgery or in a staged fashion. In the case of cloacal exstrophy this is performed along with a diverting colostomy. These children are immobilized for a period of 1 month and remain on antibiotic prophylaxis until the ureteral stents are removed.

TESTICULAR TORSION

Testicular torsion is a true surgical emergency. If testicular ischemia is not corrected, damage may develop within 4–6 h. This is followed by complete infarction within 24 h.[42] Testicular torsion occurs at a rate of 1 in 4000 males younger than 25 years of age.[43] Torsion is most often observed in pubertal boys, however, it can occur at younger ages. These patients often present with an acute onset of scrotal pain but the presentation may be more insidious. Physical examination will most often reveal a high-riding testicle, which is painful to examine. The testicle may have an abnormal transverse orientation and the cremasteric reflex may be absent. The treatment of testicular torsion includes surgical exploration and fixation of the contralateral side. Manual detorsion of the testicle can be attempted; however, this should be followed

with prompt surgical fixation. Diagnostic modalities such as testicular ultrasound and radionuclide imaging should only be performed when the diagnosis is in question, such as in the case of torsion of the testicular or epididymal appendix.

TORSION OF THE TESTICULAR APPENDAGES

The appendix testis and epididymis, although of different origins (the former being a müllerian remnant and the latter a vestige of the wolffian duct) may present in the same manner as testicular torsion. Clinically the cremasteric reflex is present and often a blue discoloration is noticed on the scrotum signaling the presence of the infarcted appendage. In these cases, a scrotal ultrasound with blood flow to the testicle eliminates the need for surgery. Treatment is supportive, consisting of non-steroidal anti-inflammatory agents for pain control.

PRENATAL TORSION

When torsion occurs prenatally, a hard painless mass is palpable in a discolored scrotum. This type of torsion (extravaginal) is due to twisting of both the tunics and the cord. The management of prenatal torsion is highly controversial. The salvage rate of these testicles in spite of prompt surgical intervention is near zero. Since the mechanism of postnatal torsion is different (secondary to a fixation defect within the tunica) there should be no need for fixation of the contralateral testicle. However, there have been reports of contralateral torsion in the newborn period, suggesting that fixation is warranted.

Although less common, prenatal torsion can occur bilaterally, again surgery in these cases rarely results in testicular salvage and observation remains the best course of treatment.[44]

REFERENCES

1. Stein JP, Kaji DM, Eastham J et al. Blunt renal trauma in the pediatric population indications for radiologic evaluation. *Urology* 1994; **44**: 406–10.
2. Mendez R. Renal trauma. *J Urol* 1977; **118**: 698–703.
3. McAleer IM, Kapalan GW, Scherz HC. Genitourinary trauma in the pediatric population. *Urology* 1993; **42**: 563–7.
4. Kuzmarov IW, Morehouse DD, Gibson S. Blunt renal trauma in the pediatric population. *J Urol* 1981; **126**: 648–9.
5. Schmidline FR, Iselin CE, Naimi A. The higher injury risk of abnormal kidneys in blunt renal trauma. *Scand J Urol Nephrol* 1998; **32**: 388–92.
6. Mee SL, McAninch JW, Robinson AL. Radiographic assessment of renal trauma: A 10 year study of patient selection. *J. Urol* 1989; **141**: 1095–8.
7. Medica J, Caldamone A. Pediatric renal trauma: special considerations. *Semin Urol* 1995; **13**: 73–6.
8. Morey AF, Bruce JE, McAninch JW. Efficacy of radiographic imaging in pediatric blunt renal trauma. *J. Urol* 1996; **156**: 2014–18.
9. Brown SL, Haas C, Dinchman KH, Elder JS, Spirnak P. Radiographic evaluation of pediatric blunt renal trauma in patients with microscopic hematuria. *World J Surg* 2001; **25**: 1557–60.
10. Carroll PR, McAninch JW. Operative indications in penetrating renal trauma. *J Trauma* 1985; **25**: 587–93.
11. Morey AF, McAninch JW. Renal trauma: principles of evaluation and management. *Trauma Quarterly* 1996; **13**: 79–94.
12. Matthews LA, Smith EM, Spirnak JP. Nonoperative treatment of major blunt renal lacerations with urinary extravasation. *J Urol* 1997; **157**: 2056–8.
13. Russell RS, Gomelsky A, McMahon DR, Andrews D, Nasrallah PF. Management of grade 4 renal injury in children. *J Urol* 2001; **166**: 1049–50.
14. Noe HN, Jenkins GR. *Genitourinary Trauma*. Philadelphia: WB Saunders, 1992.
15. Rao CR. Ureteral avulsion secondary to blunt abdominal injury. *J Urol* 1973; **110**: 188–90.
16. Bard JL, Klein FA. Ureteropelvic junction avulsion following blunt abdominal trauma. *J Tenn Med Assoc* 1990; **83**: 242–3.
17. Sivit CJ, Cutting JP, Eichelberger MR. CT diagnosis and localization of rupture of the bladder in children with blunt abdominal trauma: significance of contrast material extravasation in the pelvis. *Am J Roentgenol* 1995; **164**: 1243–6.
18. Iverson AJ, Morey AF. Radiographic evaluation of suspected bladder rupture following blunt trauma: critical review. *World J Surg* 2001; **25**: 1588–91.
19. Tarman GJ, Kaplan GW, Lerman SL, McAleer IM, Losasso BE. Lower genitourinary injury and pelvic fractures in pediatric patients. *Urology* 2002; **59**: 123–6.
20. Podesta ML, Jordan GH. Pelvic fracture urethral injuries in girls. *J Urol* 2001; **165**: 1660–5.
21. Koraitim MM. Pelvic fracture urethral injuries: evaluation of various methods of management. *J Urol* 1996; **156**: 1288–91.
22. Boone TB, Wilson WT, Husman DA. Postpubertal genitourinary function following posterior urethral disruptions in children. *J Urol* 1992; **148**: 1232–4.
23. Koraitim M. Posttraumatic posterior urethral strictures in children: a 20 year experience. *J Urol* 1992; **157**: 641–4.
24. Elliott DS, Barrett DM. Long-term follow-up and evaluation of primary realignment of posterior urethral disruptions. *J Urol* 1997; **157**: 814–16.
25. Waterhouse K, Gross M. Trauma to the genitourinary tract: a 5 year experience with 51 cases. *J Urol* 1969; **101**: 241–6.
26. El-Bahnasawy MS, El-Sherbiny MT. Pediatric penile trauma. *BJU Int* 2002; **90**: 92–6.
27. Baskin LS, Canning DA, Synder HM, Duckett JW. Surgical repair of urethral circumcision injuries. *J Urol* 1997; **158**: 2269–71.
28. Sherman J, Borer JG, Horowitz M. Circumcision: successful glandular reconstruction following traumatic amputation. *J Urol* 1996; **156**: 842–4.
29. Ozkan S, Gurpinar T. A serious circumcision complication: penile shaft amputation and a new reattachment technique with a successful outcome. *J Urol* 1997; **158**: 1946–7.
30. Hashem FK, Ahmed S, Al-Malaq A, AbuDaia JM. Successful replantation of penile amputation (post-circumcision) complicated by prolonged ischemia. *Br J Plast Surgery* 1999; **52**: 308–10.
31. Corrales JG, Corbel L, Cipolla B, et al. Accuracy of ultrasound diagnosis after blunt testicular trauma. J Urol 1993; **150**: 1834–6.
32. Weiss HB, Freidman DI, Coben JH. Incidence of dog bite injuries treated in emergency departments. *JAMA* 1998; **279**: 51–3.
33. Cline KJ, Mata JA, Venable DD. Penetrating trauma to the male external genitalia. *J Trauma* 1998; **44**: 492–4.
34. Gomes CM, Ribeiro-Filho L, Giron AM, Mitre AI, Figueira ER et al. Genital trauma due to animal bites. *J Urol* 2000; **165**: 80–3.
35. Stark H. Urinary tract infections in girls: the cost-effectiveness of currently recommended investigative routines. *Pediatr Nephrol* 1997; **11**: 174–7.
36. Winberg J, Bergstron T, Jacobsson B. Morbidity, age and sex distribution, recurrences and renal scarring in symptomatic urinary tract infection in childhood. *Kidney Int Suppl* 1975; **4 (Suppl)**: 101.
37. Abbott GD. Neonatal bacteriuria: a prospective study in 1460 infants. *BMJ* 1972; **i**: 267–9.
38. Asscher AW, McLachian MSF, Jones RV. Screening for asymptomatic urinary-tract infection in schoolgirls. *Lancet* 1973; **ii**: 1–4.
39. Spencer JR, Schaeffer AJ. Pediatric urinary tract infections. *Urol Clin North Am* 1986; **13**: 661–72.
40. Ochsner MG. Acute urinary retention. *Compr Ther* 1986; **12**: 26–31.
41. Lancaster P. Epidemiology of bladder exstrophy and epispadias: a communication from the International Clearinghouse for Birth Defects monitoring system. *Teratology* 1987; **36**: 221–7.
42. Cosentino MJ, Rabinowitz R, Valvo JR. The effect of prepubertal spermatic cord torsion on subsequent fertility in rats. *J Androl* 1984; **5**: 93–8.
43. Williamson RCN. Torsion of the testis and allied conditions. *Br J Surg* 1976; **63**: 465–76.
44. Cooper CS, Synder OB, Hawtrey CE. Bilateral neonatal testicular torsion. *Clin Pediatr* 1997; **36**: 653–6.
45. Okan S, Gurpinar T. A serious circumcision complication: penile shaft amputation and a new reattachment technique with successful outcome. *J Urol* 1997; **158**: 1946–7.

12. Emergency management of gross hematuria

Leon Lilas and Faiz Mumtaz

Massive hematuria in the emergency setting is an alarming symptom for both patients and doctors. Its management therefore demands urgent assessment to identify the underlying cause and severity. The differential diagnosis includes both glomerular and non-glomerular causes. The latter accounts for the majority of causes of massive hematuria encountered in the emergency department. Rarely, the hematuria may become intractable hematuria and, therefore, present as a life-threatening situation, whose management can be challenging. The appropriate use of history, clinical examination and diagnostic tests leads to the most efficient way of diagnosing and treating the most common causes (Figure 12.1).

From a management point of view it is useful to think of frank hematuria as being caused by upper tract or lower tract pathology. Some of the more challenging causes that may present as gross hematuria are listed in Table 12.1. It must be emphasized that gross hematuria in the absence of an evident predisposing cause

should be considered as highly suspicious of a neoplastic lesion. It has been reported that up to 40% of patients presenting to the emergency department with a history of gross hematuria will have a neoplastic pathology on further evaluation.

This chapter discusses the management of gross and intractable hematuria that may prove difficult to manage.

UPPER URINARY HEMATURIA TRACT

The management of upper urinary tract bleeding secondary to urolithiasis and trauma are discussed in detail in Chapters 4 and 6, respectively. The diagnosis and treatment is predominantly guided by a good history and appropriate imaging. The management of bleeding in these situations is linked to the management of the underlying conditions.

SPONTANEOUS RENAL HEMORRHAGE

Gross hematuria can occasionally be the presenting sign of spontaneous renal hemorrhage from benign or malignant renal neoplasms. The common causes contributing to the hematuria are renal cell (Figure 12.2) and transitional cell (Figure 12.3) carcinomas, angiomyolipoma and vascular diseases such as haemangiomas. The underlying cause is best identified by computed tomography (CT), which has an overall sensitivity and specificity of 0.57 and 0.82, respectively. The immediate management of frank hematuria secondary to malignant renal neoplasms may require embolization. This can be followed by an elective radical nephrectomy.

Angiomyolipoma may present with spontaneous bleeding (with hypotension), loin pain and gross hematuria (Figure 12.4). Massive

---

Table 12.1 Causes of gross hematuria
Upper urinary tract
• Renal trauma
• Urolithiasis
• Spontaneous: renal tumors
• Iatrogenic: Post-renal biopsy and percutaneous nephrolithotomy (PCNL)
Lower urinary tract
• Pelvic trauma
• Bladder tumors
• Bladder radiation changes
• Hemorrhagic cystitis
• Prostatic bleeding post transurethral resection of the prostate (TURP)
Renal and retroperitoneal haemorrhage

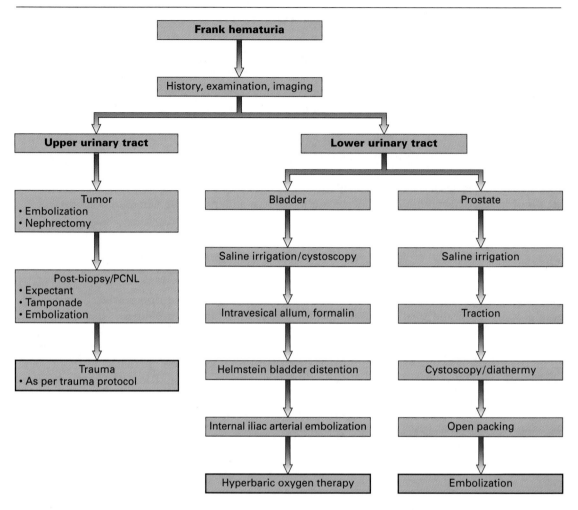

Figure 12.1

Algorithm for the emergency management of gross hematuria. PCNL, percutaneous nephrolithotomy.

retroperitoneal bleeding from angiomyolipomas (Wunderlich's syndrome) occurs in up to 10% of cases. Approximately 20% of cases of angiomyolipoma occur against a background of tuberous sclerosis syndrome, an autosomal dominant disorder characterized by mental retardation, epilepsy, and adenoma sebaceum with a female to male ratio of 2:1. In the 80% of angiomyolipomas not associated with tuberous sclerosis the female preponderance is even

more significant. The majority of symptomatic angiomyolipomas are usually more than 4 cm in diameter. CT provides the ideal imaging modality where the typical appearance of fat within tumor of the kidney (Hounsfield units ≤10) is diagnostic (Figure 12.5). Current management of renal angiomyolipomas is dependent on the size of the tumor and the clinical status of the patient. Treatment includes observation, transcatheter embolization and/or

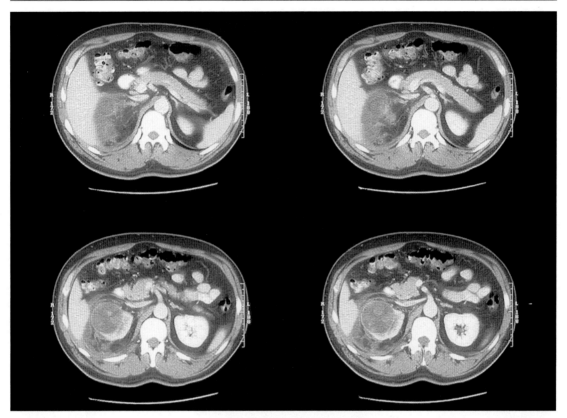

Figure 12.2

A CT scan of the abdomen in a patient with proven right-sided renal cell carcinoma. CT shows a rupture into the renal pelvis causing gross painless hematuria.

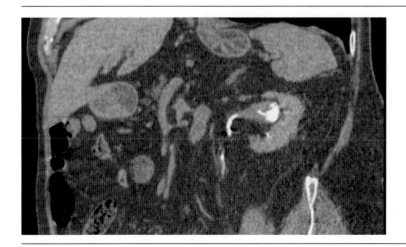

Figure 12.3

A contrast CT scan showing a large left-sided renal pelvis transitional cell carcinoma in a patient with gross painless hematuria. (Courtesy of Raj Bagree, University Hospital of Wales.)

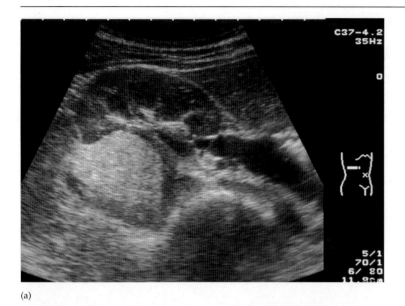

(a)

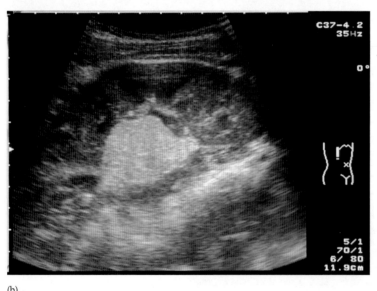

(b)

Figure 12.4

Ultrasound scan showing a focal well-defined echogenic mass in a patient with renal angiomyolipoma who presented with gross hematuria. (a) Axial view. (b) Sagittal view.

partial or total nephrectomy. If the bleeding is minimal based on clinical and radiographic assessment, bed rest and serial clinical observations may suffice. However, if bleeding is clinically significant it should initially be treated with selective arterial embolization. This approach is particularly important in cases associated with tuberous sclerosis, as these tend to be multicentric and bilateral. Long-term follow-up has shown that selective arterial embolization is effective and durable in the management of symptomatic angiomyolipomas

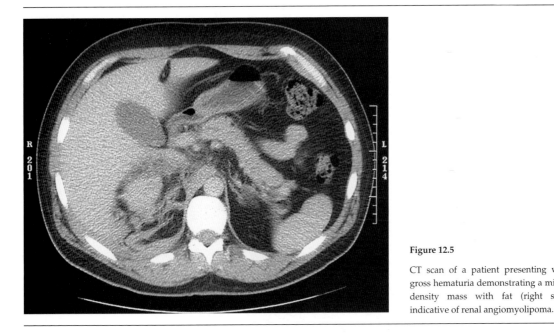

Figure 12.5

CT scan of a patient presenting with gross hematuria demonstrating a mixed density mass with fat (right side) indicative of renal angiomyolipoma.

(Figure 12.6). In addition to the general complications associated with arterial embolization (pain and fever), a minority of patients may experience sterile liquefaction of the fatty components of the angiomyolipoma. This can generally be drained percutaneously. However, some cases may require partial or total nephrectomy. If surgical exploration is warranted in the case of uncontrolled bleeding, the outcome is usually nephrectomy, although on occasions where bleeding is secondary to localized angiomyolipoma it may be treated by a partial nephrectomy.

IATROGENIC HEMATURIA

RENAL BIOPSY

Ultrasound-guided renal biopsy with an automated spring-loaded biopsy device has become the standard method for kidney biopsy. The incidence of significant hematuria (i.e. needing blood transfusion or intervention) has reportedly decreased from 7.7% to 0.36%. One suggested reason for this improvement is the reduction in size of the needle from 14 to 18 gauge. Other factors which have contributed to the decreased incidence of bleeding include: stopping aspirin or non-steroidal anti-inflammatory drugs for at least 5 days; routine checking of bleeding time; and avoiding biopsy in uncontrolled hypertensive patients. The rare cases of uncontrolled bleeding are best managed by selective embolization.

PERCUTANEOUS RENAL SURGERY

Renal hemorrhage is the most worrisome complication of percutaneous renal surgery. Reported incidence rates range from 0.3 to 2.3%. When noted intraoperatively the standard therapeutic measures include the placement of a large bore nephrostomy tube via the percutaneous tract as the initial step. The tract is then tamponaded by clamping the nephrostomy tube. Bleeding can also be controlled by the placement of a tamponade balloon catheter. If bleeding persists, the next step is to identify and localize the bleeding site by arteriography and treat by embolization. In larger series of

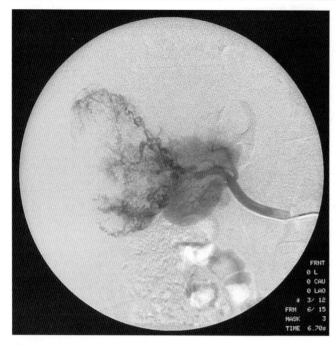

(a)

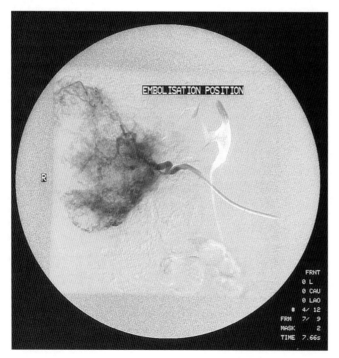

(b)

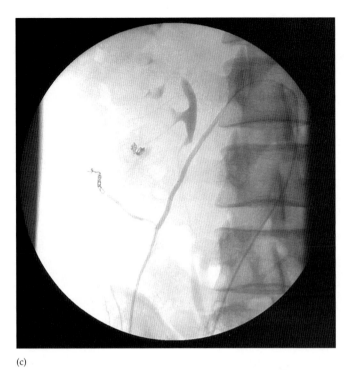

(c)

Figure 12.6

Embolization of angiomyolipoma. (a) Pre-embolization angiogram demonstating a large extravasation. (b) An embolization catheter in place at the site of bleeding. (c) Post-embolization with coils in place. (Courtesy of Andrew Wood, University Hospital of Wales.)

percutaneous renal operations, 0.8% required angiography and embolization for significant bleeding uncontrolled by the usual measures. The angiographic abnormalities identified are: arteriovenous fistula, pseudoaneurysm and lacerated renal vessels. Embolization allows definitive treatment of these lesions in the majority of cases. The failure of embolization may require a partial nephrectomy.

CONGENITAL ARTERIOVENOUS FISTULA

These can present with gross hematuria. The lesions are best assessed by color Doppler scan and treated by selective angiographic embolization (Figure 12.7).

LOWER URINARY TRACT HEMATURIA

Pelvic trauma is discussed in Chapter 7.

BLADDER HEMORRHAGE

The causes of severe bleeding arising from the bladder include bladder carcinoma (Figure 12.8), radiation cystitis, cyclophosphamide-induced cystitis and severe infection. After initial resuscitation, management consists of insertion of a large-bore three-way irrigation catheter and irrigation with saline. An ultrasound of the bladder can provide the diagnosis (Figure 12.9). If the bleeding is significant it leads to the formation of clots which makes catheter irrigation unrewarding (Figure 12.10).

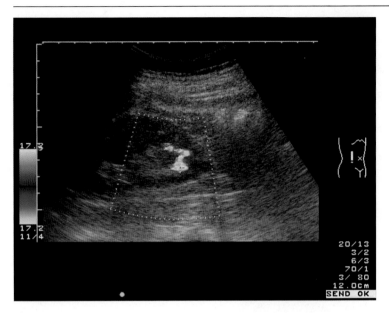

(a)

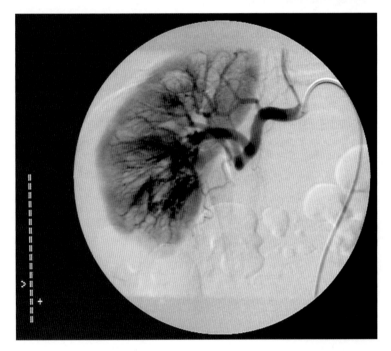

(b)

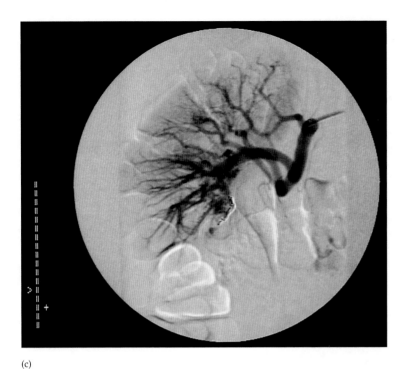

(c)

Figure 12.7

Congenital arteriovenous fistula: a 34-year-old female with recurrent severe hematuria. (a) A color Doppler showing the fistula. (b) An angiogram showing the site of the fistula in the lower pole of the kidney. (c) Post embolization.

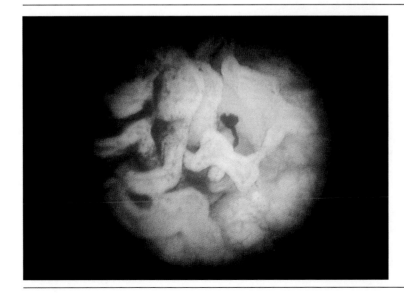

Figure 12.8

A large transitional cell carcinoma of the bladder, which presented with gross hematuria. (Courtesy of CRJ Woodhouse, UCL, London.)

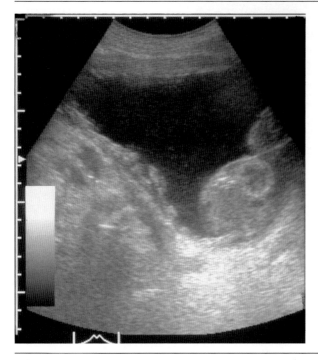

Figure 12.9

Ultrasound scan demonstrating blood clots in association with a bladder tumor.

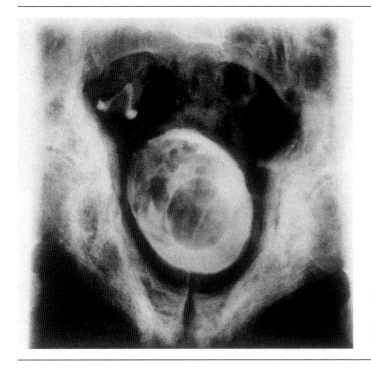

Figure 12.10

Intravenous urogram showing a large organized clot in the bladder. (Courtesy of CRJ Woodhouse, UCL, London.)

Thus, gentle evacuation of intravesical blood clots via a large bore urethral catheter could be initially carried out in the emergency department. Failure to maintain continuous irrigation and control of hemorrhage warrants an urgent cystoscopy with a large sheath (24–26 Ch) under regional or general anesthetic. This allows the efficient evacuation of clots and debris and identifies the cause of bleeding. Bladder washout in this setting is facilitated with the use of evacuators such as the Urovac™ evacuator (Boston Scientific, Watertown, MA, USA) or bladder syringes (Figures 12.11 and 12.12). Active bleeding points can then be seen and coagulated with

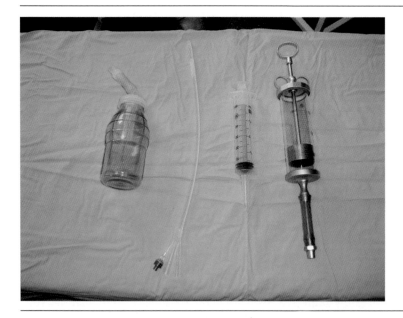

Figure 12.11

From left to right: various instruments used to evacuate blood clots. Urovac. Hematuria large bore 3-way catheter. Bladder syringe. Tomey bladder syringe.

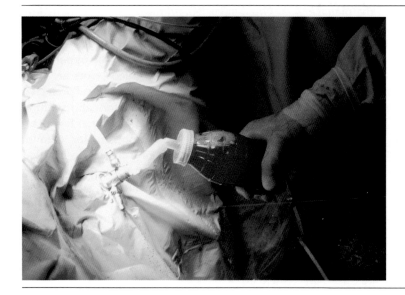

Figure 12.12

Use of urovac to evacuate blood clots from the bladder.

Table 12.2 Methods of management of intractable hematuria

Intravesical alum
Intravesical formalin
Hydrostatic pressure
Embolization
Hyperbaric oxygen
Prostaglandins
Single-dose radiation

surgical diathermy. If a bladder tumor is identified it can be resected at the same setting. If bleeding persists despite these measures, a life-threatening situation may develop, when blood transfusion fails to keep pace with the rate of blood loss. This group of patients are often elderly and unfit for cystectomy as a treatment option. In these circumstances, the management of intractable hematuria can be a challenging clinical problem. Several options for dealing with bleeding that does not settle with the initial preliminary steps have been described with varying degrees of success (Table 12.2).

INTRAVESICAL ALUM

Intravesical irrigation with 1% alum (aluminum ammonium sulfate or aluminum potassium sulfate) has been extensively used in the management of intractable bladder hematuria. Alum works by its direct astringent action on the cell surface and superficial interstitial spaces. The resultant decrease in capillary permeability, contraction of intercellular space, vasoconstriction and hardening of the capillary endothelium restores hemostasis.

One suggested regimen is 50 g of alum dissolved in 5 l of sterile water. This solution is then irrigated via a three-way catheter at a rate of 250–300 ml/h. Alum irrigation is usually well tolerated without the need for regional or general anesthesia. Alum should be carefully used in patients with renal impairment and large absorptive surface areas. Toxic accumulation (>2000 nmol/l) results in neurofibrillary degeneration. Affected patients may present with encephalopathy, lethargy, speech disorder, vomiting and convulsions. In symptomatic patients, stopping the irrigation can usually reverse these effects. In patients at increased risk (e.g. severe renal impairment) aluminum levels should be measured daily while carrying out irrigation.

INTRAVESICAL FORMALIN

Intravesical formalin has been used to control severe hemorrhage from the bladder. Though very effective (80–92%), formalin is highly toxic and needs to be given under spinal or regional anesthesia. When given intravesically, formalin causes edema, inflammation and necrosis throughout all the layers of the bladder. It also precipitates cellular proteins and has occluding and fixative actions on telangiectatic tissue and smaller capillaries. Complications are not infrequent and reports vary from 0% (1–2% solution) to 75% (10% solution). These include a small contracted bladder, urinary incontinence, vesicoureteric reflux, ureteric strictures, vesicoureteric junction obstruction with hydroureteronephrosis, acute tubular necrosis with anuria, vesicovaginal fistula, vesicoileal fistula, a toxic effect on the myocardium, bladder rupture and death.

One suggested protocol recommends a low initial concentration of 1–2% of formalin. Cystography is used to exclude reflux. Fogarty catheters can be used to protect the upper tracts in the presence of reflux. Blood clots are then evacuated and external perineal areas protected with the use of vaseline. The formalin solution can then be irrigated under gravity at low pressure (<15 cmH$_2$O or 11 mmHg) for 10 min. Alternatively, the solution can just be instilled under gravity and left intravesically for 10–15 min. More recently formalin has been applied via endoscopic placement of 10% formalin-soaked pledgets on the bleeding points for 15 min. Topical application of formalin-soaked pledgets is as effective in controlling the hemorrhage as conventional intravesical formalin instillation, with fewer complications.

HYDROSTATIC PRESSURE

There is a direct relationship between bladder blood flow and bladder pressure. Helmstein first used this principle to treat bladder tumors. Helmstein and others later used the technique to treat intractable bladder hematuria. The bladder pressure can be raised by fluid instillation or overinflation of an intravesically placed balloon. This balloon is available on specially designed catheters or can be formed using a condom tied over a Foley catheter with its tip cut off. The procedure is usually carried out under regional anesthesia. The balloon is inserted into the bladder and inflated to a pressure of 10–20 cmH$_2$O (7.4–14.7 mmHg) above diastolic. This pressure is then maintained for 6–7 h. After deflation the bladder is irrigated until the irrigant becomes clear of blood.

The most serious complication of bladder distension is bladder rupture. This is noted by sudden decrease of intravesical pressure and confirmed by an on-table cystogram. Extraperitoneal rupture can be successfully managed by urethral catheterization, whereas intraperitoneal ruptures will require an open repair. Other minor complications include nausea and vomiting, temporary incontinence and abdominal pain.

EMBOLIZATION

Embolization of the internal iliac (hypogastric) artery can also be used in the management of intractable bleeding from the bladder. Access to the internal iliac artery can be gained via the femoral or the axillary artery. A variety of substances have been used to occlude the internal iliac artery. Complications of internal iliac embolization include gluteal pain, lower limb ischemia, gangrene of the bladder and lower limb neurological compromise. Embolization has been reported to be successful in the control of significant hematuria in 92% of cases.

HYPERBARIC OXYGEN

Hyperbaric oxygen therapy has been specifically used to treat hematuria secondary to radiation-induced cystitis. The rationale of hyperbaric therapy is to reverse the radiation-induced vascular changes by causing neovascularization of the bladder wall and hence an increase in tissue oxygen tension. This increase in tissue oxygen tension is thought to reverse the radiation-induced changes and hence reduces the risk of recurrent bleeding. The protocol for hyperbaric oxygen therapy includes 20 sessions of 100% oxygen inhalation at 0.3 MPa in a multiplace hyperbaric chamber (90 min/session). The number of sessions may be increased to 40. Success has been reported in 75–90% patients treated. Serious complications are rare but this treatment is limited by lack of general availability.

INTRAVESICAL PROSTAGLANDINS FOR CYCLOPHOSPHAMIDE-INDUCED HEMORRHAGIC CYSTITIS

Cyclophosphamide is used in the treatment of B cell malignant diseases and some solid tumors, conditioning before bone marrow transplantation and in the treatment of nephrotic syndrome, rheumatoid arthritis and systemic lupus erythematosus. Cyclophosphamide results in the formation of acrolein which is excreted in the urine. Acrolein causes hemorrhage, edema, ulceration and necrosis of the urothelium. In this context, various prostaglandins have been used intravesically due to their cytoprotective effect on the urothelium. In addition, prostaglandins encourage platelet aggregation, induce vasoconstriction and cause smooth muscle contraction in mucosal and submucosal blood flow. The advantages of intravesical prostaglandins include good tolerance with no significant toxicity, no anesthetic requirement, easy bedside administration, no significant complication from vesicoureteral reflux and no formation of precipitate to the block catheters. The disadvantages include a high percentage of bladder spasms, intensive nursing supervision, cost and failure to control bleeding in all patients.

The overall incidence of cyclophosphamide-induced hemorrhagic cystitis is estimated to be between 2 and 40%.

HEMATURIA OF PROSTATIC ORIGIN

Hematuria of prostatic origin may be:

- spontaneous
- post biopsy
- post TURP
- post open prostatectomy.

Bleeding of prostatic origin is usually caused by the friable hypervascularity of the prostate, the vessels of which are easily disrupted by physical activity. Bleeding may occur in the setting of infection, benign prostatic hyperplasia or prostate cancer. Infection-related bleeding is usually diagnosed against the background of a typical history and examination. The treatment is primarily with antibiotics.

Prostate cancer can be the cause of significant bleeding in a small number of patients. Diagnosis is facilitated by digital rectal examination and measurement of serum prostate-specific antigen (PSA). Treatment in cases of significant hematuria may include catheterization and cystoscopy with a bladder washout. In selected cases limited TURP may be warranted. Hormonal therapy could also be considered as adjunctive treatment to reduce prostate vascularity.

In a large European randomized screening study the incidence of post-prostatic biopsy haematuria lasting more than 3 days was 22.6%. Hematuria correlated significantly with a larger prostate volume and an increasing transition zone volume/total prostate volume ratio. After multivariate logistic regression analysis, only prostate volume correlated significantly. No intervention was required to stop the hematuria as in all cases it settled spontaneously.

Excessive bleeding associated with TURP as defined by the need for blood transfusion, occurs in 6.4% (2.5% intraoperative, 3.9% postoperative) of cases. Bleeding usually occurs in the setting of large volume resections and capsular penetration. Contributing factors include the transurethral resection syndrome and hypocoagulable states (e.g. uncorrected pharmaceutical anticoagulation or hypocoagulation associated with metastatic disease).

Preoperatively, ensure platelet count and clotting status are optimal. In larger glands, it has been suggested that the preoperative use of finasteride may reduce the risk of excessive intraoperative bleeding. Finasteride acts by reducing gland volume and microvessel density. For optimum effect the drug would have to be given for at least 4–6 months to achieve a volume reduction of 20–25%. Microvessel density changes can be achieved histologically as early as 2 weeks. In a recent randomized controlled trial, finasteride was shown to cause a significant reduction in the loss of blood compared with the placebo group. This difference did not translate into a measurable decrease in transfusion rate. Further studies are required to determine the optimum duration of treatment.

Other techniques, which have been applied to reduce bleeding associated with TURP, include irrigation with intravesical ε-aminocaproic acid and endoscopic injection of the vasoconstrictor ornithine-8-vasopressin. The results of irrigation of a solution of 0.5% ε-aminocaproic acid have been disappointing. Endoscopic injection of ornithine-8-vasopressin into the prostate has been shown to reduce mean operative blood loss by 48–75%.

Venous bleeding associated with capsular perforation can be managed by early recognition and termination of the procedure in an expeditious manner. Direct pressure can then be applied to the prostate in the form of catheter traction with an overinflated balloon. This traction can be manual or with the aid of suitable strapping to the thigh or abdomen. Additional pressure can be applied in the form of posterior digital pressure on the prostate per rectum. Excessive or prolonged traction should be avoided, as this is associated with significant pain and the possibility of pressure necrosis.

Arterial bleeding should be recognized intraoperatively and coagulated. Postoperatively, arterial bleeding may be suspected by careful inspection of the catheter. Active pulsation can sometimes be noted in the outflow channel. Small bleeders will normally settle with the use of gentle traction. Large bleeding points usually cannot be controlled and one should not delay in returning the patient to the operating suite where the bladder can be effectively evacuated of clots (e.g. with the use of a bladder evacuator). The prostatic fossa can then be systematically inspected and bleeding points coagulated.

Rarely venous and/or arterial bleeding cannot be effectively managed as described above. These cases should undergo open packing of the prostatic fossa. The need for packing has been reported in 0.4% of cases of a large-scale clinical audit. This can be accomplished by a transvesical or retropubic approach. In selected cases significant uncontrolled bleeding/hematuria can be controlled with the use of superselective unilateral arterial embolization or bilateral hypogastric arterial occlusion.

FURTHER READING

Albi G, del Campo L, Tagarro D. Wunderlich's syndrome: causes, diagnosis and radiological management. *Clin Radiol* 2002; **57**: 840–5.

Antonsen HK, Lose G, Hojensgard JC. The Helmstein bladder distension treatment for tumours and severe bleeding. *Int Urol Nephrol* 1986; **18**: 421–7.

Bevers RF, Bakker DJ, Kurth KH. Hyperbaric oxygen treatment for haemorrhagic radiation cystitis. *Lancet* 1995; **346**: 803–5.

Choong SK, Walkden M, Kirby R. The management of intractable haematuria. *BJU Int* 2000; **86**: 951–9.

Dickinson M, Ruckle H, Beaghler M, Hadley HR. Renal angiomyolipoma: optimal treatment based on size and symptoms. *Clin Nephrol* 1998; **49**: 281–6.

Donahue LA, Frank IN. Intravesical formalin for hemorrhagic cystitis: analysis of therapy. *J Urol* 1989; **141**: 809–12.

Donohue JF, Sharma H, Abraham R et al. Transurethral prostate resection and bleeding: a randomized, placebo controlled trial of role of finasteride for decreasing operative blood loss. *J Urol* 2002; **168**: 2024–6.

Errando Smet C, Martinez De Hurtado J, Regalado Pareja R et al. [Analysis of 895 consultations for hematuria in the emergency department in an urology unit] *J Urol (Paris)* 1996; **102**: 168–71.

Fazeli-Matin S, Novick AC. Nephron-sparing surgery for renal angiomyolipoma. *Urology* 1998; **52**: 577–83.

Goswami AK, Mahajan RK, Nath R, Sharma SK. How safe is 1% alum irrigation in controlling intractable vesical haemorrhage? *J Urol* 1993; **149**: 264–7.

Kessaris DN, Bellman GC, Pardalidis NP, Smith AG. Management of haemorrhage after percutaneous renal surgery. *J Urol* 1995; **153**: 604–8.

Lojanapiwat B, Sripralakrit S, Soonthornphan S, Wudhikarn S. Intravesicle formalin instillation with a modified technique for controlling haemorrhage secondary to radiation cystitis. *Asian J Surg* 2002; **25**: 232–5.

Martin X, Murat FJ, Feitosa LC et al. Severe bleeding after nephrolithotomy: results of hyperselective embolization. *Eur Urol* 2000; **37**: 136–9

McIvor J, Willams G, Greswick Southcott RD. Control of severe vesical haemorrhage by therapeutic embolisation. *Clin Radiol* 1982; **33**: 561–7.

Michel F, Dubruille T, Cercueil JP et al. Arterial embolization for massive hematuria following transurethral prostatectomy. *J Urol* 2002; **168**: 2550–1.

Raaijmakers R, Kirkels WJ, Roobol MJ, Wildhagen MF, Schrder FH. Complication rates and risk factors of 5802 transrectal ultrasound-guided sextant biopsies of the prostate within a population-based screening program. *Urology* 2002; **60**: 826–30.

Sharifi R, Lee M, Ray P, Millner SN, Dupont PF. Safety and efficacy of intravesical aminocaproic acid for bleeding after transurethral resection of prostate. *Urology* 1986; **27**: 214–19.

Smart RF. Endoscopic injection of the vasoconstrictor ornithine-8-vasopressin in transurethral resection. *Br J Urol* 1984; **56**: 191–7.

Walker EM, Bera S, Faiz M. Does catheter traction reduce post-transurethral resection of the prostate blood loss? *Br J Urol* 1995; **75**: 614–17.

13. Urological oncological emergencies

Masood A Khan and Alan W Partin

Urological malignancies are commonly seen in daily medical practice. They may present either asymptomatically via the primary care provider or may present as an emergency with acute onset of symptoms. There are many potential emergencies associated with urological oncology. It is important to be aware of the presentation of and have a coherent plan of action to address these emergencies. To this effect, in this chapter, we will discuss some of the most common urological oncologic emergencies encountered and their management.

SPINAL CORD COMPRESSION

Bone is a common site of metastasis from prostate cancer (Figure 13.1). Bone metastasis can lead to severe bone pain, pathological fractures and if present within the vertebrae, spinal cord compression.[1,2] Clinically evident spinal cord compression develops in approximately 10% of patients with prostate cancer at some point in the course of their disease.[3] Although it is seen most often in patients with advanced, hormone-resistant disease, it may also be the first clinical manifestation of metastasis in

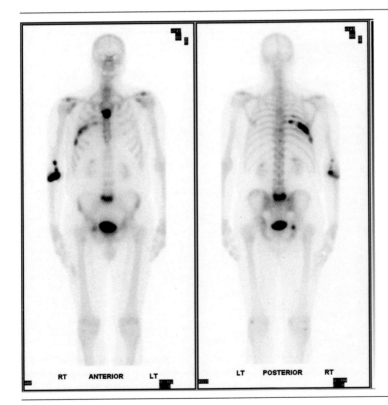

Figure 13.1

A bone scan showing multiple bony metastases as the source of acute pain in a patient with carcinoma of the prostate. (Courtesy of John Rees, University Hospital of Wales.)

patients with previously localized disease or, rarely, the presenting event in patients with previously unrecognized prostate cancer. Spinal cord compression most often occurs in the thoracic or upper lumber spine and results from either vertebral collapse from tumor invasion into the vertebral body or by extradural tumor growth anywhere along the spinal cord.[3,4]

The most common symptom is local or radicular pain. Motor weakness in the lower extremities may also arise. This weakness may be indolent and slowly progressive or, more commonly, be acute and progress rapidly to paraplegia. Sensory deficits are frequently identifiable. In addition, autonomic dysfunction, such as an atonic, painless, neurogenic bladder or unexplained acute onset of urinary incontinence, may also be evident.

Whenever spinal cord compression is suspected, evaluation must be done quickly. Neurological examination may indicate the approximate level of the lesion. In brief, the neu-rological examination should determine the tone, power and coordination of the lower and/or upper limbs. In addition, reflexes and sensation (e.g. light touch, pin-prick, two-point position and proprioception) need to be determined. Neurological examination should reveal changes consistent with an upper motor neuron defect. However, if the nerve roots are also involved, there may be a mixed pattern change demonstrating both upper and lower motor neuron defects. The presence of spinal cord compression can then be further confirmed with radiographs or a bone scan. Compression often occurs at the site of previously recognized tumor metastasis. Clear delineation of the cephalad and caudal extent of the lesion is necessary for proper therapy. Magnetic resonance imaging (MRI) provides the best detail of the spinal cord and surrounding structures.[5] Sagittal, coronal and oblique planes allow exact delineation of the level and extent of the spinal cord compression (Figure 13.2). If MRI is not

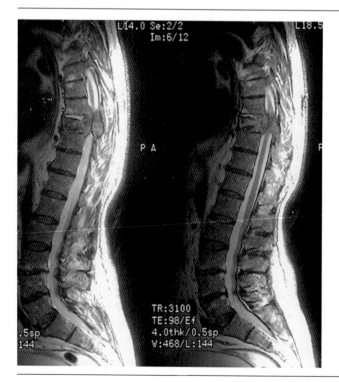

Figure 13.2

A sagittal T2-weighted magnetic resonance image showing a prostatic cancer bony metastasis of the dorsal vertebrae with compression of the spinal cord.

available, a computed tomography (CT) scan may instead be done. However, MRI has much greater resolution and is more sensitive for spinal cord lesions.

Treatment of prostatic carcinoma with spinal cord compression appears to have a relatively favorable clinical course compared with other types of tumor studied. Intervention can result in improvement of neurological symptoms in over 50% of patients; a median survival of greater than 1 year may be achieved. Overall, treatment outcome is related primarily to the patient's neurological status prior to treatment, with poor status leading to poorer post-treatment performance. Bladder dysfunction seems to be particularly ominous, as is complete para-

plegia. The duration of symptoms prior to intervention does not necessarily correlate with the degree of recovery. However, patients who have a sudden onset of paraplegia or rapid progression to paraplegia in a 24–36-h period usually have a very poor prognosis for functional recovery, regardless of treatment. In rapidly progressive cases, surgical intervention probably provides the greatest chance for limitation of neurological deficit.

The keys to successful treatment of spinal cord compression are rapid diagnosis and expedient therapy (Figure 13.3). Hence, once spinal cord compression is suspected clinically, steroids should be administered immediately in order to help reduce the edema around the

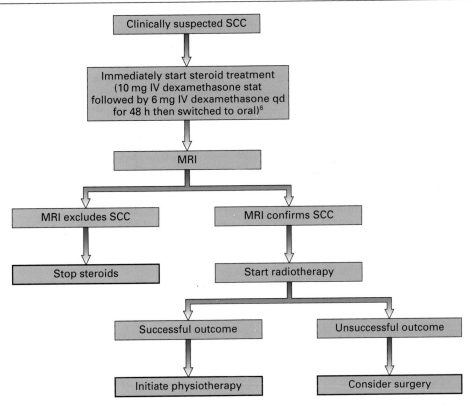

Figure 13.3

Algorithm for the management of spinal cord compression (SCC). IV, intravenous, MRI, magnetic resonance imaging; qd, once daily.

spinal cord. A typical regimen is a stat dose of 10 mg intravenous (IV) dexamethasone[6] followed by maintenance dose of 6 mg qd IV dexamethasone for the succeeding 48 h. This is then changed to oral administration once the patient is stable and the dose is tapered after a few days. One should not wait for MRI confirmation of spinal cord compression as delay in initiating treatment may worsen the prognosis. There is no clear advantage for either radiation or surgery as the next step in the definitive therapy of spinal cord compression. Numerous studies have evaluated this issue, most of them retrospectively.[7,8] Most studies have concluded that there is no distinct advantage of one therapeutic approach over the other, although both modalities can provide rapid pain relief in nearly two-thirds of patients. Hence, radiation therapy should be considered initially and surgery reserved for failed radiotherapy cases. There are a number of different radiotherapy regimens used to treat metastatic spinal cord compression. One such regimen, with proven efficacy, involves a course of 3000 cGy, which is given in 10 daily fractions of 300 cGy. Signs of recovery may be noted within a few days of starting radiotherapy. However, full ambulatory recovery may take many weeks. Surgery, which usually involves decompressive laminectomy, is associated with high mortality (3–14%) and morbidity (5–30%).[9] Hence, surgery should only be considered if vertebral stabilization is required or there is the presence of bone impingement on the cord from vertebral body collapse or radiotherapy has already been given to the affected area.

Approximately 75–100% of patients who are ambulatory at the time of treatment remain so.[9,10] However, only 14–35% of non-ambulatory patients and 5% of paraplegic patients regain useful function after treatment.[10,11]

It is imperative to be always aware of the possibility of spinal cord compression in patients with advanced prostate cancer as early diagnosis and management has a great influence on prognosis. Missing such a disorder can be associated with adverse patient outcome.

UREMIA SECONDARY TO URETERIC OBSTRUCTION

Malignant ureteric obstruction is a common late manifestation of advanced pelvic and/or retroperitoneal malignant disease. This is frequently associated with either advanced bladder or prostate cancer.[12,13] although advanced gynecological malignancies, such as cervical cancer, and malignant retroperitoneal fibrosis may instead be the cause. Ureteric obstruction may arise from either direct tumor spread or due to metastasis.

In bilateral ureteric obstruction or unilateral obstruction affecting the only functional kidney, patients will present acutely with symptoms arising from uremia, hyperkalemia and metabolic acidosis. These symptoms consist mainly of malaise, lethargy, tiredness, shortness of breath on exertion, pruritus, anorexia, nausea and vomiting.[14] These patients need to be treated urgently to avoid further complications of uremia such as coma and also to avoid potential cardiac complications of hyperkalemia, namely, cardiac arrest (Figure 13.4).

Patients presenting with symptoms suggestive of ureteric obstruction need an urgent ultrasound scan of the renal tract and bladder to confirm the presence of hydroureteronephrosis and help rule out bladder outlet obstruction (Figure 13.5). Once this is established, despite associated poor prognosis, urgent urinary diversion is required to avoid the devastating effects of uremia and, if appropriate, allow further treatment of the underlying malignancy. As urinary diversion can be very difficult and usually represents a short-lived option in this group of patients, the concept of actively treating these patients with any form of surgery raises important moral and ethical issues that are beyond the scope of this chapter. Urinary diversion is usually carried out by means of a percutaneous nephrostomy, which can be performed safely with low morbidity (Figure 13.6).[15,16] Although percutaneous nephrostomies are effective in

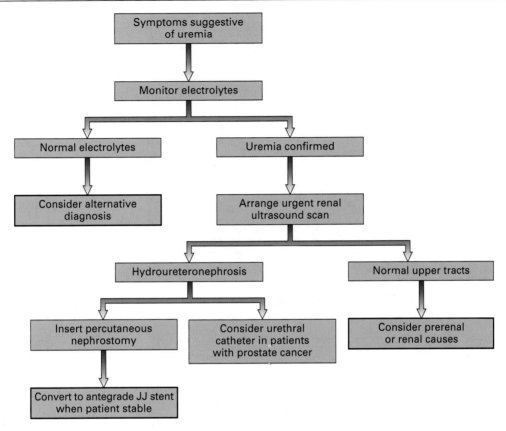

Figure 13.4

Algorithm for the management of uremia secondary to ureteric obstruction.

relieving ureteric obstruction they are considered as only a temporary measure as they have a tendency to displace or fall out. Hence, once the patient is stabilized, an antegrade ureteric stent is inserted and the nephrostomy tube is removed (Figure 13.7).

There are different types of stents available, including single or double-ended pigtail stents (more commonly known as JJ stents). Stents can also be made up of various materials. Silicone stents are less irritating and more resistant to encrustation, hence, are usually the first choice.

An alternative mode of management is retrograde ureteric JJ stent insertion as the initial procedure. However, this requires either a general or spinal anesthetic. As these patients are usually very ill with metabolic abnormalities, this is not a realistic option for the majority of cases. Furthermore, bladder cancer results in ureteric obstruction both extrinsically, by exerting pressure on the ureters, and intrinsically, by invading the ureteral orifices. Under these conditions, the ureter is very difficult to divert endoscopically with JJ stents as the ureteral orifices are either difficult to visualize or have been invaded by the cancer.

On rare occasions, in the presence of complete ureteric obstruction, it may not be possible to

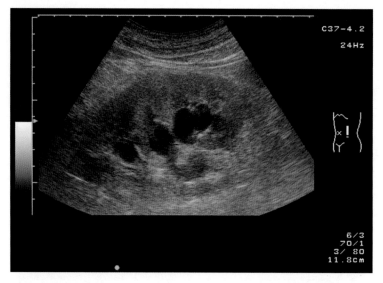

(a)

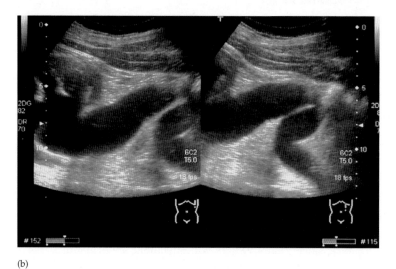

(b)

Figure 13.5

(a) Ultrasound scan showing early hydronephrosis in a patient with advanced carcinoma of the prostate. (b) Ultrasound scan showing significant hydroureteronephrosis in a patient with advanced carcinoma of the prostate.

pass a guide wire either antegrade or retrograde. In this situation a combined antegrade and retrograde approach may be required (rendezvous procedure). Briefly, the obstructed area is delineated radiographically by simultaneous antegrade and retrograde pyelograms. Ureteroscopes are then passed simultaneously in antegrade and retrograde directions and the two opposing ends of the ureter are localized using fluoroscopy. A guide wire is then passed from one end of the ureter, through the stricture, to the other lumen, using a combination of both direct vision and fluoroscopy. Once the guide wire is successfully passed across the stricture, the stricture is dilated and a stent is subsequently placed over the guide wire.

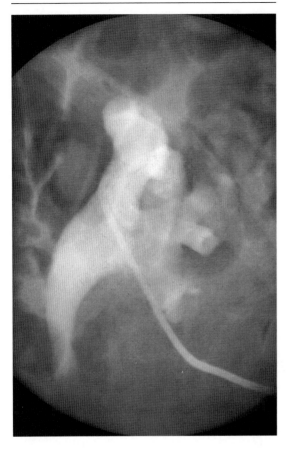

Figure 13.6

Antegrade nephrostogram in a patient with advanced carcinoma of the prostate presented with obstructed kidney. Image taken at the time of insertion of the nephrostomy tube to relieve obstruction. (Courtesy of David Rees, University Hospital of Wales.)

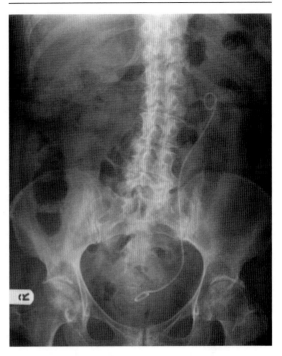

Figure 13.7

Nephrostomy tube changed to an internal stent.

Despite the initial effectiveness of JJ stents, Docimo and Dewolf[17] have reported that in 55% of patients with extrinsic ureteric obstruction, the stents become ineffective within the first month of insertion. Hence, recently, multiple simultaneous stent insertion procedures have been tried and there has been the development of extraanatomical ureteric bypass stents that are tunneled subcutaneously between the bladder and the renal pelvis. The early data appear promising but it has only been used in a small number of patients in a few centers.[12,13]

Finally, if a patient with known prostate cancer presents with uremic symptoms and ultrasound scan confirms bilateral hydro-ureteronephrosis, one should initially consider inserting a urethral catheter. If this does not result in any improvement, a nephrostomy will become necessary.

HYPERCALCEMIA

The normal calcium level is 2.2–2.6 mg/dl and treatment for hypercalcemia is usually recommended when the level reaches 3 mg/dl. There are many non-malignant causes of hypercalcemia such as use of thiazide diuretics, milk alkali syndrome, excessive vitamin D ingestion and sarcoidosis. However, hypercalcaemia may also arise as a consequence of bony metastasis from prostate or renal cell carcinoma. Furthermore, it may also be part of a paraneoplastic syndrome. To this effect, hypercalcemia is thought to occur in up to 20% of patients with renal cell carcinoma[12]. In these cases, renal cell carcinomas may produce parathyroid hormone-related peptide, which mimics the effects of parathyroid hormone. This, in turn, leads to a change in the normal calcium homeostasis and, hence, hypercalcemia. Other factors, such as, tumor necrosis factor, transforming growth factor-α and osteoclast-activating factor may also contribute to hypercalcemia.[18]

Hypercalcemia is usually asymptomatic and may be discovered by routine laboratory tests. However, it may also present as an emergency with nausea, vomiting, constipation, dehydration, anorexia, abdominal pains, renal stones, pathological fractures, depression, psychosis, delirium and confusion. Hence, one should think of the expression 'bones, stones, groans and moans' when hypercalcemia is considered. These clinical findings, reflective of hypercalcemic crisis normally present with serum calcium levels usually greater than 14 mg/dl. Hypercalcemia is also associated with electrocardiographic changes, namely, QT interval shortening.

The first step in the management of severe hypercalcemia is hydration with IV normal saline, which not only achieves volume expansion but also induces urinary calcium excretion (Figure 13.8). Patients may require up to 4 l a day for the first 48 h. Once hydration is achieved, therapy needs to be directed towards decreasing bone resorption and increasing urinary excretion of calcium. Thiazide diuretics increase renal tubular reabsorption of calcium. Hence, these must be stopped. Furosemide, a loop diuretic, on the other hand, promotes urinary excretion of calcium, and should, therefore, be given. Bisphosphonates are the mainstay therapy for severe hypercalcemia. Pamidronate (30–90 mg) is the preferred agent as it is effica-

cious and can be administered intravenously.[19] Other possible treatments include calcitonin (4–8 IU/kg every 12 h),[20] which is a rapidly acting inhibitor of osteoclast-induced bone resorption and is given either subcutaneously or intramuscularly. Slow IV infusion of gallium nitrate (100–200 mg/m^2 daily)[21] is also available for the treatment of severe hypercalcemia. However, due to its nephrotoxic side-effects, it should be avoided in patients with serum creatinine levels greater than 2.5 mg/dl. Other mainstay treatments, including oral prednisone (5–60 mg daily in 2–4 divided doses)[22] and i.v. plicamycin (25 μg/kg daily)[23] may also be considered (Figure 13.8). Due to the complexity involved in the management of hypercalcemia it is prudent to seek early assistance from an endocrinologist in order to optimize and avoid delay in patient care.

PATHOLOGICAL FRACTURES

Prostate cancer bone metastases are a common problem with the axial skeleton being the usual site, within which the lumbar spine is the most frequently implicated. The next most common sites in decreasing order are the proximal femur, pelvis, thoracic spine, ribs, sternum, skull and humerus.[24] Vertebral body involvement extending into the epidural space can result in cord compression, as discussed above. Bone metastases are also commonly seen in patients with renal cell carcinoma. As such, it has been reported that up to 30% of patients with renal cell carcinoma may present with bone pain amongst other symtpoms.[25] With the routine use of CT and ultrasound scanning, renal tumors are being increasingly detected incidentally. Hence, the older literature descriptions of renal cell cancer presentation may no longer be accurate.

Pathological fractures are more commonly associated with malignancies that lead to osteolytic bony metastasis, such as bowel cancer (Figure 13.9). This is due to the resultant weak-

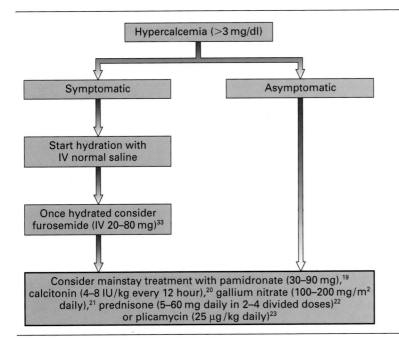

Hypercalcemia (>3 mg/dl)

Symptomatic

Asymptomatic

Start hydration with
IV normal saline

Once hydrated consider
furosemide (IV 20–80 mg)[33]

Consider mainstay treatment with pamidronate (30–90 mg),[19]
calcitonin (4–8 IU/kg every 12 hour),[20] gallium nitrate (100–200 mg/m²
daily),[21] prednisone (5–60 mg daily in 2–4 divided doses)[22]
or plicamycin (25 μg/kg daily)[23]

Figure 13.8

Algorithm for the management of hypercalcemia.

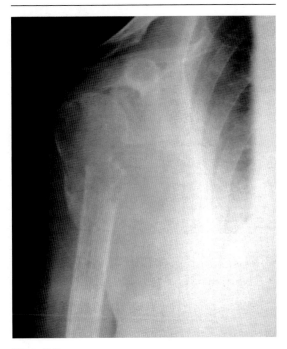

Figure 13.9

Pathological fracture of the humerus.

ening of the bone by the invading tumor. However, prostate malignancy typically produces osteoblastic lesions, which do not weaken the bone to the same extent as osteolytic lesions. Nonetheless, with the disruption of the normal bone architecture, the weight-bearing bones become vulnerable and this may lead to the development of pathologic fractures from sclerotic lesions.

Patients presenting with symptoms of pathologic fractures need radiographs of the symptomatic areas need to confirm these and a bone scan to detect any other potential sites of bone metastasis. The initial management involves patient stabilization with analgesia, IV fluids and blood products (if required). Subsequently, attention should be given to the management of the fracture. If the fracture is stable, the first line of management is radiotherapy.[26,27] In contrast, unstable fractures, such as fractures of the long bones, or stable fractures that fail to respond to radiotherapy need to be surgically treated.[26–28] For fractures of the long bones, this usually involves internal fixation by intramedullary

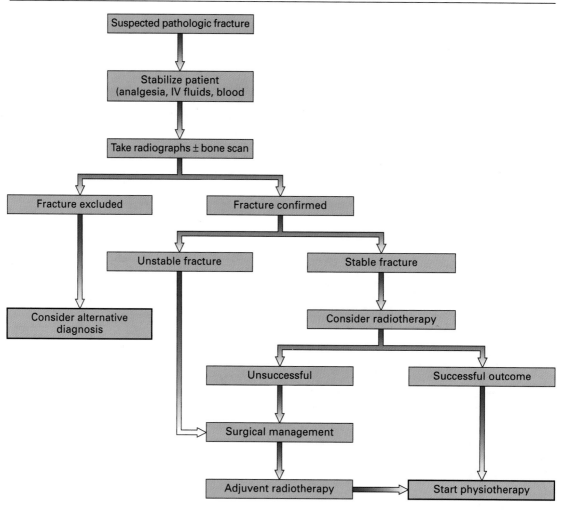

Figure 13.10

Algorithm for the management of pathologic fractures.

devices. Fixation of upper or lower limb long bone fractures are usually accomplished with minimal blood loss and morbidity.[27] However, acetabular fractures require extensive joint reconstruction or total replacement, with associated increased likelihood of morbidity and complications.[27] Once stabilization is achieved, referral to radiation therapy is required for definitive management of the pathological fracture (Figure 13.10).

ACUTE PAIN

Acute pain is a common problem requiring hospitalization in patients with advanced malignant disease and those with advanced urogenital malignancies are no exception. With multidisciplinary care, it is possible to control pain in up to 90% of patients with advanced malignant disease.[29] It is important to address all aspects of the patient's pain – the physical, psychological, social and spiritual. There is a variety of treatment modalities available to treat pain. These include pharmacotherapy, radiotherapy, radiopharmacotherapy and holistic medical therapy.

Acute bone pain is a common presentation in patients with advanced hormone-resistant metastatic prostate cancer. It presents classically as localized pain, which is frequently continuous and unrelenting. Although the pain produced by bone metastasis is not well understood, it is thought that periosteal membrane irritation and/or release of biologic mediators, such as cytokines, may play a role. The presence of bone metastasis can be diagnosed by physical examination, plain radiographs and bone scans (Figure 13.1).

Focal bone metastases can be treated with radiotherapy. There are a number of regimens available, including a single-fraction dose of 800 cGy. Radiotherapy has been associated with response rates ranging from 85 to 100%.[30] It is, however, is much less efficacious in patients with pain arising from diffuse bone metastases. In this situation, pharmacotherapy is the treatment of choice (Figure 13.11). The intensity of pain is assessed to determine the appropriate initial pharmacologic agent to use. The World Health Organization Analgesic Ladder, a repeatedly validated method for controlling pain in patients with cancer,[31] recommends starting with non-opioid agents for mild pain (step 1) and adding other agents, including opioids, for moderate pain (step 2) or severe (step 3) pain. After starting pain medication, repeated assessment of pain intensity is required to enable dose adjustments according to the patient's needs. When patients are prescribed opioids it is also necessary to add a laxative to avoid developing constipation, which can be quite distressing. In addition, it is also important to provide a back-up dose of a short-acting opioid for unexpected breakthrough pain. This dose should be equivalent to 10% of the total daily opioid dose that is normally used.

It is important to remember that patients with chronic pain may not demonstrate the physiologic (e.g. tachycardia and increased blood pressure) or emotional signs that are usually exhibited by patients presenting with acute pain. Hence, the only reliable way of determining their level of pain is by asking them. To this effect, several validated pain assessment scales are available that can provide an accurate measure of the level of pain experienced.[32] These include a verbal numerical scale, a word scale and visual scale.

Finally, as stated above, the management of acute pain in patients with metastatic cancer requires a multidisciplinary approach. Hence, it is prudent to seek the assistance of palliative care physicians from the start. This will help to hasten institution of optimal patient care.

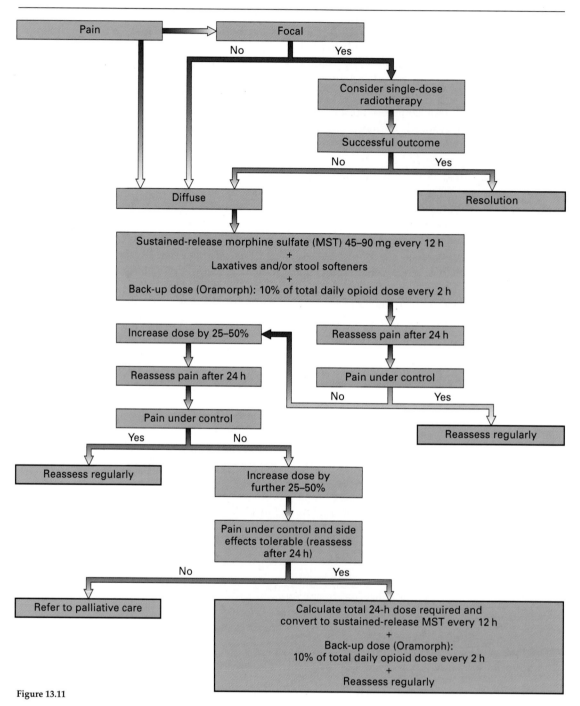

Figure 13.11

Algorithm for the management of cancer associated pain. (Reproduced from Abrahm. *Ann Intern Med* 1999; **131**: 37–46[29] with permission from the American College of Physicians.)

REFERENCES

1. Rubens RD, Fogelman I. *Bone metastases: Diagnosis and Treatment*. London: Springer-Verlag, 1991.
2. Smith JA, Soloway MS, Young MJ. Complications of advanced prostate cancer. *Urology* 1999; **54**: 8–14.
3. Kuben DA, El-Mahdi AM, Sigfred SV et al. Characteristics of spinal cord compression in adenocarcinoma of prostate. *Urology* 1986; **28**: 364–9.
4. Rubin H, Lome LG, Presman D. Neurological manifestation of metastatic prostate cancer. *J Urol* 1974; **111**: 799–802.
5. Modic MT, Masaryk T, Paushter D. Magnetic resonance imaging of the spine. *Radiol Clin North Am* 1986; **24**: 229–45.
6. American Society of Health-System Pharmacists 2002; 2926–7.
7. Young FR, Post EM, King GA. Treatment of spinal epidural metastases. *J Neurosurg* 1980; **53**: 741–8.
8. Constans JP, de Divitiis E, Donzelli R et al. Spinal metastases with neurological manifestations. *J Neurosurg* 1983; **59**: 111–18.
9. Maranzono E, Latini P. Effectiveness of radiation therapy without surgery in metastatic spinal cord compression: final results from a prospective trial. *Int J Radiat Oncol Biol Phys* 1995; **32**: 959–67.
10. Zelefsky MJ, Scher HI, Krol G et al. Spinal epidural tumor in patients with prostate cancer. *Cancer* 1992; **70**: 2319–25.
11. Kim RY, Spencer SA, Meredith RF et al. Extradural spinal cord compression: analysis of factors determining functional prognosis – prospective study. *Radiology* 1990; **176**: 279–82.
12. Tekin MI, Aytekin C, Aygun C, Peskircioglu L, Boyvat F, Ozkardes H. Covered metallic ureteral stent in the management of malignant ureteral obstruction: preliminary results. *Urology* 2001; **58**: 919–23.
13. Rotariu P, Yohannes P, Alexianu M et al. Management of extrinsic compression of the ureter by simultaneous placement of two ipsilateral ureteral stents. *J Endourol* 2001; **15**: 979–83.
14. Neild GH. Chronic renal failure. In: Mundy AR, Fitzpatrick JM, Neal DE, George NJR (eds). *The Scientific Basis of Urology*. Oxford: ISIS Medical Media, 1999: 205–15.
15. Zadra JA, Jewett MAS, Keresteci AG et al. Nonoperative urinary diversion for malignant ureteral obstruction. *Cancer* 1987; **60**: 1353–7.
16. Ekici S, Sahin A, Ozen H. Percutaneous nephrostomy in the management of malignant ureteral obstruction secondary to bladder cancer. *J Endourol* 2001; **15**: 827–9.
17. Docimo SG, DeWolf W. High failure rate of indwelling ureteral stents in patients with extrinsic obstruction: experience at 2 institutions. *J Urol* 1989; **142**: 227–9.
18. Muggia FM. Overview of cancer-related hypercalcaemia: epidemiology and etiology. *Semin Oncol* 1990; **17**: 3–9.
19. American Society of Health-System Pharmacists 2002; 3697–9.
20. American Society of Health-System Pharmacists 2002; 3072.
21. American Society of Health-System Pharmacists 2002; 3659.
22. American Society of Health-System Pharmacists 2002; 2935.
23. American Society of Health-System Pharmacists 2002; 1124.
24. Saitoh H, Hida M, Shimbo T et al. Metastatic patterns of prostate cancer: correlation between sites and number of organs involved. *Cancer* 1984; **54**: 3078–84.
25. Skinner DG, Colvin RB, Vermillion CD, Pfister RC, Leadbetter WF. Diagnosis and management of renal cell carcinoma: a clinical and pathologic study of 309 cases. *Cancer* 1971; **28**: 1165–77.
26. Janjan N. Bone metastases: approaches to management. *Semin Oncol* 2001; **28**: 28–34.
27. Harrington KD. Orthopedic surgical management of skeletal complications of malignancy. *Cancer* 1997; **80**: 1614–27.
28. Bohm P, Huber J. The surgical treatment of bony metastases of the spine and limbs. *J Bone Joint Surg (Br)* 2002; **84**: 521–9.
29. Abrahm JL. Management of pain and spinal cord compression in patients with advanced cancer. *Ann Intern Med* 1999; **131**: 37–46.
30. Madsen E. Painful bone metastases: efficacy of radiotherapy assessed by the patient – a randomised trial comparing 4 Gy × 6 vs 10 Gy × 2. *J Radiat Oncol Biol Phys* 1983; **9**: 1775–9.
31. Zech DF, Grond S, Lynch J, Hertel D, Lehmann KA. Validation of World Health Organization Guidelines for cancer pain relief: a 10-year prospective study. *Pain* 1995; **63**: 65–75.
32. Ingham J and Portenoy RK. The measurement of pain and other symptoms. In: Doyle D, Hanks GW, MacDonald N, (eds). *Oxford Textbook of Palliative Medicine*, 2nd edn. Oxford: Oxford University Press, 1997; 203–19.
33. American Society of Health-System Pharmacists 2002; 2567.

Index